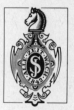

Content Analysis of Verbal Behavior

Significance in Clinical Medicine and Psychiatry

Editors: L.A. Gottschalk F. Lolas L.L. Viney

Springer-Verlag
Berlin Heidelberg New York Tokyo

Louis A. Gottschalk, M.D., Ph.D., Professor of Psychiatry and Director
Psychiatric Consultation and Liaison Division
Department of Psychiatry and Human Behavior
University of California, Irvine, CA 92717, USA

Fernando Lolas, M.D. Associate Professor
Psychophysiology Unit, Faculty of Medicine
University of Chile, P.O. Box 70055, Santiago 7, Chile

Linda Louise Viney, Associate Professor
University of Wollongong, Department of Psychology
P.O. Box 1144, Wollongong, N.S.W. 2500, Australia

ISBN 3-540-16322-0 Springer-Verlag Berlin Heidelberg New York Tokyo
ISBN 0-387-16322-0 Springer-Verlag New York Heidelberg Berlin Tokyo

Library of Congress Cataloging in Publication Data
Content analysis of verbal behavior.
Bibliography: p.
Includes index.
1. Verbal behavior. 2. Content analysis
(Communication) 3. Sick-Language. I. Gottschalk,
Louis A. II. Lolas Fernando. III. Viney, Linda L.
BF 455.C679 1986   616.8'9'075   86-6476
ISBN 0-387-16322-0 (U.S.)

Typesetting, printing and bookbinding: Appl, Wemding
2119/3140-543210

Table of Contents

Some Applications of Verbal Behavior Analysis to the Clinical Sciences

Contributors

Stephan Ahrens, Professor Dr. med. Dr. rer. soc.
Abteilung für Psychotherapie und Psychosomatik, Universitätsklinik Eppendorf,
Martinistraße 52, 2000 Hamburg 20, Federal Republic of Germany

Susana Aronsohn, B.S. Instructor
Psychophysiology Unit, Faculty of Medicine, University of Chile, P.O. Box 137-D,
Santiago, Chile

Birgitte Bechgaard, Ph.D.
Psychological Institute, Kommunehospitalet, 1399 Copenhagen K, Denmark

Paulo Belmonte De Abreu, M.D.
Assistant Professor and Clinical Supervisor, Hospital Universitario da Pontificia,
Universidade Católica, Instituto de Psiquiatria Compreensiva, Rua Florencio Ygartua,
208, 90.000 Porto Alegre, RS, Brasil

Robert E. Cole, Ph.D., Assistant Professor
Department of Psychiatry (Psychology), School of Medicine and Dentistry, University
of Rochester, 300 Crittenden Boulevard, Rochester, NY 14642, USA

Gerhard Deffner, Ph.D.
Fachbereich Psychologie, Universität Hamburg, Von-Melle-Park 5, 2000 Hamburg 13,
Federal Republic of Germany

Britta Faber, M.D.
Psychological Institute, Kommunehospitalet, 1399 Copenhagen K, Denmark

Thomas E. Gift, M.D., Associate Professor
Department of Psychiatry, School of Medicine and Dentistry, University of Rochester,
300 Crittenden Boulevard, Rochester, NY 14642, USA

Louis A. Gottschalk, M.D., Ph.D., Professor of Psychiatry and Director
Consultation and Liaison Service, University of California, Irvine, Medical Center,
College of Medicine University of California, Irvine, CA 92717, USA
and
Supervising and Emeritus Training Analyst, Southern California Psychoanalytic
Institute Los Angeles, CA.

Julia Hoigaard, M. A.
Department of Psychiatry and Human Behavior, College of Medicine, University of
California, Irvine, CA 92717, USA

Jimmie C. Holland, M. D., Professor
Department of Psychiatry, Cornell University Medical College and Chief, Psychiatry
Service, Memorial Sloan-Kettering Cancer Center, 1275 York Avenue New York,
NY 10021, USA

Bjørn Jacobsen, M. D.
Psychological Institute, Kommunehospitalet, 1399 Copenhagen K, Denmark

Lennart Jansson, M. D.
Psychological Institute, Kommunehospitalet, 1399 Copenhagen K, Denmark

Eva Kasell, B. A.
Mailman Research Center, McLean Hospital,
115 Mill Street, Belmont, MA 02178, USA
and
Harvard Medical School

Dennis K. Kinney, Ph. D.
Laboratories for Psychiatric Research, Mailman Research Center, McLean Hospital,
115 Mill Street, Belmont, MA 02178, USA
and
Department of Psychiatry, Harvard Medical School

Uwe Koch, M. D., Ph. D.
Albert-Ludwigs-Universität, Psychologisches Institut, Lehrstuhl für
Rehabilitationspsychologie, Belfortstraße 16, 7800 Freiburg i. Br., Federal Republic of
Germany

Hans Kordy, M. D., Dipl.-Math.
Psychosomatische Klinik, Universität Heidelberg, Thibautstr. 2, 6900 Heidelberg,
Federal Republic of Germany

Allen H. Lebovits, Ph. D., Assistant Professor
Department of Psychiatry, Mount Sinai School of Medicine, 1 Gustave L. Levy Place,
New York, NY 10029, USA

Fernando Lolas, M. D., Associate Professor and Head
Psychophysiology Unit, Faculty of Medicine, University of Chile, P. O. Box 70055
Santiago 7, Chile

Arturo Manns, D. D. S., Associate Professor
Laboratory of Oral Physiology, Faculty of Medicine, University of Chile, P. O. Box
137-D, Santiago, Chile

Erhard Mergenthaler, Ph.D., Dr.rer. biol. hum.
Computer Scientist (Diplom.-Informatiker) Sektion für Psychoanalytische Methodik,
Universität Ulm, Am Hochsträss 8, 7900 Ulm, Federal Republic of Germany

Rodolfo Miralles, D.D.S., Assistant
Laboratory of Oral Physiology, Faculty of Medicine, University of Chile, P.O. Box
137-D, Santiago, Chile

Carol Preston
University of Wollongong, P.O. Box 1144, Wollongong N.S.W. 2500, Australia

Michael von Rad, M.D., Professor of Psychosomatic Medicine, Director, Institut und
Poliklinik für Psychosomatische Medizin, Psychotherapie und Medizinische
Psychologie der TU München, Langerstraße 3, 8000 München 80
and
Abteilung für Psychosomatische Medizin und Psychotherapie des Städtischen
Krankenhauses Bogenhausen, Englschalkinger Straße 77, 8000 München 81, Federal
Republic of Germany

Donna Lou Udelman, Ph.D., FAPM, FAOA
President, Biomedical Stress Research Foundation, LTD 45 E. Osborn Road, Phoenix,
AZ 85012
and
Research Department, Camelback Hospitals Phoenix and Scottsdale, AZ

Harold D. Udelman, M.D., FAPA, FAPM
Chairman, Biomedical Stress Research Foundation, LTD, 45 E. Osborn Road, Phoenix,
AZ 85012, USA
and
Research Department, Camelback Hospitals, Phoenix and Scottsdale, AZ

Regina L. Uliana, Ph.D.
Staff Psychologist, Metropolitan State Hospital, 11400 Norwalk Boulevard, Norwalk,
CA 90650, USA

Linda L. Viney, Ph.D., Associate Professor and Chairman
Department of Psychology, University of Wollongong, P.O. Box 1144, Wollongong
N.S.W. 2500, Australia

Mary T. Westbrook, Ph.D.
Senior Lecturer in Psychology, Department of Behavioural and General Studies,
Cumberland College of Health Sciences, Lidcombe, N.S.W., 2141, Australia

Lyman Wynne, M.D., Ph.D., Professor
Department of Psychiatry, School of Medicine and Dentistry, University of Rochester,
300 Crittenden Boulevard, Rochester, NY 14642, USA

Introduction

1 Content Analysis:
Overview of a Measurement Method

Louis A. Gottschalk, Fernando Lolas, and Linda L. Viney

This book involves a collaboration between editors representing a wide geographical area, the United States of America (Louis A. Gottschalk), Chile (Fernando Lolas), and Australia (Linda L. Viney). The actual contributors come from a wider range of areas than is included in these locations. There are authors from West Germany – specifically from Freiburg, Hamburg, Heidelberg, Kiel, Munich, and Ulm. From South America the contributors are from Porto Alegre, Brazil and Santiago, Chile. From Australia the contributors are from Wollongong and Lidcombe. There are four authors from Copenhagen, Denmark. From the United States of America there are contributors from Irvine, CA; San Francisco, CA; Phoenix, AZ; Kansas City, MO; Boston, MA; Rochester, NY; New York, NY; and many other cities. What brings together these diverse and geographically widely distributed authors is the common use of content analysis of verbal behavior in research, linking the psychosocial and biomedical sciences.

The type of content analysis focused on in this volume originated with a method developed by Louis A. Gottschalk and Goldine C. Gleser [1–4]. It provides a model for content analysis which can be modified, built upon, and extended in many directions. Some of the contributors in this volume have made innovative and useful contributions to and departures from the Gottschalk-Gleser model.

Some of the papers included in this volume have been previously published or are in press in professional journals. All the papers selected for this collection contribute important information on the application of the analysis of verbal behavior to clinical medicine and psychiatry. We have tried to arrange them in an order and in groups into which they naturally seem to fall.

The paper we have placed in a lead position in the section dealing with theoretical considerations is by Fernando Lolas and is entitled "Behavioral Text and Psychological Context: On Pragmatic Verbal Behavior Analysis" for it deals with the broad issue of the place of verbal behavior and its content analysis in the basic and clinical sciences. Lolas begins his paper by formulating some of the problems posed by the content analysis method for studying verbal behavior within the wider context of psychological and medical research. He distinguishes between an experimental and a clinical tradition, each possessing an intuitive-empathic and a scientific-analytic dimension, illustrated by way of examples. Speech is viewed as part of a "total" human communication system which becomes a behavioral "text" when perceived by an observer, who also endows it with meaning by means of a pragmatic metalanguage of so-called *psychic structures*. These constructions provide guiding clues for diagnosis, research, and prediction and may be considered the interpretative *context* for the behavioral text. The author also discusses different forms of meaning (or content) analysis, emphasizing some features of the method illustrated in this volume. He underscores the advantages of an assessment procedure which relies on undistorted natural speech over traditional paper-and-pencil psychometric testing.

The next three papers are concerned with presenting a modern historical development of certain basic and clinical science applications of the Gottschalk-Gleser content analysis method in the English, German, Spanish, Portuguese, and Danish languages. In so doing, they provide evidence toward construct validation of many of these content analysis scales. The first of these two papers, entitled "Research. Using the Gottschalk-Gleser Content Analysis Scales in English Since 1969" by Louis A. Gottschalk, was prepared, in an earlier version, at the request of Uwe Koch and Gert Schofer to be translated into German so as to serve as an updating chapter in a German book they have edited involving the use of these content analysis scales [5]. The version prepared for this volume has been modified and further updated. The paper entitled "Studies Proving the Validity of the Gottschalk-Gleser Content Analysis Scales in German-Speaking Countries" was first read by its author, Uwe Koch, at the VII World Congress of the International College of Psychosomatic Medicine at Hamburg, Germany, in July, 1983. It reports on many clinical trials confined to the Gottschalk-Gleser Anxiety and Hostility Scales, and, in so doing, it contributes to the construct validity of these specific scales. A paper that belongs with these two papers was written by Linda L. Viney entitled "Assessment of Psychological States Through Content Analysis of Verbal Communications" and has been published elsewhere [6]. It is included in this collection because it provides cogent arguments and evidence supporting the important place of verbal content analysis in data gathering for the behavioral and clinical sciences as well as describing applications of the many new content analysis, scales developed by Viney and her associates.

The next four papers have in common some technical, procedural, or other original contribution to the Gottschalk-Gleser method of measurement. The first of this tetrad, by Thomas Gift, Robert Cole, and Lyman Wynne, is entitled "An Interpersonal Measure of Hostility Based on Speech Context." It describes a useful variant for eliciting relevant verbal communication on marital relationships. This new approach results in verbal content findings that one would well expect from women in dyads having marital discord in comparison to women from more congenial marital pairs. The paper, "Microcomputers as Aids to Avoid Error in Gottschalk-Gleser Rating" by Gerhard Deffner, offers a time- and error-saving small computer approach to recording, coding, tabulating, and scoring speech samples. The paper by Louis A. Gottschalk and Julia Hoigaard entitled "A Depression Scale Applicable to Verbal Samples" offers a theoretical formulation, normative data, and a set of validation studies on a new depression scale – with seven subscales – applicable to verbal samples. The paper entitled "Content Analysis of Verbal Behavior in Psychotherapy Research: A Comparison Between Two Methods" by Fernando Lolas, Erhard Mergenthaler, and Michael von Rad presents a comparison between the clause-based Gottschalk-Gleser method and the word-based Anxiety Topics Dictionary (ATD) developed at the University of Ulm, West Germany. Both procedures were applied to the same speech samples and the comparison, largely confined to anxiety assessment, yields interesting perspectives regarding operationalization of psychological constructs and implementation of machine analysis programs.

The next group of papers reports on applications of content analysis scales to medical and psychiatric disorders. They each constitute little gems, in themselves, and their titles well reveal their subject matter.

The paper entitled "Use of the Gottschalk-Gleser Verbal Content Analysis Scales with Medically Ill Patients" by Allen H. Lebovits, and Jimmie C. Holland, reviews ten papers utilizing the Gottschalk-Gleser Content Analysis Scales with medically ill patients, and, in so doing, illustrates that the Gottschalk-Gleser approach is a versatile instrument that measures many states of considerable relevance to the medically ill.

The paper entitled "Affective Content of Speech and Treatment of Outcome in Bruxism" by Susan Aronsohn, Fernando Lolas, Arturo Manns, and Rodolso Miralles shows that the Gottschalk-Gleser method provides a differentiated probing of psychological characteristics related to somatic illness, indeed much more accurate than the one permitted by conventional psychometric testing for the purpose of describing psychological profiles in bearers of pathological conditions.

The paper entitled "Psychological States in Patients with Diabetes Mellitus" by Linda L. Viney and Mary T. Westbrook is one of a growing series of creative studies by a group of researchers from Australia investigating ways in which the objective assessment of the content of verbal communications can be used to characterize the personal reactions of people with acute or chronic disease and to explore healthy and unhealthy ways of coping with such disease. Patients with diabetes mellitus, similarly to patients with other chronic disease, were observed to have significantly more anxiety, depression, and anger than healthy individuals.

The paper entitled "Emotional Impact of Mastectomy" by Louis A. Gottschalk and Julia Hoigaard compares content analysis data obtained from five participating institutions studying many psychosocial dimensions of four groups of women: (1) women who had unilateral mastectomy for stage I or II breast cancer, (2) women who had a biopsy for benign breast disease, (3) women who had a cholecystectomy, and (4) healthy women who had no major surgical treatment over the preceding 2 years. The collaborating institutions were: Montifiore Hospital, the Bronx, New York; Peter Bent Brigham Hospital, Boston, Massachusetts; Midwest Research Institution Kansas City, Missouri; West Coast Cancer Foundation; San Francisco, California; and Stanford Research Institute International, Menlo Park, California. The study reveals significantly different emotional responses derived from the content analysis of 5-min speech samples obtained from these four groups of women. Moreover, by following the responses of these women 12 months after the initial personality assessment, a reduction in the emotional distress of the mastectomy group was demonstrated, but they remained, even then, more emotionally disturbed than the other groups of women.

The 60 drug-users, 43 men and 17 women, studied in the paper "Some Sources of Alienation for Drug Addicts" by Linda L. Viney, Mary T. Westbrook, and Carol Preston had been addicted to some combination of heroin, Methadone, barbiturates, LSD, Pethedine, or amphetamines, and when interviewed only 14 had been drug-free for more than 2 or 3 days. Their deep sense of alienation, when compared to a group of university students from the same Australian city, is clearly revealed by a Sociality Scale applicable to verbal communications and developed by Linda L. Viney and Mary Westbrook.

The study entitled "Content Analysis of Speech of Schizophrenic and Control Adoptees and Their Relatives: Preliminary Results" by Dennis K. Kinney, Bjørn Jacobsen, Birgitte Bechgaard, Lennart Jansson, Britta Faber, Eva Kasell, and Regina Uliana involving the Gottschalk-Gleser social alienation-personal disorganization scores, derived from speech samples of 20 Danish schizophrenic adoptees, 26 control adoptees, and their respective biological and adoptive relatives, supports the evidence that high scores on this scale may be associated with a genetic liability for schizophrenia.

In the study from Kiel, West Germany entitled "Alexithymia and Affective Verbal Behavior of Psychosomatic Patients and Controls" by Stephan Ahrens, the emotional reactions to silent films of three groups of patients – somatic, psychosomatic, and psychoneurotic – were studied. Psychosomatic patients were not found to be alexithymic, that is, they were found to have the same kind of sensitive emotional responses to affect-laden silent films as the other two groups of patients when affects were assessed by the Gottschalk-Gleser content analysis procedure. When a different method of measurement was used – a self-report (adjective check list method) – the psychosomatic group appeared to be alexithymic. The author offers an explanation for why there are different results evoked by different measurement methods.

In the paper entitled "Expression of Positive Emotion by People Who Are Physically Ill: Is it Evidence of Defending or Coping?" by Linda L. Viney, content analysis scales were used to explore whether the expression of positive emotion by a sample of 507 hospitalized medical patients was evidence of defending or coping. Positive emotions were found to constitute a predictor of favorable psychosocial and biological coping with medical illness.

The last group of four papers involves the application of content analysis to the psychotherapy and/or pharmacotherapy of psychiatric patients. The first of this series is entitled "Affective Content of Speech as a Predictor of Psychotherapy Outcome" by Fernando Lolas, Hans Kordy, and Michael von Rad. This collaboration of Fernando Lolas with two co-investigators from Heidelberg indicates, as other studies have, that certain Gottschalk-Gleser scores might provide early indicators relevant to prognosis or outcome of therapeutic interventions. In this specific study, evidence was collected, from examining the treatment outcome of a sample of 98 patients heterogeneous with regard to diagnosis or form of psychotherapy, that certain patients with pretreatment anxiety and hostility scores 0.5 standard deviations above or below the mean scores for a normative sample of German subjects had significantly poorer outcome following psychotherapy. For example, patients with high pretreatment overt-hostility-outward, ambivalent-hostility, guilt, or shame anxiety scores had significantly poorer ($P < 0.02$) outcome after treatment. The results of these researchers seem to be at variance with those reported by the Menninger Clinic group in that they reported finding a better treatment outcome among those patients with a higher pretreatment anxiety. This calls attention to the principle underlying operationalization of psychological constructs in psychotherapy research. A method such as the Gottschalk-Gleser content analysis might constitute a good instrument for bridging the gap between workers of different theoretical persuasions since its basic principles and implemention are eclectic in nature.

The paper entitled "Aggressiveness in Psychotherapy and Its Relationship with the Patient's Change: An Adaptation of the Gottschalk-Gleser Hostility Scales to the Portuguese Language" by Paulo Belmonte de Abreu is an ingenious and successful attempt to examine the hostile content of patient statements and therapist interpretive comments and to follow the extent to which the content of these communications are predictive of psychotherapeutic outcome.

The article entitled "A Preliminary Report on Antidepressant Therapy and Its Effect on Hope and Immunity" by Donna Lou and Harold Udelman introduces the reader to the new frontier of psychoneuroimmunology. It is an initial attempt to determine whether an antidepressant psychoactive drug, in combination with psychotherapy, can enhance immune competence in depressed psychiatric outpatients. In this study, hope is assessed from the analysis of content of speech, and hope scores are considered a marker of a mental state favorable to a good immune response. Although at this point the findings are inconclusive with respect to whether an antidepressant drug is capable of preventing impairment of immune function sometimes brought on by a mental depression or bereavement, there is some preliminary suggestive evidence that hope scores may be a predictor of some types of favorable immune responses.

The final chapter in this collection "The Pharmacokinetics of Some Psychoactive Drugs and Relationships to Clinical Response" by Louis A. Gottschalk illustrates the application of verbal behavior analysis in the assessment of clinical responses to the scientific arena of neuropsychopharmacology by reviewing the findings of a series of investigations in this area, carried out in the Department of Psychiatry and Human Behavior, University of California at Irvine, covering the decade from 1975 to 1985.

References

1. Gottschalk LA, Gleser GC (1969) The measurement of psychological states through the content analysis of verbal behavior. University of California Press, Berkeley
2. Gottschalk LA, Winget CN, Gleser GC (1969) Manual of instructions for using the Gottschalk-Gleser content analysis scales: anxiety, hostility, and social alienation-personal disorganization. University of California Press, Berkeley
3. Gottschalk LA (ed) (1979) The content analysis of verbal behavior: further studies. Spectrum, New York
4. Gottschalk LA, Winget CN, Gleser GC, Lolas F (1984) Analisis de la Conducta-verbal. University of Chile Press, Santiago
5. Koch U, Schofer G (eds) (1986) Sprachinhaltsanalyse in der psychosomatischen Forschung: Grundlagen und Anwenderstudien mit den Affektskalen von Gottschalk und Gleser. Beltz, Weinheim
6. Viney LL (1983) The assessment of psychological states through content analysis of verbal communication. Psychol Bull 44: 542–563

Theoretical Issues
and Modern Historical Development

2 Behavioral Text and Psychological Context: On Pragmatic Verbal Behavior Analysis

Fernando Lolas*

2.1 "Introspection" and "Verbal Report"

Although it is generally accepted that psychology is the study of behavior, specifications of the meaning of behavior vary considerably. To record an action potential in a cell is different from observing an organism in its environment. General functional principles can be formulated in both cases and be predictive of further occurrences of the phenomena under study. Basic mechanisms discovered in simplified preparations or simple organisms could operate also at more complex levels of organization. This does not, however, make data relevant, interpretable, or applicable.

A truly scientific approach demands methods appropriate to the particular level of observation and to the purposes of the investigation. Recognition of this fact calls for relevant and "level fair" methodological strategies.

This is particularly true for human symbolic behavior, from time immemorial a distinctive feature of human nature. Concern for it has been institutionalized in literature, education, and academic disciplines, such as sociology, anthropology and psychology, and shaped by several ancient disciplines, such as philosophy and art. It has also been influenced by developments in political, economic, and scientific thought.

Even within the scientific tradition, the study of this aspect of human behavior has been more metaphorical than empirical. Early psychological theorizing spread speculative nets over wide areas of human endeavors, attempting to explain everything by means of limited observations and *ad hoc* explanatory principles.

During the early phases of scientific psychology a widely employed method for studying human behavior was *introspection,* characteristic of the psychological schools called *structuralism* and *functionalism* [46]. The main objectives of men like Wundt and Titchener were to analyze consciousness into its elements and to explain how experience develops and is constituted. They placed emphasis on the unelaborated mental content – free of inference. Wundt's analysis distinguished between two kinds of elementary conscious experiences: sensations, which seem to come to us from the outside, and feelings, which seem to belong to ourselves. One of the preferred experimental procedures for studying them was the so-called *method of impression*. The subject was confronted with a stimulus and requested to report on the sensations it aroused. This method yielded much of the data employed by psychophysicists in their theorization.

* Psychophysiology Unit, Faculty of Medicine, University of Chile, PO Box 70055 – D, Santiago 7, Chile.

For functionalists and structuralists, introspection was closer to experience and thus helped to understand the workings of consciousness. They did not reject physiological data or behavioral observation. However, as Titchener expressed it, a science of behavior would belong to biology – concerned with the relationships between organism and environment – rather than to psychology – dealing with processes within the organism [47].

Even before the behaviorist era, many writers had questioned the validity of data obtained through introspection. Von Feuchtersleben (as quoted by Altschule [2]) wrote that "we do not observe the springs of our psychical functions when they are in active operation, but only when they are quiescent and cannot be investigated." Broussais expressed that "it will be impossible to assert, after this inspection of the interior, a single fact that will not require to be verified by the senses" (quoted by Altschule [2]). In spite of these and other criticisms, methods dependent upon introspection reached virtually the status of experimental procedures during the nineteenth century.

Another method for acquiring psychological knowledge was *free association,* intended to elicit unconscious thoughts. It had been used as a literary device in the late eighteenth century by Friedrich Schiller, the German poet, who also was a physician. In psychiatry and psychology, both Kraepelin and Jung advocated its use.

The behaviorist movement explicitly attempted a reformulation of the methods and aims of psychology. According to Watson [50]:

> Psychology, as the behaviorist views it, is a purely objective experimental branch of natural science. Its theoretical goal is the prediction and control of behaviour. Introspection forms no essential part of its methods, nor is the scientific value of its data dependent upon ... interpretation in terms of consciousness ... The time seems to have come when psychology must discard all reference to consciousness; when it needs no longer delude itself into thinking that it is making mental states the subject of observation ... Our quarrel is not with the ... structural psychologist alone ... The difference between functional psychology and structural psychology, as the functionalists have so far stated the case, is unintelligible. The terms sensation, perception, affection, emotion, volition are used as much by the functionalist as by the structuralist ... We advance the view that behaviourism is the only consistent and logical functionalism.

In addition to redefining psychology as the science of behavior, Watson was interested in comparing work on the human being with work on animals. He stressed prediction and control, not explanation. Any reference to "mentalist" constructs was unnecessary. Although structural psychologists accepted that overt behavior was valuable if it threw light on conscious experience and others suggested that behavior should be studied through the consciousness of the individual *and* by external observation (e. g., [35]), for Watson introspection was inaccurate. No agreement could be found, even among trained observers. Introspective reports pretended to deal with something "not objectively observable" supposedly going on within the organism. Watson did not demand that *all* behavior *must* be observable. His concept of "implicit behavior" acknowledged the existence of *potentially* observable behavior, suggesting that phenomena "under the skin" (physiological processes) were of the same kind as overt, observable behavior. According to Tolman [48], Watson referred in fact to two possible definitions of behavior: on the one hand, to "its strict underlying physical and physiological details" (the "molecular" definition). On the other, he regarded behavior as more than and different from the sum of its parts, as an "emergent" phenomenon with defining and descriptive properties of its own. Tolman himself stressed its goal-seeking, purposive, and cognitive aspects [48].

These considerations are relevant considering the radical treatment Skinner gave to human language. In 1934, trying to convert the philosopher Alfred North Whitehead to behaviorism, he was challenged to show how human speech could be fitted into the behaviorist's deterministic scheme. Skinner's *Verbal Behavior* attempted to demonstrate that verbal behavior, like other operant behaviors, is determined by stimuli and reinforcements. In his theorization, the *mand* is the speaker's response to an internal or aversive stimulus calling on the listener for attention or help and the *tact* is the speaker's response to an external stimulus. During development, differential reinforcement by the "verbal community" establishes meaningful associations. Skinner accepted the existence of "intraverbal" behavior, accounting for the development of word associations and syntactic structures. Thought would be simply behavior [42].

It is interesting to note that Skinner relaxed the taboo against introspection in many places of his work. He pointed out, among other things, that the problem of subjective terms does not coincide exactly with that of private stimuli, but that there is a close connection. We must know the characteristics of verbal responses to private stimuli to approach the operational analysis of subjective terms. Although we usually *infer* the private event, "this is opposed to the direction of inquiry in a science of behavior in which we are to predict response through, among other things, an independent knowledge of the stimulus" [41].

Spence [43], observing that many varieties of behaviorism had little in common with the particular pattern of assumptions advanced by Watson, commented that the majority of American psychologists in the 1940s took for granted the basic postulates of the behaviorist formulation. This was different from classical structuralism in that structuralism took sensations, emotions, and thoughts as *"observable aspects of direct experience,"* whereas behaviorists, like physicists, inferred systematic constructs from immediate experience without assuming that they were "real" in the sense of being accessible *per se* [43]. "Scientific empiricism", wrote Bergmann and Spence in 1944, "holds to the position that all sciences, including psychology, deal with the same events, namely, the experiences or perceptions of the scientist himself" [4]. Immediate experience, the initial matrix out of which all sciences develop, is no longer considered a matter of concern for the scientist qua scientist. Although in this schema the experiences of the observing scientist do indeed have a privileged, even unique position, the empirical scientist should realize that his behavior, symbolic or otherwise, does not lie on the same methodological level as the responses of his subjects, and consequently he should not, in reporting the latter, use any mentalist terms which have not been introduced from a basis of physicalistic meaning. This amounts to saying that all scientific terms in psychology should be defined behavioristically.

With the demise of extreme positivism in the 1930s and the change in emphasis from radical or metaphysical behaviorism to logical or methodical behaviorism, many social and experimental psychologists were willing to make inferences about internal processes. The long-standing debate between behaviorists and humanists focused on "internalism" versus "externalism" [33]. Homme [20] argued that private events were not wholly unobservable if one acknowledges that they can be scrutinized by their owner (i. e., the person experiencing them).

From this vantage point, behaviorism means nothing else than a form of operational analysis of traditional mentalist concepts, as Skinner formulated it [41]. The task of the behavioral scientist is to bring order and meaning into the particular realm of events he studies.

These considerations are important for the study of verbal behavior. As the historian E.G.Boring remarked, although the word "introspection" has "dropped out of use" the method "is still with us, doing business under various aliases, of which *verbal report* is one" [5]. This is as valid today as it was in 1953.

The "cognitive turn" in behavioral research gave new impetus to the traditional quest for a unified treatment of language and mind. Research on verbal report, with the problem it poses for subjective data (a remnant of the introspectionist attempt at grasping *real* immediate experience), faces the challenge of avoiding tautological conjectures about the "inner world" and reductive fallacies devoid of practical significance.

The experimental traditions of introspectionism and behaviorism face, in spite of their differences, one and the same problem: to achieve a lawful description of verbal behavior, finding the "empirical referents" of "internal" states or events and accounting for their use and maintenance.

2.2 The Clinical Tradition: Language-in-Context

Alongside with the introspectionist and the behaviorist traditions, a different stream of concerns with verbal report evolved. While the first two traditions can be labeled experimental, in that the emphasis was placed on more or less controlled observations, this one can be called clinical. Clinical means essentially a practical aim – diagnosis or therapy – but also a particular form of approach which can be subsumed under the rubric *"language-in-context."* From the very beginnings of psychotherapy, the immense power of words in the relation between people has been recognized. Language behavior in a dyadic or group situation is different from verbal reports elicited by the method of impression (vide supra) or in response to behavioral experiments. Speech has both communicative and expressive functions, not always considered jointly in the experimental traditions. They are accorded a different status in those approaches concerned with the pragmatic aim of knowing something about subjects in the role of patients.

We are also justified in regarding this a separate tradition because it has been less systematic in its conclusions and its results have been couched in different concepts. The stance taken by many clinicians dealing with verbal reports in the dyadic therapeutic situation resembles literary narrative and may be exemplified in the following quotation from Freud [6]:

I have not always been a psychotherapist. Like other neuropathologists, I was trained to employ local diagnosis and electroprognosis, and it still strikes me myself as strange that the case histories I write should read like short stories and that, as one might say, they lack the serious stamp of science. I must console myself with the reflection that the nature of the subject is evidently responsible for this, rather than any preference of my own. The fact is that local diagnosis and electrical reactions lead nowhere is the study of hysteria, whereas a detailed description of mental processes such as we are accustomed to find in the work of imaginative writers enables me, with the use of a few psychological formulas, to obtain at least some kind of insight into the course of that affection.

It is interesting to note that the "talking cure" Freud developed on the basis of verbal report was not directly linked to the introspectionist psychology of his time. It could have been expected that psychoanalysts and functionalists might early have found some common ground of interest; the fact is that there was little interchange between the theorists of the laboratory and the theorists of the consulting room. The distrust was, and still is, mutual. The psychoanalyst is skeptical of the practical value of the laboratory approach. The experimentalist is scornful of what he considers undisciplined theorizing by the analyst (or, for that matter, any clinician dealing with verbal reports). The differences refer to the purposes and theoretical bias which determine what data to collect, how to collect them, and disparate emphases on individual differences (idiographic approach, more akin to the clinical enterprise) or on general principles (nomothetic approach). Clinicians working with words have seldom spoken the same language as researchers.

The often imprecise character of the clinical "method" can be attributed to its reliance upon insight, its practical commitment, and the humanistic attempt to "understand" the person in its subjectivity. This means devoting attention not only to the communicative aspects of language but to its expressive aspects as well, to its self-depicting function. In psychotherapy, language is not only conversation. It is conversation plus comment on the imagined or real interpersonal transactions (relations) embedded in connotative meaning. The person of the trained observer is given an equal status in the construction of shared meaning. This interactional character of the "clinical" verbal report is both an advantage and a weakness. While scientific empiricism recognizes that experiences and perceptions of the observer are the raw material for description, inference, and prediction, these operations are guided by *explicit* rules. The clinician relies upon *implicit* principles or rules. Intermediate steps in the argumental chain may be lost, and many of the conclusions cannot be accounted for in terms of precisely defined, step-by-step operations. It is difficult to imagine the roles of researcher and clinician combined in a single person. Proximity and detachment seem to constitute divergent basic attitudes.

This opposition has been stressed by those who contend that human beings possess a type of knowledge enabling them to share "states of mind" with other persons. This knowledge is distinct from the kind of perception gleaned from tests and statistics. It is related to "empathic" understanding or "imaginative reconstruction" and strives at "meaning," conceived of as distinct from causal-functional relationships. This particular form of understanding has characterized phenomenological approaches focusing on the experiences of the patient or client as the medium through which movement or behavior change occurs. As Jaspers [21] wrote:

Our chief help ... comes from the patient's own self descriptions, which can be evoked and tested out in the course of personal conversation. From this we get our best defined and clearest data ... An experience is best described by the person who has undergone it. Detached psychiatric observation with its own formulation of what the patient is suffering is not a substitute for this.

The particular type of understanding implied in the German word *Verstehen,* applicable to human behavior in the context of interpersonal relations, is the ability, on the part of the observer, to parallel an observed or assumed connection with something we know through self-observation. While not being a method of verification or a scientific tool of analysis, clinical *Verstehen* can aid in setting up hypotheses about a given subject [1, 27]. It can also help in preliminary explorations of "emotional syllogisms" (or self-evident connections between verbal report and feeling) formulated on the basis of our own experiences as observers.

Most of the criticisms against this form of clinical intuition derive from the difficulty of ascertaining whether its data are "true" or "false" independent, "objective" confirmations [25]. This is a reflection of the scientist's prejudice against immediate experience and "tacit knowledge" [36], that is, knowledge that cannot be accounted for in terms of physical operations of measurement.

Language-in-context, the domain of clinical expertise, is also a distinguishing feature of psychoanalysis, a discipline anchored in intersubjectivity as evinced in language. This tradition has elaborated the distinction, common to other approaches relying on experience, between expert and layman. The former, due to his/her training, possesses a sort of "categorical perception" of events and can name them with the aid of labels provided by a theory. The analytical situation demands that one participant (the patient) speaks to the other (the analyst) in an unrestrained manner. The analyst, in turn, is in possession of a "third ear" glued to a "psychic stethoscope which magnifies the otherwise unheard stirrings of the unconscious" [40]. It is assumed that the analyst's floating attention can, aided by a set of theoretical principles, grasp hidden meanings and formulate the "rules" of the subject's conversation.

Psychoanalysis, perhaps more than other theories of human behavior, has carefully specified the position and characteristics of the observer as well as the conditions for observation. It "reconstructs" psychic reality with the aid of language, like phenomenological *Verstehen,* but on different methodological and theoretical assumptions, more removed from naive common sense. It implies self-experience, but guided by a normative theoretical foundation which helps shape the process of data acquisition and inferential reconstruction. The importance ascribed to language is well described by Edelheit [9], who wrote that the *ego* may be regarded as a vocal/auditory organization – a language-determined and language-determining structure which functions as the characteristic human organ of adaptation. Despite the widespread acceptance of these basic tenets by most analysts, the clinical method ends up by sharply contrasting what Spence [44] called "private competence" versus "normative competence". The contrast resembles that between idiographic versus nomothetic approaches. Attention is paid to the peculiarities of the individual, on the one hand, and reliance upon general principles, on the other. Subjective experience, reflected in verbal report, continues to be elusive without an appropriate framework for retaining it while making it scientifically acceptable. Many attempts in quantitative research in psychoanalysis have been directed precisely at this, with varying degrees of success [31]. The same holds true for research in cognitive or behavioral psychotherapy.

2.3 Communicative Structures and Psychic Structures

As Woodworth and Sheehan [51] wrote, "the history of psychology could be written on the theme of the small dash that connects stimulus with response in the "S-R symbol." Watson contended that the task of the student of behavior was to predict responses knowing the stimuli and, given the responses, specify the effective stimuli. Later, the O in the S-O-R symbol was designed to account for any nonlinearity between inputs and outputs.

In the present discussion, the O is of primary interest for it is the unobservable link about which we wish to obtain knowledge or make predictions. Classical behaviorism, according to Polanyi [36], depended for its credibility on covertly alluding to the mental states which it set out to eliminate. Skinner [41] observed that behaviorism never finished an acceptable formulation of the verbal report. "The conception of behavior which it developed could not convincingly embrace the 'use of subjective terms'". He suggested: "A considerable advantage is gained from dealing with terms, concepts, constructs and so on, quite frankly in the form in which they are observed – namely, as verbal responses."

Language behavior, as verbal report, has never been excluded from psychological research. Graham [16] referred to the scientific treatment of such "raw data" as one of the "major problems of psychology":

> In particular, the problem of analysis and classification of responses does not involve accepting them as understandable conversation, but is one of formulating their uniformities and rules in a system where they are taken *as* behaviour. This sort of analysis provides the anomaly that conversation is not viewed as such, but is considered in terms of other words or symbols – that is, scientific description that formulates the rules of the subject's conversation.

This categorization of raw data is the essence of scientific description. The peculiar difficulties posed by verbal report stem from the tacit knowledge everybody has obtained from experiences with persons other than verbal exchanges. A discrepancy may ensue between language and our perception of the other's behavior, since language is only part of a "complete system of human communication." Even considering verbal behavior as a verbal response to external or internal stimuli, how to make predictions about persons on its basis is an open question. As Spence [43] put it, there are essentially four types of empirical relationships or laws in which psychologists have been interested:

1. $R = f(R)$, laws of association of behavioral properties based on correlations between responses
2. $R = f(S)$, laws of the effects of present or past environments (in learning, perception, and so on)
3. $R = f(O)$, laws on response properties derived from organismic conditions or features
4. $O = f(S)$, laws on organismic properties derivable from stimulus conditions

Spence meant by O essentially physiological processes. He observed that psychologists interested in "mediational" problems have concerned themselves with type 3 and type 4 laws. Laws of the type $O = f(R)$ are not discussed; for many behaviorists such a relationship would amount to a tautology, much as a relationship of the form $O = f(O)$ would.

For a science of behavior dealing with subjectivity, intersubjectivity is the only means of being "objective" (objective here meaning to imply methods and theories adequate to the intended level of analysis). In this regard, the oral/aural mode (spoken language) has one specific quality, the simultaneity of "inner" and "outer". Symbols conveyed through language are anchored on "external" and "internal" reality simultaneously, and no other perceptual/operational mode shows so clearly the type and intensity of immediate feedback which allows for self-representation and communication in one single act. I cannot see my eyes "seeing" but I can hear my voice "speaking." To a certain extent, communication, that is, the *intentional* operation of sending and receiving messages, is possible by this monitorization of their emission and reception and is more developed in this than in any other channel [8]. This does not tell us whether the message is true or not, but even when it deceives, speech seems to be closer to subjectivity than other behaviors. As the locus of intersubjectivity, language behavior not only permits inferences about individuals, it also shows the societal dimensions of mind by relating inner experience to overt behavior.

Every act of communication exhibits what Freedman and Grand [11] labeled "communicative structures," meaning the "manifest vehicles of communication through which messages are transmitted." The inner (or "mental") organization of experience upon which communication rests may be generically termed "psychic structure."

The "mentalist" flavor of these constructs is designed to stress that in dealing comprehensively with verbal reports we should take advantage of both the experimental and the clinical approach. We have discussed two main varieties of each: the intuitive-empathic and the scientific-analytic. One important difference between them is precisely the treatment of verbal data. Introspectionism and phenomenology conceive verbal products as "givens." (Phenomenology, from this viewpoint, could be labeled extrospectionism.) Behaviorism and psychoanalysis take verbal reports as referents, or facts, which must be theoretically organized to become data. Each of these points of view, irrespective of their experimental or clinical origin, strives for knowledge, that is, *organized information*. Organized information "makes sense" – is meaningful – only when incorporated into a wider network of assumptions (a theory) that takes into account the level at which to make predictions, the position and characteristics of the observer, and the conditions under which observation, prediction, and control are possible. The task of dealing with verbal report seems to be more than purely scientific, in the traditional sense. It should follow the canons of science, enlarging at the same time the possibilities of scientific awareness through acceptance of the observer's own creative sensibility for other forms of comprehension.

In their analysis of "intervening variables" and "hypothetical constructs" in psychology, MacCorquodale and Meehl [34], after observing that some "tough-minded" psychologists use words such as unobservable and hypothetical in an essentially derogatory manner, proposed a linguistic convention. They restricted the phrase "intervening variables" to the original use implied by Tolman. Such a variable:

> will then be simply a quantity obtained by a specified manipulation of the values of empirical variables, it will involve no hypothesis as to the existence of nonobserved entities or the occurrence of unobserved processes, it will contain … no words which are not definable either explicitly or by reduction sentences in terms of the empirical variables; and the validity of empirical laws involving only observables

will constitute both the necessary and sufficient conditions for the validity of the laws involving these intervening variables.

Examples are Tolman's *demand,* Hull's *habit strength* and Lewin's *valence.* In other disciplines, concepts such as solubility or resistance meet the same criterion, namely, their definition is not a wholly arbitrary and conventional matter.

As a second linguistic convention, the authors [34] proposed that the term "hypothetical construct" be used to designate theoretical concepts which do not meet the requirements for intervening variables in the strict sense. These constructs:

> involve terms which are not wholly reducible to empirical terms; they refer to processes or entities that are not directly observed (although they need not be in principle unobservable); the mathematical expression of them cannot be formed simply by a suitable grouping of terms in a direct empirical equation; and the truth of the empirical laws involved is a necessary but not a sufficient condition for the truth of these conceptions.

Examples are Allport's *biophysical traits* and most theoretical constructs in psychoanalytic theory.

This clarification of terms is needed in the present context to emphasize that "psychic structures" can be either intervening variables or hypothetical constructs. Our main concern is whether at all, and if so, in which systematical position, verbalizations should be used for the definition of psychological constructs. Some "psychic structures" might meet the criteria for intervening variables and others not. It is of importance to underline the fact that the term communicative structure in its present usage does not mean *stimuli* or *responses* but *stimulus-response networks* realized in the linguistic system. We will not enter into the debatable definitions of stimulus and response. Even within the behaviorist tradition, each of these concepts is usually defined in terms of the other. Communicative structure underscores the "embeddedness" of stimulus and response in the matrix of the communicative *act* (or, for that matter, the speech act).

In addition, the use of these terms should make it clear that the approach to verbal report espoused here, while intending to retain the analytic-scientific imprint, should not neglect empathic-intuitive knowledge. The latter inevitably belongs to the "tacit knowledge" [36] experts and laymen use when dealing with language. The weaknesses inherent to "less than pure" science in this domain can be turned into advantages when the observer is aware of their existence and accepts them beyond fallacious prejudices.

Our main contention is more an axiom than a theorem: there is a link between communicative structures and psychic structures. The nature of it can only be disclosed after a brief methodological discussion on methods of dealing with verbal reports that offer prospects of being comprehensive and useful.

2.4 Meaning Analysis and Behavior Texts

From a pragmatic point of view we are interested in the relation between language and its user. The conditions under which messages are emitted and their effects both in sender and receiver are the main concern of the behavioral scientist. In the study of communicative transactions, "language" itself is a concept open to various interpretations and definitions. We want to analyze and understand not just its internal morphologico-syntactic and phonological structure as a conveyor of meaning, but also its relationship with the biological characteristics of the individual, his state of health, his ways of life, his personality, and his behavior in society. Since speech cannot be treated isolated from the total behavior stream, its position in a "total human communication system" must be ascertained. Poyatos [37] distinguished between interactive and noninteractive forms of communication within a culture and discussed a framework for the study of verbal and nonverbal aspects of behavior. Research on kinesics, proxemics, bodily communication, paralanguage, gestures, and human ethology has demonstrated that nonlanguage behavior conveys information and serves expressive functions [10, 18, 37]. There are reservations, nonetheless, as to the independence of communication channels and their mutual influence. As a matter of fact, even when dealing with nonlanguage behavior, the investigator converts the information to some form of verbal statement so that the linguistic structuration of experience could be said to be universal. We have employed the dichotomy explicit-implicit to refer to different aspects of the total human communication system, according to the availability of shared codes of meaning and the functions of the behavioral elements under consideration [28].

It must be explicitly stated that focusing on verbal report does not imply neglect of other sources of information, i.e., physiological data or nonlanguage behavior. The main thrust of this presentation is on the methodological assumptions that should be made for rendering verbal behavior useful in terms of pragmatic concerns in behavioral science. The kind of relationships that could be established between verbal and nonverbal data is an interesting question, but from the point of view pursued here, this question artificially separates integral parts of the behavior stream. What we know of and can observe are always "acts." Some acts carry weight in the oral/aural mode, are more linguistically organized, and connote suprapersonal rules. These "speech acts" lead to the production of *meaning,* which in the present context refers to "rule of use." In a communicative structure, meaning is derived from the set of possible predictions concerning the behavior of language users inside or outside the limits of the verbal system. Meaning refers thus to a dispositional attribute of the user of the language.

As we have already observed, meaning can be derived from verbal reports in two main forms. Either it can be achieved through intuitive judgmental processes of the empathic understanding sort or it can be arrived at by definable step-by-step operations. Both forms are represented within the experimental and the clinical traditions, as the examples provided above suggest, but the main problem remains meaning. For our practical purpose, the *meanings of communicative structures* are *psychic structures.* In communicative structures, we find a complex network of stimuli and responses related to contexts on which sense-reading and sense-giving operations are performed. The nature of these operations varies according to theoretical persuasion and spontaneous preferences, but their result is the constitution of organized knowledge about individuals, which we coin in psychic structures. These are, in the words of Polanyi [36]:

> boundary conditions [which] harness the principles of a lower level in the service of a new, higher level … The higher comprehends the workings of the lower and thus forms the meaning of the lower. As an example, a vocabulary sets boundary conditions on the utterance of the spoken voice; a grammar harnesses words to form sentences; and the sentences shaped into a text which conveys meaningful information.

In dealing with the "behavior texts" constituted on the basis of communicative structures by an observer, we are interested in the sources of their meaning, that is, the psychic structures underlying them. Behavioral particulars in the behavior text receive meaning *from* them.

There are many questions that can be raised before applying the axiom that communicative structures are related to psychic structures. One of them is how this relation is to be conceived of. The other is how truthful it is, in the sense of univocal relations between communicative structures and psychic structures. The problems of deception, the unreliability of verbal report, the existence of interindividual and intercultural differences, and experimenter (observer) bias all seem to militate against a reasonable link between behavioral "hypotheticals" and behavioral "results". As we shall argue, the "existence" or "reality" of a given "hypothetical" (psychic structure) is an interesting but in this context irrelevant concern. The emphasis should be placed on their usefulness, that is, their suggestive and heuristic power.

2.4.1 From Text to Context

Behavioral texts (verbal reports among them) can be studied in an endless variety of ways. A text is an array of symbols and signs that turns into a message when an observer becomes aware of its symbolic-representational nature. The observer may also become aware of constraints imposed on the message by the medium of communication (channel) and take them into account. He may, in addition, be aware of the global and dynamic interdependencies that exist between different parts of the behavior text, such as transitional probabilities from one event to the next or the influence of past experience. Much of what any given observer considers the meaning of a message may also be affected by his/her biases or knowledge besides the text as such. This knowledge about persons or situations might lead to unreproducible results and make these less reliable, but it does not lessen the importance of the relationship between data (communicative structures) and psychological meaning (psychic structures). All and each of these features of sense-reading and sense-giving operations have been stressed, at one time or the other, by different researchers of theorists. The pragmatic concern outlined above leaves out of discussion hermeneutical and empathic approaches. We are not interested in texts as such but in *behavior texts,* produced by persons and converted into messages by an observer who can understand them in terms of a pragmatic metalanguage of psychic structures. On the other hand, valuable as any empathic *Verstehen* is, unavoidable perhaps as "tacit knowledge" regarding persons, we shall approach the topic (discussion) from the vantage point of systemic and reproducible methods for making inferences from (behavior) texts to their (psychological) contexts. In the realm of verbal report, most of the available techniques would fall under the rubric of *content analysis*.

2.4.2 Content Analysis

Although *content analysis* might not be the most adequate designation, it has become an umbrella term for many different techniques for dealing with verbal reports. As an already venerable method of naturalistic documentary research, it has excited great enthusiasm as to its possibilities for use in social and behavioral science and also considerable rejection as to its reliability and validity. In general terms, content analysis might be said to be concerned with ways of treating verbal data as symbolic communications. A classic definition by Berelson [3] defined it as "a research technique for the objective, systematic and quantitative description of the manifest content of communication." Aside from its unclear ("manifest") or restrictive ("quantitative") character, the chief objection to Berelson's definition is, according to Krippendorf [24], "that it does not spell out what 'content' is or what the object of a content analysis should be." Some researchers have resorted to counting; others have suggested that it is a method for "extracting" content from the data as if it were objectively "contained" in them. As Krippendorf [24] put it, "content analysis is a research technique for making replicable and valid inferences from data to their context." He made the reservation that messages do not have a single meaning and that meaning need not be shared. He also made the point that messages and symbolic communication are about phenomena other than those directly observed. This "vicarious nature" of symbolic communications forces the use of inference from sensory data to "portions" of the "empirical environment" of the receiver. It is this empirical environment that he referred to as context of the data. The author also pointed out that the technique of content analysis has been generalized and can be applied to nonlinguistic forms of communication where patterns in data are interpreted as *indices and symptoms*.

Stone et al. [45] presented their definition of content analysis as "a research technique for making inferences by systematically and objectively identifying specified characteristics within a text." What is absent from this definition is the need for relating what is gained from the study of the text to other aspects of behavior, a prerequisite for its behavioral meaningfulness. Psychological validity can obtain only when the inferences made through content analysis are tested on different grounds and with other methods.

It should be stressed that content analysis is a research technique for making inferences. It does go beyond mere description, as the equivalence between *coding* and content analysis might suggest [7]. The reader is referred to authoritative reviews for further information regarding the general principles of content analysis [3, 7, 13, 15, 19, 22, 24, 26, 32, 45].

2.5 Psychological States and Traits and Content Analysis

Marsden [32] distinguished three models of content analysis that have been applied in psychology. The *classical model,* best exemplified in Berelson's work [3], "places a premium on objectivity" and is designed so that "a worker with minimal special training can perform the analysis, maximizing his ability to specify just what configuration of data led to the investigator's inferences." The classical model restricts the analysis from the pragmatic aspect, approachable only after the units are coded and with additional validation procedures. In the *pragmatic model,* the pragmatically relevant inference is made initially, at the time of coding, and is the basis of the coding. In addition to these two, Marsden considered a *nonquantitative model,* lacking methodological homogeneity, but free of the "frequency theorem" of the quantitative classical and pragmatic models. According to this assumption, the *frequency of occurrence* of units in a category is highly correlated with the *intensity* of that category in the communication.

Among the main advantages of content analysis (or, as we would prefer, *meaning* or *symbolic* analysis), it could be mentioned at this point that it is an unobtrusive technique which can be applied both to structured and unstructured material collected under a wide variety of situations. Data collection is not time-consuming, requires simple equipment, and there are practically no limits to the volumes of data that can be analyzed. On the theoretical side, Viney [49] pointed out that, as a method, it may be applied by researchers of different theoretical perspectives. Data collection, as in any scientific procedure, may be influenced by personal biases (for instance, when selecting a sample of subjects or situations), but it may be kept independent of the inferential process itself so that the same "text" may be studied by different researchers or by the same researcher in different moments. In most pragmatic methods, the need for an accurate definition of the aspect to be studied forces the investigator to employ a more adequate operationalization of terms and to devise validational procedures (psychophysiological, psychoanalytical, and sociological) that eventually foster interdisciplinary communication. Properly developed procedures may be appropriate for dealing with other aspects of the "behavioral text" (i.e., nonlinguistic) [38].

Most of the studies presented in this book are based on a pragmatic model of content analysis eclectic as to its basic assumptions, but strongly influenced by psychoanalytic thinking. Carefully defined psychological constructs can be quantitated through language behavior by trained technicians. A provision is made for weighting according to personal participation of the speaker and "centrality" with regard to the construct explored. In standardized situations, the projective aspect may be maximized, thus allowing for a psychological probing of psychological attributes that resembles an experimental analogue of clinical, dyadic situations [13, 15].

It is important to emphasize some features of this approach. The method depends heavily upon the specification of the content characteristics to be measured and the proper identification of empirical referents (verbal behavior markers). The first must be theoretically justified. While this also holds true for the second, at this stage empirical validation aspects should be considered. Replication in this field is more a function of the "analysis program" (the set of operations for identifying and recording the characteristics when they occur in the text) than of the "objectivity" or "validity" of the constructs studied. Objectivity refers to intersubjective aspects of meaning structures. Validity should be ascertained by convergent evaluations of the same data or testing some criterion result derived from the theory justifying (or supporting) the construct under study. Understandable rules and clear-cut operationalization are thus preconditions for the reliable use of the method but are independent of validation.

In the Gottschalk-Gleser and Viney-Westbrook Scales, as examples of pragmatic methods, the coding unit is the grammatical clause. It constitutes the minimal element in the text that conveys meaning. This is at variance with other methods that operate on the basis of more elementary coding units, such as words or frequencies of word combinations. While one could argue about advantages and limitations of each of these approaches, caution should be exercised in extrapolating results from one technique to another, particularly if they employ similar labels to characterize the constructs under study. In comparisons between the Gottschalk-Gleser method and the Anxiety Topics Dictionary (ATD) developed at the University of Ulm – a word-based method implemented by computer – a fair degree of agreement has been found in anxiety scores, particularly in shame and separation anxiety [17, 29], a finding suggestive of convergent validity in some of the constructs investigated. Both methods, like different staining procedures in histology, might be sensitive to the same or different aspects of the message and tell something about how representative the empirical referents (coding units) in fact are. This comparison of methods should be made, whenever possible, in the texts to be analyzed.

There is, however, another aspect that merits consideration: the situation in which verbal data are collected. The same comparison between the ATD and Gottschalk-Gleser anxiety categories, when made on verbal exchanges during medical visits in an internal medical setting and not in a psychotherapeutic one, yielded almost complete lack of correlation between scores [17].This fact could be taken to imply a strong situational dependency, demonstrated for the Gottschalk-Gleser method, [23] and leads to differing degrees of stability for the "Affect" Scales (Anxiety and Hostility). The last study also investigated stability over time, which, being rather low for some scales, can be brought to bear on the discussion about trait and state measurement [23]. While some writers insist that the method is sensitive to state-dependent factors [15, 49], the complex interactions between trait, state, and situation should be explored in more detail than hitherto has been the case. This is all the more important considering that applications of these techniques range from psychopharmacological effects and cognitive performances to nosological differentiations [12, 13, 15, 30, 39, 49].

Despite extensive validation and comparison studies, there is a paucity of theoretical elaboration of the basic assumptions. This, along with empirical studies on the relationships between nonverbal and verbal behavior, remain challenging areas for research. The same holds true for automatic content analysis by computer, easily implemented in word-based methods but difficult to apply to clause-based ones. The promising efforts of Gottschalk and co-workers in this direction [14] should be expanded considering the higher direct relevance of their pragmatic categories to clinical questions. Word-based methods, while easily implemented and able to rapidly produce large volumes of data, need a further validation step between "dictionary" and inference that a more comprehensive method could avoid. At present, the difficulties associated with computarization of some of the Gottschalk-Gleser Scales can only be resolved by a closer collaboration with language scientists and by attention to syntactic and semantic aspects. This will probably give rise to a method of truly psycholinguistic import, reaching beyond the study of the *parole* (speech) to the study of the *langage* (language). It is to be hoped that the pragmatic relevance and practical applicability of the method are not lost in the process.

Other needed expansion concerns the progressive incorporation of other aspects of the "total human communication system." A truly integrative approach to biopsychosocial medicine demands that the methods employed attempt an at least asymptotic approximation to the joint consideration of complementary sources of information. The "behavior text" to be deciphered in communicative structures consists not solely of speech, but of physiology and motor behavior as well. The "psychic structures" to be formulated – from which the behavior text derives its meaning – will be more useful the larger the observational field they summarize and express.

Granted that this might be possible in principle, the reification of psychic structures so constructed should be avoided. The type of empirical law might look like $O = f(R)$ if we want to formulate it in the language of logical behaviorism, that is, O (organism = psychic structures) should be a function of recordable R_s (responses, but understood here as *stimulus-response networks*) without implying a causal connection between them. Psychic structures (be they traits, states, emotions, etc.) do not "cause" communicative structures. They help give them meaning by an observer. They aid in prediction and control. They are not true or false. They should be useful.

Finally, it should be remarked that psychic structures are not "contained" (in a physical sense) in the empirical observables of the communicative structures. Meaning analysis is by definition not a method for discovering but a method for organizing facts, or better, for converting facts into organized, meaningful knowledge. The radical individuality of all behavior calls for an equilibrated analysis of idiosyncratic, individual subjects expressing themselves through supraindividual means and general and lawful formulations of "models of man."

In content (meaning) analysis, we have a method for combining the intuitive clinical approach with the rigor of experimental science.

2.6 Concluding Remarks

The main conclusion of this chapter is that content (meaning) analysis of speech might be developed as a technique integrating the intuitive-empathic and the scientific-analytic dimensions present in both the experimental and the clinical approach. Speech is part of a behavioral text which, considered as *communicative structures,* can be given meaning in terms of a pragmatic metalanguage of *psychic structures.* Psychological states and traits, emotions, attitudes, and other constructs so defined serve as guiding clues for further research, for diagnosis, and for prediction. They constitute the (psychological) context for the interpretation of the (behavioral) text. This, made up of behavioral particulars, receives its meaning from it. Psychic structures are stimulus-response networks encompassing both dispositions on the part of the subject observed and characteristics of the observer. In this sense, their main value should be sought after in their usefulness, not in their reification as "realities" endowed with causal properties. They do not explain behavior. They rather help in organizing knowledge about persons and situations, rendering them understandable and predictable.

The proper place of content analysis of verbal behavior in a comprehensive program of studies of the "total" human communication system is yet to be ascertained. Different techniques, diverse theoretical foundations, and disparate aims characterize the field. Decisions regarding applications and methodology depend on the investigator wishing to combine the objective and the subjective in his/her approach to human subjects. The basic axioms and theorems underlying content analysis of verbal behavior, as well as its relationships with other domains of inquiry, are illustrated in the different chapters of this book, which represents an array of examples of research centered around a common methodology. As it will be seen, there are grounds to believe that ecologically valid formulations about human beings can be developed when intuitive-empathic understanding is associated with rigorous experimental measurement.

References

1. Abel T (1953) The operation called Verstehen. In: Feigl H, Brodbeck M (eds) Readings in the philosophy of science. Appleton-Century-Crofts, New York, pp 677–687
2. Altschule MD (1977) Origins of concepts in human behavior. Halsted-Wiley, New York
3. Berelson BR (1954) Content analysis. In: Lindsey G (ed) Handbook of social psychology, vol 1. Addison-Wesley, Reading
4. Bergmann G, Spence KW (1944) The logic of psychophysical measurement. Psychol Rev 51: 1–24
5. Boring EG (1953) A history of introspection. Psychol Bull 50: 169–189
6. Breuer J, Freud S (1916) Studien über Hysterie, 3rd edn. Deuticke, Leipzig
7. Cartwright D (1953) Analysis of qualitative material. In: Festinger L, Katz D (eds) Research methods in the behavioral sciences. Holt Rinehart and Winston, New York
8. Dance FEX (1977) Acoustic trigger to conceptualization. A hypothesis concerning the role of the spoken word in the development of higher mental processes. Health Comm Inform 5: 203–213
9. Edelheit H (1969) Speech and psychic structure. J Am Psychoanal Assoc 17: 342–381
10. Eibl-Eibesfeldt I (1967) Grundriß der vergleichenden Verhaltensforschung-Ethologie. Piper, München
11. Freedman N, Grand S (1977) Prologue: a gesture toward a psychoanalytic theory of communication. In: Freedman A, Grand S (eds) Communicative structures and psychic structures. Plenum, New York
12. Gottschalk LA (ed) (1979) Pharmacokinetics of psychoactive drugs: further studies. Spectrum, New York
13. Gottschalk LA (ed) (1979) The content analysis of verbal behavior. Further studies. Spectrum, New York
14. Gottschalk LA, Bechtel RJ (1982) The measurement of anxiety through the computer analysis of verbal samples Compr Psychiatry 23: 364
15. Gottschalk LA, Gleser GC (1969) The measurement of psychological states through the content analysis of verbal behavior. University of California Press, Berkeley
16. Graham CH (1958) Sensation and perception in an objective psychology. Psychol Rev 65: 65–76
17. Grünzig HJ, Mergenthaler E (in press) Computerunterstützte Ansätze. Empirische Untersuchungen am Beispiel der Angstthemen. In: Koch U (ed) Sprachinhaltsanalyse in der psychosomatischen und psychiatrischen Forschung. Grundlagen und Anwendungsstudien mit den Affektskalen von Gottschalk und Gleser. Beltz, Weinheim
18. Hinde R (ed) (1972) Non-verbal communication. Cambridge University Press, Cambridge
19. Holsti OR (1969) Content analysis for the social sciences and humanities. Addison – Wesley, Reading
20. Homme LE (1965) Perspectives in psychology. XXIV. Control of coverants, the operants of the mind. Psychol Rec 15: 501–511

21. Jaspers K (1968) General psychopathology, 7th edn. University of Chicago Press, Chicago
22. Kerlinger FN (1964) Foundations of behavioral research. Holt, Rinehart and Winston, New York
23. Kordy H, Lolas F, Wagner G (1982) Zur Stabilität der inhaltsanalytischen Erfassung von Affekten nach Gottschalk und Gleser. Z Klin Psychol Psychother 30: 202–213
24. Krippendorf K (1980) Content analysis. An introduction to its methodology. Sage, Beverly Hills
25. Lieberman DA (1979) Behaviorism and the mind. Am Psychol 34: 319–333
26. Lisch R, Kriz J (1978) Grundlagen und Modelle der Inhaltsanalyse. Rowohlt, Reinbeck
27. Lolas F (1979) Anthropological psychiatry and melancholia; a critical appraisal. J Phenomenol Psychol 10: 139–149
28. Lolas F, Ferner H (1978) Zum Begriff des impliziten Verhaltens. Z Klin Psychol Psychother 26: 223–233
29. Lolas F, Mergenthaler E, von Rad M (1982) Content analysis of verbal behaviour in psychotherapy research: a comparison between two methods. Br J Med Psychol 55: 327–333
30. Lolas F, von Rad M, Scheibler H (1981) Situational influences on verbal affective expression of psychosomatic and psychoneurotic patients. J Nerv Ment Dis 169: 619–623
31. Luborsky L, Spence DP (1978) Quantitative research on psychoanalytic therapy. In: Garfield SL, Bergin AE (eds) Handbook of psychotherapy and behavior change. Wiley, New York
32. Marsden G (1971) Content analysis studies of psychotherapy: 1954 through 1968. In: Bergin HE, Garfield SL (eds) Handbook of psychotherapy and behavior change. Wiley, New York
33. Matson FW (ed) (1973) Without/within: behaviorism and humanism. Brooks-Cole, Monterey
34. Mac Corquodale K, Meehl PE (1953) Hypothetical constructs and intervening variables. In: Feigl H, Brodbeck M (eds) Readings in the philosophy of science. Appleton-Century-Crofts, New York
35. Pillsbury WB (1911) Essentials of psychology. Macmillan, New York
36. Polanyi M (1969) Knowing and being. In: Grene M (ed) Essays. University of Chicago Press, Chicago
37. Poyatos F (1976) Language in the context of total body communication. Linguistic 168: 49–62
38. Russell RL, Stiles WB (1979) Categories for classifying language in psychotherapy. Psychol Bull 86: 404–419
39. von Rad M, Drücke M, Knauss W, Lolas F (1979) Alexithymia: a comparative study of verbal behavior in psychosomatic and psychoneurotic patients. In: Gottschalk LA (ed) The content analysis of verbal behavior. Further studies. Spectrum, New York
40. Shevrin H (1977) Some assumptions of psychoanalytic communication: implications of sublimal research for psychoanalytic method and technique. In: Freedman N, Grand S (eds) Communicative structures and psychic structures. Plenum, New York
41. Skinner BF (1953) The operational analysis of psychological terms. In: Fergl H, Brodbeck M (eds) Readings in the philosophy of science. Appleton-Century-Crofts, New York, pp 585–595
42. Skinner BF (1957) Verbal behavior. Appleton-Century-Crofts, New York
43. Spence KW (1953) The postulates and methods of "behaviorism." In: Frigl H, Brodbeck M (eds) Readings in the philosophy of science. Appleton-Century-Crofts, New York, pp 571–584
44. Spence D (1981) Psychoanalytic competence. Int J Psychoanal 62: 113–124
45. Stone PJ, Dunphy DC, Smith MS (1966) The general inquirer: a computer approach to content analysis. MIT, Cambridge, Mass

46. Titchener EB (1899) Structural and functional psychology. Philos Rev 8: 290–299
47. Titchener EB (1929) Systematic psychology: prolegomena. Macmillan, New York
48. Tolman EC (1949) Purposive behavior in animals and men. University of California Press, Berkeley
49. Viney L (1983) The assesment of psychological states through content analysis of verbal communications. Psychol Bull 94: 542–563
50. Watson JB (1914) Behavior: an introduction to comparative psychology. Holt, Rinehart and Winston, New York
51. Woodworth RS, Sheehan MR (1964) Contemporary schools of psychology, 3rd edn. Ronald, New York

3 Research Using the Gottschalk–Gleser Content Analysis Scales in English Since 1969

Louis A. Gottschalk*

3.1 Scope of the Content Analysis Method

3.1.1 Development and Applications of the Gottschalk–Gleser Method: An Overview

In *The Measurement of Psychological States Through the Content Analysis of Verbal Behavior* [1], authors Gottschalk and Gleser thoroughly discussed the theoretical bases for qualifying and quantifying psychological states through content analysis of speech. They outlined their theoretical approaches to content analysis in general, the method of eliciting verbal behavior, and the effect of the method of elicitation used on the data obtained, assessing intensity, scale development, and validation. While providing a detailed description of their theories concerning the measurement of anxiety, hostility, and social alienation/personal disorganization, they also supplied guidelines on how to develop procedures for measuring other psychological states from verbal samples.

Since publication of that volume in 1969, further investigation has been performed on several scales mentioned then only briefly. Additional validation studies have been performed on a scale designed to measure hope [2] and on another designed to measure cognitive-intellectual impairment [3–7]. Results of research on the "Hope" Scale suggested that scores are capable of predicting longevity in terminal cancer patients who are receiving total- or half-body irradiation [8], predicting favorable outcome in patients at a mental health crisis clinic [9], and predicting which patients are likely to follow through on recommendations to continue psychiatric treatment [10].

Results of work with the Gottschalk–Gleser Cognitive Impairment Scale indicate that transient impairment of cognitive function occurs with total- or half-body irradiation [8], on exposure to sensory overload (especially in individuals who are field dependent) [11], and on smoking marijuana (as compared with placebo) [12]. Gottschalk et al. [13–16] have also shown that certain types of cognitive defect, as determined by the Gottschalk–Gleser Cognitive Impairment Scale, occur in the schizophrenic syndrome and that these verbal cognitive defects can be improved when phenothiazines are administered. In addition, cognitive impairment scores in the pathological range, as determined by a battery of neurological tests which include the Halstead-Reitan Tests [17–19] and the Gottschalk–Gleser Cognitive Impairment Scale [1, 4, 13–15], occur

---

* Department of Psychiatry and Human Behavior, UCI-California College of Medicine, University of California at Irvine, Irvine, CA 92717

with chronic alcoholism [20]. A number of investigations [15, 16, 21] have independently provided more evidence that the Gottschalk-Gleser Social Alienation/Personal Disorganization Scale differentiates schizophrenic individuals from nonschizophrenic individuals.

Wooley et al. [22] used a somewhat modified form of the Gottschalk-Gleser content analysis method to measure achievement orientation and complaints in individuals who had been patients on the psychosomatic ward of a large metropolitan hospital. At the 1-year follow-up evaluation, an analysis of trends showed a significant ($P < .05$) effect of family status in the pattern of changes in both dimensions; patients with intact families had treatment successes and those without intact families had treatment failures. This finding was based on the manifest content of their verbal samples.

Gottschalk and Hoigaard-Martin [23] have developed a scale that measures depression from verbal samples, and Cleghorn at McMaster University in Canada has been developing a similar scale derived in part from the Gottschalk-Gleser method (personal communications, 1978).

Discrepancies among different test results have been noted when investigators use rating scales, self-report scales, and content analysis scales to measure psychological states. For this reason, Gottschalk et al. [24] performed a study comparing scores when the same patients were evaluated with the Gottschalk-Gleser Content Analysis Scales, the Hamilton Anxiety Rating Scale, the Physician Questionnaire Rating Scale, and the Hopkins Symptom Checklist. The results showed low correlations among the tests in the measurement of anxiety and hostility. However, when all the subcomponents of the different scales are intercorrelated, significant correlations are often found, indicating that the developers of these different measurement procedures incorporated different compositions of dimensions in each of their constructs of anxiety and histility. These measurement problems have been described elsewhere [25]. Gottschalk and Uliana [26] have attempted to clarify the extent to which the Gottschalk-Gleser Anxiety, Hostility, and Social Alienation/Personal Disorganization Scales measure psychological states as opposed to psychological traits.

3.1.2 Content Analysis in Children

An individual's knowledge and use of language undergoes developmental changes that begin with the onset of speech in infancy, and Gottschalk felt that the speech of younger children – especially those under age 10 – was noticeably different from that of older children and adults. Therefore, before his content analysis procedure could be used to measure psychological states in children, Gottschalk realized that it would first be necessary to revalidate the "adult" scales for a number of psychological dimensions.

Because criterion measures capable of independently assessing psychological states in children are unavailable, Gottschalk has approached construct validation with younger children carefully, and he is still engaged in the systematic validation of the scales for children in general. He has, however, published normative scores for children that are stratified by school grade and sex and has also reported on the differences in speech content between boys and girls in the age range of 6–16 years [27, 28].

Uliana [29] has used the Anxiety and Hostility Scales to measure the affective states in black children. Scores were also stratified by grade and sex. In addition, she has examined the effect of the interviewer's race on the affective states, which were also measured by the Gottschalk-Gleser method. Gleser et al. [30] conducted a study using the Gottschalk-Gleser Anxiety and Hostility Scales to evaluate the effectiveness of psychotherapy on adolescents. The study showed that the beneficial effects of supervision of psychotherapy were significantly greater than psychotherapy without supervision. Silbergeld et al. [31] have used the Anxiety and Hostility Scales in group studies of adolescents.

3.2 Scoring and Illustrating Scores in Content Analysis

Certain problems attend scoring in content analysis, a procedure that is performed by content analysis technicians. To maintain test precision, the accuracy of scoring must periodically undergo reliability checks. Scoring is also time-consuming, even though obtaining the speech samples is simple and rapid. A computerized system for scoring would solve these problems. A feasibility study [32] showed that scores on the Gottschalk-Gleser Hostility-Outward Scale obtained by human experts could be roughly approximated by computer analysis. Other studies in progress are concerned with developing a computer system that will measure psychological reactions from verbal samples according to the Gottschalk-Gleser method.

Marsden [33] raised the issue as to whether the use of percentage scores to control for productivity of speech in verbal content analysis can yield erroneous conclusions. Gleser and Lubin [34] have addressed many of his objections as they might pertain to the scoring of Gottschalk-Gleser Scales.

Two papers [26, 35] contain suggestions on ways of diagnostically illustrating scores obtained with the Gottschalk-Gleser Scales. In one paper, Gottschalk and Uliana presented a system whereby scores obtained with children on 17 content analysis scales may be compared graphically to the scores of a normative group of children, either white or black, through the use of T scores. Twelve of these 17 content analysis scales are the Anxiety and Hostility Scales plus their subscales.

3.3 Neuropsychopharmacological Studies

3.3.1 Effects of Psychoactive Drugs or Chemical Substances on Language Content

Propranolol, a beta-adrenergic blocking agent, was reported to have reduced the anxiety scores of relatively nonanxious subjects as well as to lower the fasting plasma free fatty acid levels associated with these scores. However, propranolol did not prevent a significant rise in anxiety scores that were evoked by a stress interview. It was found that, when not on propranolol, the subjects' anxiety scores correlated positively ($+0.70$) with average plasma free fatty acid level, but when the subjects were on propranolol, anxiety scores correlated negatively (-0.55), and the average pulse rate was significantly reduced. To explain this observed antianxiety effect of propranolol, it was suggested that basal or resting anxiety may be maintained by peripheral afferent autonomic biofeedback and that the latter can be reduced by beta-adrenergic blocking agents [36]. In support of this, Gottschalk [37] has found that the magnitude of anxiety aroused through a stress interview is mediated more through the central than peripheral nervous system.

Gardos et al. [38] investigated the effect of oxazepam (45 mg/day) and chlordiazepoxide (30 mg/day) on hostility and anxiety. Hostility was evaluated from 10-min written verbal samples that were scored according to the Gottschalk-Gleser method. Anxiety was measured by the Shier and Cattell Eight Parallel Anxiety Battery. Compared with placebo, both drugs tended to increase hostility: in highly anxious subjects, chlordiazepoxide significantly increased ambivalent hostility scores, while oxazepam significantly increased hostility-directed-inward scores. After administration for 1 week, both drugs significantly reduced anxiety. The results of the study indicated that the initial level of anxiety played an important role in determining the degree and direction of change in hostility resulting from drug administration.

The effects of smoking either marijunana or placebo marijuana on the psychological states and psychophysiological cardiovascular functioning of angina patients were studied. Although the effects of the marijunana on anxiety and hostility scores varied, significant increases in social alienation/personal disorganization and cognitive-intellectual impairment scores did occur. These findings were associated with observed adverse effects on cardiovascular functioning [12, 39].

A study was carried out on a sample of 108 college students to investigate the influence of the doctor's mental set on a patient's response to psychoactive medication. After reading one of three cards suggesting what effect to expect from the drug they were about to take, 10-min written verbal samples were collected from subjects before and 45–60 min after ingesting either 10 mg of racemic amphetamine sulfate, 10 mg of secobarbital, or placebo. The amphetamine set was: "This drug will probably make you feel more peppy and energetic and cheerful." The secobarbital set was: "This drug will probably make you feel less anxious and more relaxed. It might even make you feel a bit sleepy." The noncommital placebo set was: "It is not known exactly what effect this drug will have on you as an individual." Subjects were randomly assigned to one of nine possible drug/mental set combinations. Although no significant effect of mental set on anxiety scores was detected, mean achievement strivings scores were significantly higher with the amphetamine drug/amphetamine mental set combination [40]. Another study [41] explored the effect of amphetamine or chlorpromazine on achievement strivings scores obtained by content analysis. Scores were found to be significantly increased with amphetamine.

In a double-blind study, Silbergeld et al. [42] examined the effects of an oral contraceptive [norethynodrel with mestranol; Enovid (USA)] or placebo on the affect changes that had been previously observed [43, 44] in speech samples collected during different phases of the menstrual cycle. The oral contraceptive was found to suppress the cyclical changes in affect that occurred with the menses.

In other neuropsychopharmacological research, verbal cognitive impairment scores were found to be increased with nitrous oxide intoxication [45]. The chronic administration of diphenylhydantoin to prisoners was not found to have any significant effect on anxiety and hostility scores [46], while lorezepam, a potent new benzodiazepine, was found to significantly reduce anxiety scores [47]. The effects of a stressful film on the anxiety and hostility scores of alcoholic and nonalcoholic subjects have also been studied [48].

3.3.2 Neuropsychiatric Syndromes, Psychoactive Drugs, and Language Characteristics

Gottschalk et al. [14] studied 74 chronic schizophrenic patients for 8 weeks to evaluate the effect of first withdrawing and then readministering their phenothiazine medication. During the first 4 weeks all patients were given placebo. During the next 4 weeks, half continued on placebo and half were given thioridazine. Five-minute speech samples were obtained at least twice weekly for 8 weeks, and the samples were scored for anxiety, hostility, and social alienation/personal disorganization according to the Gottschalk-Gleser method.

The following results were obtained:
1. Average scores for social alienation/personal disorganization increased significantly over the first 4 weeks, indicating that psychopathological processes increased in these patients when their phenothiazine medication was withdrawn.
2. The patients who continued on placebo showed little increase in social alienation/ personal disorganization scores, whereas those who were given thioridazine showed a nonsignificant decrease.
3. Using multiple correlation techniques with the scores for social alienation/personal disorganization averaged over the first 4 weeks, it was possible to predict response to phenothiazine withdrawal.

Using factor scores of psychotism and disorientation from the Mental Status Schedule of Spitzer et al. [49, 50], a score of 7 or more in either factor scale was used as the criterion to divide the patients into two groups: those whose social alienation/personal disorganization scores got increasingly higher while they were on placebo, and those whose scores showed practically no change. Initial scores of 2 or less on the Social Alienation/Personal Disorganization Scale were predictive of those who would not react to phenothiazine withdrawal or readministration, and initial scores of 2 or more were predictive of those who would react to phenothiazine withdrawal with exacerbation of the schizophrenic syndrome or to readministration with a reduction in the severity of the symptom complex. Covert hostility-outward scores, i.e., statements about others being hostile to others, tended to be predictive of those who would not be disoriented 4 weeks after their tranquilizer had been withdrawn ($r = -0.28$, $P < 0.05$). This finding suggested that the more the schizophrenic patient verbalized about the hostility among others, the more likely it was to be a sign of relative alertness to external events and, hence, an index of the capacity to test reality.

Gottschalk [13] has examined the use of language by schizophrenic patients in greater detail, demonstrating that cognitive defects, as measured by the Gottschalk-Gleser Cognitive Impairment Scale, are associated with the schizophrenic syndrome. In schizophrenia, these defects are typically accompanied by signs of social alienation that can be detected in the content of speech, and they tend to be improved in many patients with the administration of a phenothiazine derivative [51, 52]. Similar signs of cognitive defects appear in children between the ages of 6 and 10, but they decrease significantly with age and are not associated with verbalization of psychosocial withdrawal or alienation [13, 27].

Psychotomimetic drugs administered to normal subjects can bring out these cognitive defects but not the other speech characteristics of schizophrenic patients [1, 13]. Similar cognitive defects are evident in the speech of normal subjects shortly after inhaling 40% nitrous oxide [45]. Also, benzodiazepine derivatives can produce anterograde amnesic effects and transient verbal cognitive defects. These effects and defects may take the form of a significantly higher incidence of remarks that are inaudible, not understandable, or are incomplete phrases or clauses [53, 54].

Further validation of the ability of the Gottschalk-Gleser Cognitive Impairment Scale to measure impairment of brain function by evaluating speech samples has been obtained from a number of investigations [4–7] that are ongoing. These studies use the scores from a battery of 18 neuropsychological tests as their criterion measures in concurrent validation research. Multiple regression (predictor) formulas have been developed. The independent variables in these formulas are the verbal category scores that were previously found to correlate with each separate neuropsychological test score at a 0.05 level or better. The dependent variable is the neuropsychological test score. Two sets of formulas that can be applied to scores obtained from 5-min speech samples have been derived. One set uses only verbal category scores and their frequency of use per 100 words as independent variables. The other set uses verbal category scores plus the subject's age and educational level (both of which are related to cognitive function) as independent variables. For most of the 18 tests, the correlation with these predictor formulas is significant.

These 18 neuropsychological tests would ordinarily take 3–5 h per subject to administer and an even longer time to score. It would be impossible to generate sets of these test scores on an hourly basis for many subjects if the tests were administered in the usual fashion. However, by incorporating the frequency of use of certain verbal categories found in 5-min speech samples into a multiple regression formula, this new method of assessing changes in cognitive function enables one to observe the progression of these changes under various conditions.

3.3.3 Psychoactive Drugs: Pharmacokinetics and Clinical Response

Subjects' values for blood concentration of chlordiazepoxide after a single oral dose have been found to occupy a broad range, and significant decreases in anxiety scores, which were determined through Gottschalk-Gleser content analysis, were found to occur only in those subjects whose blood drug concentration was above a certain level [15, 55–58]. A similar variation in blood drug concentration has been noted with both oral and intramuscular administration of meperidine, and the decrease in anxiety or hostility level after a single dose has also been found to be related to the blood drug concentration [59].

Single-dose studies [51, 55] in which thioridazine (4 mg/kg) or mesoridazine (2 mg/kg) was administered to acute schizophrenic patients have revealed wide variation in the values for pharmacokinetic variables among these individuals. Reduction in social alienation/personal disorganization scores and other measures of the schizophrenic syndrome was found to be related to these variables. There is also evidence that a favorable change in social alienation/personal disorganization scores in response to a single dose of one of these phenothiazines is strong indication that there will be a favorable response upon continued phenothiazine (thioridazine) administration. Single-dose pharmacokinetics of thioridazine can also be used as predictors of the steady-state blood drug concentration during continuous daily drug administration [60].

Single-dose studies [3, 50] with the benzodiazepines have shown that there is a significant correlation between blood drug concentration and a favorable clinical response. This correlation is not found when administration is continuous, probably because of increasing tolerance to the drug and increasing metabolic breakdown of it by activated hepatic level enzymes.

In an unsuccessful attempt to hasten improvement in their cognitive function within a 4-h period, diazepam or haloperidol was administered intramuscularly to individuals who were intoxicated with alcohol. Among the tests used to evaluate speech samples was the Gottschalk-Gleser Cognitive Impairment Scale. The scores of other psychological tests that were used were derived through multiple regression formulas that involved the frequency with which various verbal categories had been used in 5-min speech samples produced over the 4 h following drug administration [20].

3.3.4 Problems in Measuring Psychological States

Several works dealing with problems in measuring and assessing psychological states include discussion of the Gottschalk-Gleser Content Analysis Scales. The use of behavior rating scales, self-report scales, and content analysis scales in psychopharmacological research has been described, and the advantages and shortcomings of each method of assessing the magnitude of psychological reactions have been discussed [24, 25, 61, 62]. The use of these different methods in research that does not involve psychoactive drugs has also been reviewed [63, 64].

One paper [26] presents scoring forms that permit diagnostic illustration and comparison of the content analysis scores of children with normative scores derived from large samples of white and black children. Empirical data concerning the extent to which various affect and other content analysis scales that use the Gottschalk-Gleser method measure psychological states as opposed to psychological traits are also presented. Other works [50, 51] describe the use of discriminant function formulas that incorporate verbal categories from the Social Alienation/Personal Disorganization Scale to distinguish between the schizophrenic patients likely to be placebo-responders, those likely to be phenothiazine-responders, and those likely to be phenothiazine-nonresponders. Another innovative use of verbal content or form categories involves incorporating selective verbal categories into multiple regression correlations. This procedure predicts the score of any one of more than a dozen neuropsychological tests that measure cognitive-intellectual impairment [5].

3.4 Studies of Psychophysiological and Psychosomatic Phenomena

Certain methods of indicating and quantifying emotions have been used in various psychophysiological and psychosomatic studies. These methods have been reviewed [64, 65]. The studies [36, 37] that focused on the relationship between anxiety scores and changes in the concentration of fasting plasma free fatty acids have shown that the slight pain associated with a venipuncture elevates the plasma free fatty acid level in fasting subjects. In addition, verbal anxiety scores were found to be directly related to fasting plasma free fatty acid level, except when the subject is taking propranolol.

The arousal of anxiety and/or hostility in free-associative speech was found to trigger petit mal electroencephalographic paroxysms in a susceptible patient [66]. Silbergeld et al. [67] demonstrated that the anxiety scores derived from speech samples correlate significantly with changes in serum dopamine beta-hydroxylase, especially in women. This finding substantiates the results of other studies [36, 37, 46, 53, 68] that have shown a strong relationship between scores of the Gottschalk-Gleser Anxiety Scales and arousal of the sympathetic nervous system.

Muscle reflexes in the scrotal sac were found to correlate with anxiety scores derived from the subjects' dreams, the contents of which were evaluated by the Gottschalk-Gleser method [69, 70]. Such use of the Anxiety-Scales has been corroborated by the results of other research that indicated fasting plasma free fatty acids (which are markers of catecholamine secretion) become significantly more elevated during 15 min of rapid-eye-movement (REM) sleep, i. e., during dreaming, when more anxiety is occurring during these dreams [68]. Karacan et al. [71] have shown that penile erections are reduced during dreams whose content, as evaluated by Gottschalk-Gleser analysis, revealed higher anxiety. A different kind of dream-content study examined the relationship of the mother's manifest dream content to duration of childbirth in primiparae; the results showed that the greater the anxiety in dreams occurring during the last trimester of pregnancy, the less likely it was that labor would be prolonged [72]. This finding suggests that, under certain circumstances, the arousal of anxiety and the catecholamine system have adaptive functions in preparing humans to carry out stressful tasks.

3.5 Somatopsychic Studies and Studies of Environmental Effects on Psychological Processes

The effect of total- or half-body irradiation on the cognitive and emotional processes of terminal cancer patients was mentioned earlier (Sect. 3.1.1). Individual differences in the affective responses to such irradiation were observed, but there seemed to be a uniform transient increase in cognitive impairment scores, which were obtained by the Gottschalk-Gleser method [8]. In another investigation [11] of the effects of the environment on psychological reactions, subjects were exposed to sensory overload by having them watch a specially made movie. This 43-min film was composed of unusual combinations of colors and lights that were accompanied by cacophonous sound. Affective responses varied among individuals, and significant increases in the average scores for social alienation/personal disorganization were seen. These effects were more notable in the field-dependent subjects. The results of a subsequent study [73] corroborated these findings.

Taub and Berger [74] reported that the Affective Adjective Checklist registered more homogeneous diurnal mood changes, e.g., fatigue decreased from morning to noon and increased from noon to evening, when compared with scores derived from Gottschalk-Gleser content analysis. However, the importance of individual variation in diurnal mood changes was disregarded. The assumption seemed to be that all individuals have similar diurnal mood changes, which is probably erroneous.

3.6 Studies of Psychokinesic Phenomena

The interest in nonverbally communicating emotions and feelings through bodily movement has been gradually increasing in the United States. Deutsch [75], a pioneer in this area, approached kinesics by searching for meaning in every gesture. To a large extent, he perceived a one-to-one relationship between gesture and some underlying drive. Scheflen [76] regarded the relationships between body movement and psychological state as being more complex. He maintained that rarely and only in the simplest cases is the meaning of a single gesture clear. He noted complex patterns of communication in which body language was one element, and, for it to be understood, it must be considered within its complex interaction with the patient's verbal behavior.

Haggard and Isaacs [77] singled out micromomentary facial expressions as a kinesic variable of interest. They observed that three-fourths of the time these micromomentary expressions can be adjudged to be incompatible with the contextual affect expression. More recently, there have been investigations [78–82] using the Gottschalk-Gleser Content Analysis Scales to measure the psychological reactions associated with body movement.

Steingart et al. [78] videotaped the hand movements of 16 male chronic schizophrenic patients and correlated them with anxiety scores derived from a 10-min segment from each of their clinical interviews. A significant correlation was found between highly communicative manual behavior and what the authors termed the "anxiety function" factor, which was obtained by factor analysis of the Gottschalk-Gleser Anxiety Scale scores. This factor had a high positive loading of *guilt anxiety* and a high negative loading of *diffuse anxiety*. *Diffuse anxiety* was viewed as nonsignal anxiety in which there is no cognition as to what the anxiety is all about and *guilt anxiety* as signal anxiety that is relatively independent of situational determinants. The conclusion from these findings was what one might expect: marginally adjusted patients, such as chronic schizophrenics, will have extreme difficulty in the function (or information processing) of anxiety and will tend to not differentiate the different kinds of anxiety within themselves or others.

Another investigation [79] examined the relationship of body movements to different kinds of hostility as evaluated by Gottschalk-Gleser content analysis. Hand movements directed away from the body, or "object-focused" movements, correlated significantly with overt-hostility-outward scores ($r = 0.49$), and hand movements in the direction of the body, or "body-focused" movements, were strongly associated with covert-hostility-outward scores ($r = 0.53$).

Certain observations were made during the psychoanalysis of a patient who periodically stroked his lips. By synchronizing the content of this patient's free associations and his lip-touching, it was apparent that he made references to women and to positive feelings during lip-caressing [82]. These observations inspired investigation into the effect of lip-caressing on hope scores, oral references, and various psychological states including shame anxiety and hostility, all as expressed in the content of speech. Among other findings, subjects who had evidence of early social deprivation showed a greater increase in hope scores during lip-caressing than subjects who had no evidence of such deprivation [80, 81].

Gottschalk [63] has reviewed some of the applications of the Gottschalk-Gleser content analysis method in psychotherapy research. Two papers [9, 83] report on the use of these scales as a predictive tool; one evaluates their ability to predict change in a community mental health training program, and the other measures their ability to predict outcome of therapy in a mental health crisis clinic. The results of the second paper showed that higher hope and social alienation/personal disorganization scores derived from the patients' pretreatment speech samples indicated greater likelihood of a favorable outcome of therpy.

Lewis [84] has written extensively on the necessity of differentiating shame and guilt anxiety in neurosis, and she has used the Gottschalk-Gleser Content Analysis Scales to make this differentiation. In teaching psychotherapy, Kepecs [85] has used somewhat modified versions of the scales to analyze the content of process notes from psychiatric interviews.

3.7 Psychodynamic and Other Studies

Witkin et al. [86] observed the affective reactions and patient-therapist interactions of field-dependent and field-independent patients early in their psychotherapy. It was found that shame-anxiety scores tended to be higher among the field-dependent patients and guilt-anxiety scores higher in the field-independent patients. Also, the correlation between guilt-anxiety scores and histility-outward scores was found to be high, and the correlation between shame-anxiety scores and hostility-inward scores was significant. This finding was corroborated by Gottschalk and Gleser [1]. Goodenough et al. [87] used Gottschalk-Gleser content analysis to investigate the effect of repression, interference, and field dependence on dream-forgetting. This same group [88] looked at the effects of stress and movies on dream affect. They noted that stressful movies increased the affects detected in the verbal reports of the subjects' dreams.

A study of the psychodynamic changes in women with depression conducted by Klerman and Gershon [89] afforded an opportunity to test the psychoanalytic, psychodynamic theory that there is a reciprocal relationship between hostility and depression. Three women, each hospitalized for depression, were studied before and during treatment with imipramine. (It is known from research and clinical observation that imipramine mobilizes hostility, and it is this psychodynamic action that constitutes the drug's therapeutic value.) Hostility-directed inward and hostility directed outward were measured using the Gottschalk verbal sample technique. No significant differences between the pretreatment and treatment periods were found, even though there was significant clinical improvement during the drug treatment period. There are many different kinds of depression, some stemming from separation and loss, some from shame, and some from guilt. Only the kind that stems from guilt would be expected to have a reciprocal relationship with hostility directed outward.

The speech samples of psychiatric emergency room patients who were likely to respond favorably to recommendations for psychotherapy had higher hope scores than did the speech samples of the patients who did not follow through on this recommendation [10]. When Viney et al. [90] explored the role played by defense mechanisms in the expression of anxiety, Gottschalk-Gleser content analysis was found to be more capable of tapping deeper levels of conciousness in measuring anxiety than were three self-report measures.

3.8 Psychopolitics

Tolz [91] has written on paranoia and the politics of inflammatory rhetoric after evaluating the speeches of campaigning politicians by Gottschalk-Gleser analysis.

3.9 Content Analysis Research Outside the United States

Use of the Gottschalk-Gleser Content Analysis Scales to measure psychological states and traits from verbal behavior in languages other than English has been promoted by Gottschalk, the scales' principal developer. The successful application of the scales to several languages other than English is evidence of the validity and universality of the procedure and is an indication that the bases of neuropsychiatric syndromes and emotional phenomena of individuals from different national and cultural backgrounds have common denominators.

Although the various kinds of literature from different countries have been successfully translated from one language into another, some writers maintain that it is impossible to do this precisely when connotations of words are ambiguous. This contention is unsupported. However, even if it were the least bit true, the present level of accuracy in translating is still adequate to effectively communicate scientific information.

The successful application of these content analysis scales to languages other than English requires that the administrator be bilingual and well-acquainted with both the idiom of American English and that of the subject language. Many people are qualified to this extent, but there are relatively few who, in addition, appreciate the scientific value of a psycholinguistic investigation, possess the educational background to fully understand its implications, and also have the professional expertise and motivation to perform this kind of undertaking.

Schofer and Koch in Germany are two who meet all the above criteria. Both are widely published on the use of the Gottschalk-Gleser Content Analysis Scales in German [92–99]. Schofer has translated key portions of books by Gottschalk and co-workers [1, 100], and one of his early works [96] is an example of the successful application of the scales in German. He has applied the scales innovatively and in sophisticated ways to the clinical setting and in research involving psychosomatic disorders. His content analysis studies, some of which have been published in the United States [92–94], include landmark research on the measurement of psychological states and traits. Other studies describing or using this content analysis method include trials conducted in Portuguese [101], Danish [102], Spanish [103, 104], and other works in German [105, 106].

Non-American studies conducted in English include two Canadian investigations; one is a psychopharmacological trial [107], and the other is the ongoing investigation by Cleghorn mentioned earlier (Sect. 3.1.1). In Australia, the emotional response of husbands to suicide attempts by their wives was studied [108], while Viney [109] has reviewed and appraised the verbal content analysis method of psychological states assessment. Her review suggests applications of the Gottschalk-Gleser Scales in personality, developmental, social, clinical, community, and health psychology.

3.10 Conclusion

The broad application of the Gottschalk-Gleser Content Analysis Scales to basic and clinical research in the behavioral sciences and psychiatry in English has been reviewed. These scales are very popular in the United States among graduate students, and their use as measuring tools is documented in these student's dissertations. Systematic review of graduate monographs is difficult because bibliographic access to them is limited. Because of this limitation, the present review does not include many current uses of the scales in the United States.

The continued use and development of these content analysis scales in many languages is anticipated.

References

1. Gottschalk LA, Gleser GC (1969) The measurement of psychological states through the content analysis of verbal behavior. University of California Press, Berkeley
2. Gottschalk LA (1974) A hope scale applicable to verbal samples. Arch Gen Psychiatry 30: 779–785
3. Gottschalk LA, Cohn JB (1978) The relationship of diazepam und ketazolam blood levels to anxiety and hostility in chronic alcoholics. Psychopharmacol Bull 14: 39–43
4. Gottschalk LA, Eckardt MJ, Feldman DJ (1979) Further validation studies of a cognitive-in-

tellectual impairment scale applicable to verbal samples. In: Gottschalk LA (ed) The content analysis of verbal behavior: further studies. Spectrum, New York, Chap 2

5. Gottschalk LA, Eckardt MJ, Pautler CP, Wolf RJ, Terman SA (1983) Cognitive impairment scores derived from verbal samples. Compr Psychiatry 24: 6–19

6. Gottschalk LA, Eckardt MJ, Hoigaard-Martin JC, Gilbert RL, Wolf RJ, Johnson W (1983) Neuropsychological deficit in chronic alcoholism: early detection and prediction by analysis of verbal samples. Subst Alcohol Actions Misuse 4: 45–58

7. Gottschalk LA, Hoigaard-Martin JC, Eckardt MJ, Gilbert RL, Wolf RJ (1983) Cognitive impairment and other psychological scores, derived from the content analysis of speech, in detoxified male chronic alcoholics. Am J Drug Alcohol Abuse 9: 447–460

8. Gottschalk LA, Kunkel RL, Wohl T, Saenger E, Winget CN (1969) Total and half body irradiation: effect on cognitive and emotional processes. Arch Gen Psychiatry 21 : 574–580

9. Gottschalk LA, Fox RA, Bates DE (1973) A study of prediction and outcome in a mental health crisis clinic. Am J Psychiatry 130: 1107–1111

10. Perley J, Winget CN, Placci C (1971) Hope and discomfort as factors influencing treatment continuance. Compr Psychiatry 12: 557–563

11. Gottschalk LA, Haer JL, Bates E (1972) Effect of sensory overload on psychological state. Arch Gen Psychiatry 276: 451–457

12. Gottschalk LA, Aronow WW, Prakash R (1977) Effect of marijuana and placebo-marijuana smoking on psychological states and on psychophysiological cardiovascular functioning in anginal patients. Biol Psychiatry 12: 255–266

13. Gottschalk LA (1978) Cognitive defect in the schizophrenic syndrome as assessed by speech patterns. In: Serban G (ed) Cognitive defects in the development of mental illness. Brunner-Mazel, New York, pp 314–350

14. Gottschalk LA, Gleser GC, Cleghorn JM, Stone WN, Winget CN (1970) Prediction of changes in severity of the schizophrenic syndrome with discontinuation and administration of phenothiazines in chronic schizophrenic patients. language as a predictor and measure of change in schizophrenia. Compr Psychiatry 11: 123–140

15. Gottschalk LA, Biener R, Noble EP, Birch H, Wilbert DE, Heiser JF (1975) Thioridazine plasma levels and clinical response. Compr Psychiatry 16: 323–337

16. Gottschalk LA, Dinovo E, Beiner R, Birch H, Syben M, Noble EP (1976) Plasma levels of mesoridazine and its metabolites and clinical response in acute schizophrenia after a single intramuscular dose. In: Gottschalk LA, Merlis S (eds) Pharmacokinetics of psychoactive drugs: blood levels and clinical response. Spectrum, New York, pp 171–189

17. Halstead WC (1947) Brain and intelligence. University of Chicago Press, Chicago

18. Reitan RM (1966) A research program on the psychological effects of brain lesions in human beings. In: Ellis NR (ed) International review of research in mental retardation, vol 1. Academic, New York

19. Reitan RM (1955) The relation of the trailmaking test to organic brain damage. J Consult Clin Psychol 19: 393–394

20. Gottschalk LA, Cohn JB (1979) Studies of cognitive function as influenced by administration of haloperidol or diazepam in detoxification of acute alcoholics. Methods Find Ex Clin Pharmacol 1: 51–61

21. Mozdzierz GJ, Krauss HH, Finch B, Reisinger C (1974) Discriminating between schizophrenics and normals with the social alienation-personal disorganization scale. J Clin Psychol 30: 85–87

22. Wooley SC, Blackwell B, Winget CN (1978) A learning theory model of chronic illness behavior: theory, treatment, and research. Psychosom Med 40: 379–401

23. Gottschalk LA, Hoigaard JC (1986) A depression scale applicable to verbal samples. Psychiatry Res (to be published)

24. Gottschalk LA, Hoigaard-Martin JC, Birch H, Rickels K (1976) The measurement of psycho-

logical states: relationship between Gottschalk-Gleser content analysis scores and Hamilton anxiety rating scale scores, Physician questionnaire rating scale scores, and Hopkins symptom checklist scores. In: Gottschalk LA, Merlis S (eds) Pharmacokinetics of psychoactive drugs: blood levels and clinical response. Spectrum, New York, pp 61–113

25. Gottschalk LA, (1975) Drug effects in the assessment of affective states in man. In: Essman WB, Valzelli L (eds) Current developments in psychiatry, vol 1. Spectrum, New York, pp 263–299

26. Gottschalk LA, Uliana RL (1979) Profiles of children's psychological states derived from the Gottschalk-Gleser analysis of speech. J Youth Adolesc 8: 269–282

27. Gottschalk LA (1976) Children's speech as a source of data towards the measurement of psychological states. J Youth Adolesc 5: 11–36

28. Gottschalk LA (1976) Differences in the content of speech of girls and boys ages six to sixteen. In: Siva-Sankar DV (ed) Mental health in children, vol 3. PDJ, New York, pp 351–379

29. Uliana RL (1979) Measurement of black children's affective states and the effect of interviewer's race on affective states as measured through language behavior. In: Gottschalk LA (ed) Content analysis of verbal behavior: further studies. Spectrum, New York, Chap 7

30. Gleser GC, Winget CN, Seligman R, Rauh JL (1979) Evaluation of psychotherapy with adolescents using content analysis of verbal samples. In: Gottschalk LA (ed) Content analysis of verbal behavior: further studies. Spectrum, New York, Chap 8

31. Silbergeld S, Manderscheid RW, O'Neill PH (1975) Free association anxiety and hostility: view from a junior high scholl. Psychol Rep 37: 495–504

32. Gottschalk LA, Bechtel RJ (1982) The measurement of anxiety through the computer analysis of verbal samples. Compr Psychiatry 23: 364–369

33. Marsden G, Kalter N, Ericson WA (1974) Response productivity: a methodological problem in content analysis studies in psychotherapy. J Consult Clin Psychol 42: 224–230

34. Gleser GC, Lubin A (1976) Response productivity in verbal content analysis: a critique of Marsden, Kalter, and Ericson. J Consult Clin Psychol 44: 508–510

35. Lolas F, von Rad M (1977) The Gottschalk-Gleser affective profile. Res Commun Psychol Psychiatry Behav 2: 231–234

36. Stone WN, Gleser GC, Gottschalk LA (1973) Anxiety and beta-adrenergic blockage. Arch Gen Psychiatry 29: 620–622

37. Gottschalk LA, Stone WN, Gleser GC (1974) Peripheral versus central mechanisms accounting for anti-anxiety effect of propranolol. Psychosom Med 36: 47–56

38. Gardos G, DiMascio A, Saltzman C, Shader RI (1968) Differential actions of chloridazepoxide and oxezepam on hostility. Arch Gen Psychiatry 18: 757–760

39. Prakash R, Aronow WS, Warren M, Laverty W, Gottschalk LA (1975) Effect of marijuana and placebo marijuana smoking on hemodynamics in coronary disease. Clin Pharmacol Ther 18: 90–95

40. Gottschalk LA, Gleser GC, Stone WM, Kunkel RL (1969) Studies of psychoactive drug effects on nonpsychiatric patients: measurement of affective and cognitive changes by content analysis of speech. In: Evans WO, Kline NS (eds) Psychopharmacology of the normal human. Thomas, Springfield, pp 162–188

41. Gottschalk LA, Bates DE, Waskow IE, Katz MM, Olson J (1971) Effect of amphetamine or chlorpromazine on achievement strivings scores derived from the content analysis of speech. Compr Psachiatry 12: 430–435

42. Silbergeld S, Brast N, Noble EP (1971) The menstrual cycle: a double-blind study of mood, behavior, and biochemical variables with Enovid and a placebo. Psychosom Med 33: 411–428

43. Gottschalk LA, Kaplan SM, Gleser GC, Winget CN (1962) Variations in the magnitude of emotions: a method applied to anxiety and hostility during phases of the menstrual cycle. Psychosom Med 24: 300–311

44. Ivey MH, Bardwick JM (1968) Patterns of affective fluctuation in the menstrual cycle. Psychosom Med 30: 336–348
45. Atkinson RM (1979) Measurement of subjective effects of nitrous oxide: validation of past drug questionnaire responses by verbal content analysis of speech samples collected during intoxication. In: Gottschalk LA (ed) Content analysis of verbal behavior: further studies. Spectrum, New York, Chap 17
46. Gottschalk LA, Covi L, Uliana RL, Bates DE (1973) Effects of diphenylhydantion on anxiety and hostility in institutionalized prisoners. Compr Psychiatry 14: 503–511
47. Gottschalk LA, Elliott HW, Bates DE, Cable CG (1972) Analysis of speech samples to determine effect of lorezepam on anxiety. Clin Pharmacol Ther 13: 323–328
48. Parker ES, Alkana RL, Noble EP (1979) A laboratory study of emotional reactions to a stressful film in alcoholic and nonalcoholic subjects. In: Gottschalk LA (ed) Content analysis of verbal behavior: further studies. Spectrum, New York, Chap 15
49. Spitzer RL (1966) The mental status schedule: potential use as a criterion measure of change in psychotherapy research. Am J Psychol 20: 156
50. Spitzer RL, Fleiss JL, Kernohan W, Lee JC, Baldwin IT (1967) Mental status schedule. Arch Gen Psychiatry 16: 479–493
51. Gottschalk LA (1979) A preliminary approach to the problem of relating the pharmacokinetics of phenothiazines to clinical response with schizophrenic patients. In: Gottschalk LA (ed) Pharmacokinetics of psychoactive drugs: further studies. Spectrum, New York, Chap 5
52. Gottschalk LA, Cohn JB, Mennuti SA (1979) Thioridazine plasma levels and clinical response in five schizophrenic patients receiving daily oral medication: correlations and the prediction of clinical responses. In: Gottschalk LA (ed) Pharmacokinetics of psychoactive drugs: further studies. Spectrum, New York, Chap 6
53. Gottschalk LA, Elliott HW (1976) Effects of triazolam and flurazepam on emotions and intellectual function. Res Commun Psychol Psychiat Behav 1: 575–595
54. Gottschalk LA (1977) Effects of certain benzodiazepine derivatives on disorganization of thought as manifested in speech. Curr Ther Res 21: 192–206
55. Gottschalk LA, Kaplan SA (1972) Chlordiazepoxide plasma levels and clinical responses. Compr Psychiat 13: 519–527
56. Gottschalk LA, Noble EP, Stolzoff GE, Bates DE, Cable CG, Uliana RL, Birch H, Fleming EW (1973) Relationships of chlordiazepoxide blood levels to psychological and biochemical responses. In: Garattini S, Mussini E, Randall LO (eds) The benzodiazepines. Raven, New York, pp 257–280
57. Gottschalk LA (1978) A preliminary approach to the problems of relating the pharmacokinetics of phenothiazines to clinical response with schizophrenic patients. Psychopharmacol Bull 14: 35–39
58. Gottschalk LA (1978) Pharmacokinetics of the minor tranquilizers and clinical response. In: Killam KS, Lipton MA, DiMascio A (eds) Psychopharmacology: a generation of progress. Raven, New York, pp 975–986
59. Elliott HW, Gottschalk LA, Uliana RL (1974) Relationship of plasma meperidine levels to changes in anxiety and hostility. Compr Psychiatry 15: 249–254
60. Gottschalk LA, Dinovo C, Biener R, Birch H (1975) Pharmacokinetics of chlordiazepoxide, meperidine, thioridazine and mesoridazine and relationships with clinical response. World J Psychosyn 7: 23–27
61. Gottschalk LA (1978) Content analysis of speech in psychiatric research. Compr Psychiatry 19: 387–392
62. Gottschalk LA (1984) Measurement of mood, affect, and anxiety in cancer patients. Cancer 53: 2236–2242
63. Gottschalk LA (1974) The application of a method of content analysis to psychotherapy research. Am J Psychother 28: 488–499

64. Gottschalk LA (1974) Quanitfication and psychological indicators of emotions: the content analysis of speech and other objective measures of psychological states. Int J Psychiatry Med 5: 587–610
65. Gottschalk LA (1972) An objective method of measuring psychological states associated with changes in neural function. J Biol Psychiatry 4: 33–49
66. Luborsky L, Docherty J, Todd T, Knapp P, Mirsky A, Gottschalk LA (1975) A content analysis of psychological states prior to petit mal EEG paroxysms. J Nerv Ment Dis 160: 282–298
67. Silbergeld S, Manderscheid RW, O'Neill PH, Lamprect F, Lorentz KY (1975) Changes in serum dopamine-beta-hydroxylase activity during group therapy. Psychosom Med 37: 352–359
68. Gottschalk LA, Stone WN, Gleser GC, Iacono JM (1966) Anxiety levels in dreams: relation to changes in plasma free fatty acids. Science 153: 654–657
69. Bell A, Stroebel CF, Prior DD (1971) Interdisciplinary study of the scrotal sac and tests correlating psychophysiological and psychological observations. Psychoanal Q 40: 415–434
70. Bell A (1975) Male anxiety during sleep. Int J Psychoanal 56: 455–464
71. Karacan I, Goodenough DR, Shapiro A, Starker S (1966) Erection cycle during sleep in relation to dream anxiety. Arch Gen Psychiatry 15: 183–189
72. Winget CN, Kapp FT (1972) The relationship of the manifest content of dreams to duration of childbirth in primiparae. Psychosom Med 34: 313–320
73. Bates DE (1975) The effect of sensory overload on behavioral and biochemical measures. Diss Abst Int 36: 6349
74. Taub JM, Berger RJ (1974) Diurnal variations in mood as asserted by self-report and verbal content analysis. J Psychiatry Res 10: 83–88
75. Deutsch F (1966) Some principles of correlating verbal and nonverbal communication. In: Gottschalk LA, Auerbach AH (eds) Methods of research in psychotherapy. Appleton-Century-Crofts, New York, pp 170–184
76. Scheflen AE (1966) Natural history method in psychotherapy: communicational research. In: Gottschalk LA, Auerbach AH (eds) Methods of research in psychotherapy. Appleton-Century-Crofts, New York, pp 263–288
77. Haggard EA, Isaacs KS (1966) Micromomentary facial expressions as indications of ego mechanisms in psychotherapy. In: Gottschalk LA, Auerbach AH (eds) Methods of research in psychotherapy. Appleton-Century-Crofts, New York, pp 154–165
78. Steingart I, Grand S, Margolis R, Freedman N, Buchwald C (1976) A study of the representation of anxiety in chronic schizophrenia. J Abnorm Psychol 85: 535–542
79. Freedman N, Blass T, Rifkin A, Quitkin F (1973) Body movements and the verbal encoding of aggressive affect. J Pers Soc Psychol 26: 72–85
80. Gottschalk LA, Uliana RL (1976) A study of the relationship of nonverbal to verbal behavior: effect of lip-carressing on hope and oral references as expressed in the content of speech. Compr Psychiatry 17: 135–152
81. Gottschalk LA, Uliana RL (1977) Further studies on the relationship of nonverbal behavior: effect of lip-caressing on shame, hostility, and other variables as expressed in the content of speech. In: Freedman N, Grand S (eds) Communicative structures and psychic structures: a psychoanalytic interpretation of communication. Plenum, New York, pp 311–330
82. Gottschalk LA (1974) The psychoanalytic study of hand-mouth approximations. In: Goldberger L, Rosen VN (eds) Psychoanalysis and contemporary science, vol 3. International Universities Press, New York
83. Gottschalk LA, deGroot C, Whitman M (1969) An evaluation of a program of continuing education in community mental health. Compr Psychiatry 10: 423–441
84. Lewis HB (1971) Shame and guilt in neurosis. International Universities Press, New York
85. Kepecs JG (1977) The teaching of psychotherapy by use of brief typescripts. Am J Psychother 31: 383–393

86. Witkin HA, Lewis HB, Weil E (1968) Affective reactions and patient-therapist interactions among more differentiated and less differentiated patients early in therapy. J Nerv Ment Dis 146: 193–208
87. Goodenough DR, Witkin HA, Lewis HB, Koulack D, Cohen H (1974) Repression, interference, and field dependence as factors in dream forgetting. J Abnorm Psychol 83: 32–44
88. Goodenough DR, Witkin HA, Koulac D, Cohen H (1975) The effects of stress films on dream affect and on respiration and eye-movement activity during rapid-eye-movement sleep. Psychophysiology 12: 313–320
89. Klerman GL, Gershon ES (1970) Imipramine effects upon hostility in depression. J Nerv Ment Dis 150: 127–132
90. Viney L, Manton M, MacQuarie U (1974) Defense mechanism preferences and the expression of anxiety. Soc Behav Pers 74: 50–55
91. Tolz RD (1979) Paranoia and the politics of inflammatory rhetoric. In: Gottschalk LA (ed) Content analysis of verbal behavior: further studies. Spectrum, New York, Chap 56
92. Schofer G, Balck F, Koch U (1979) Possible applications of the Gottschalk-Gleser content analysis of speech in psychotherapy research. In: Gottschalk LA (ed) Content analysis of verbal behavior: further studies. Spectrum, New York, Chap 48
93. Schofer G, Koch U, Balck F (1979) The Gottschalk-Gleser content analysis of speech: a normative study (the relationship of hostile and anxious affects to sex, sex of interviewer, socioeconomic class, and age). In: Gottschalk LA (ed) Content analysis of verbal behavior: further studies. Spectrum, New York, Chap 4
94. Schofer G (1979) Test criteria of the Gottschalk-Gleser content analysis of speech: objectivity, reliability, validity in German studies. In: Gottschalk LA (ed) Content analysis of verbal behavior: further studies. Spectrum, New York, Chap 5
95. Koch U, Schofer G (eds) (1986) Sprachinhaltsanalyse in der Psychosomatischen und Psychiatrischen Forschung: Grundlagen und Anwendungsstudien mit den Affektskalen von Gottschalk und Gleser. Beltz, Weinheim
96. Schofer G (1977) Gottschalk-Gleser method: verbal content analysis to measure aggressive and anxious affects. Z Psychosom Med Psychoanal 23: 86–102
97. Schofer G (1980) Sprachinhaltsanalyse Theorie und Technik. Studien zur Messung Ängstlicher und Aggressiver Affekte. Beltz, Weinheim
98. von Rad M, Drucke M, Knauss W, Lolas F (1979) Alexithymia: a comparative study of verbal behavior in psychosomatic and psychoneurotic patients. In: Gottschalk LA (ed) Content analysis of verbal behavior: further studies. Spectrum, New York, Chap 36
99. Gottschalk LA (1986) Foreword. In: Koch U, Schofer G (eds) Speech analysis in psychosomatic and psychiatric research: fundamental and applied studies with the affect scales of Gottschalk and Gleser. Beltz, Weinheim (in German)
100. Gottschalk LA, Winget CN, Gleser GC (1969) Manual of instructions for using the Gottschalk-Gleser content analysis scales. University of California Press, Berkeley
101. de Abreu PB (1986) Aggressiveness in psychotherapy and its relationship with the patient's change: an adaptation of the Gottschalk-Gleser hostility scales to the Portuguese language. This volume, Chap 19
102. Kinney DK, Jacobsen B, Bechgaard B, Jansson L, Faber B, Kasell E, Uliana RL (1985) Content analysis of speech of schizophrenic and control adoptees and their relatives: preliminary results. Soc Sci Med 21: 589–593
103. Lolas F, Gottschalk LA (1978) El metodo de analisis de contenido de Gottschalk y Gleser en la investigacion psyquiatrica. Acta Psiquiatr Psicol Am Lat 24: 247–256
104. Gottschalk LA, Winget CN, Gleser GC, Lolas F (1984) Analisis de la conducta verbal. Editorial Universitaria, Santiago
105. Flegel H (1967) Erfassung Schizophrener Morbiditätsverläufe mit Gottschalk's Verbaler

Stichprobe, Verglichen mit Wittenborns Rating Scales und der BPRS. Z Psychother Med Psychol 5: 186–194

106. Flegel H (1967) Sprachmerkmale bei Chronischen Schizophrenien. Forum der Psychiatrie, No.19. Problematic, Therapie und Rehabilitation der Chronischen Endogenen Psychosen. Enke, Stuttgart, pp 208–221

107. Cleghorn JM, Peterfy G, Pinter EJ, Pattee CJ (1970) Verbal anxiety and beta-adrenergic receptors: a facilitating mechanism? J Nerv Ment Dis 151: 266–272

108. Bennett MDJ (1973) The emotional response of husbands to suicide attempts by their wives. Thesis, University of Sydney, Sydney

109. Viney LL (1983) Assessment of psychological states through content analysis of verbal communications. This volume, Chap 5

4 Studies Proving the Validity of the Gottschalk-Gleser Content Analysis Scales in German-Speaking Countries*

Uwe Koch

I would like to review the studies conducted in German-speaking countries that have used the content analysis method first introduced by Gottschalk and Gleser. The various possible uses and the value of this instrument will be discussed. In the last 10 years approximately 30–40 studies have been conducted in German-speaking countries that employ this technique, most of which have been done by a research group of the Sonderforschungsbereich 115 in Hamburg. One member of this group, G. Schofer, has translated the Gottschalk-Gleser Scales for German usage. As in the early studies conducted by Gottschalk, these studies concentrated on the Anxiety and Hostility Scales and omitted the later content analysis scales developed by these investigators [1–4]. First, let me review a series of basic research investigations, and then I would like to discuss some clinical studies that have employed this method.

4.1 Basic Research

Schofer, Koch and Balck [5, 6] assessed 406 subjects, who were randomly selected from, and thus representative of, the population of Hamburg, using the Gottschalk-Gleser Scales. We investigated the relationship between Anxiety and Hostility Scales, on the one hand, and such variables as sex, socioeconomic status, and age on the other.

Among the Hostility Scales, the Hostility-Directed-Inward Scale showed a relationship to sex, whereas more substantial correlations were evident for the Anxiety Scales (separation, diffuse anxiety, and total anxiety) (woman showing more anxiety). Socioeconomic status appeared to play an even more important role in the hostility and anxiety scores. The trend we found suggested that persons of lower socioeconomic status tend to report more anxiety and hostility. The age dependency on the Anxiety and Hostility Scales was not substantial and did not lead to unequivocal interpretation (the highest scores were found for the age group between 40 and 49 years).

Further findings of this study were:
1. The average rate of refusal to participate was 14%.
2. The interrater reliability averaged between $r = 0.82$ and 0.94.
3. To determine the temporal stability of the Gottschalk-Gleser method, the scores of

---

* Paper presented at the VIIth World Congress of the International College of Psychosomatic Medicine, July 17-July 22, 1983, Hamburg, Federal Republic Germany.

two speech samples that were evoked within an hour were compared. The low correlation coefficients we found (under 0.20) agree with Gottschalk's contention that the scales assess states that fluctuate considerably over short periods of time.

4. Split-half reliability was tested by splitting up the speech segments using the odd-even method. The average correlation that resulted was 0.60.

Kordy, Lolas and Wagner [7] investigated the stability of the Gottschalk scores by employing the speech-sampling method. They considered the first 1000 words of an interview, the responses to a TAT picture, and the content of a complete-the-story test. These authors concluded that some scales exhibit a certain amount of stability over time and situations, for example, the Hostility-Directed-Inward and Shame Scales.

Bruhn, Stemmler and Koch [8] investigated the influence of different instructions on the Gottschalk scores. The instructions were either the standard version or a variation that contained cues for anxiety and hostility. We found that even slight variations from the standard instructions elicited considerable changes in the affect scores. In the same study, we investigated the effect of experimental manipulation on the affect scores by analyzing the subsequent speech segments. Hostility, anxiety, and joy were experimentally induced. A considerable increase in the anxiety scores was evident following experimental manipulation for the anxiety condition. The magnitude of this difference was, however, less than that induced by a variation in the instruction set.

In several studies [6, 9], we tested the influence of the interviewer's sex during the interviews. The findings suggested that the interaction between the interviewer's sex and the sex of the subject was important. The same-sex combination yielded higher scores on a number of scales compared to the opposite-sex combination.

Stemmler, Thom and Koch [10] and Muthny [11] looked at the relationship between the Gottschalk-Gleser affect scores and a series of psychophysiological variables. The results pointed to a modest to low covariation between these variables. In contrast, Gottschalk et al. [12] and Gottlieb et al. [13] in the United States found a significant correlation in anxiety scores and a decrease in skin temperature over the time interval during which the speech sample was obtained. Stegie [14] also reported negative results concerning a possible relationship between patients' transcripts of dreams and Gottschalk-Gleser anxiety and hostility scores. While dreaming, various psychophysiological variables were recorded, and it was attempted to relate these to the anxiety and hostility scores, without much success.

Gottschalk et al. [15], however, reported finding a significant positive correlation between anxiety scores derived from 15 min of rapid-eye-movement dreaming and increases in plasma free fatty acids (an indirect measure of adrenergic secretion).

Correlations between the Gottschalk-Gleser scores and questionnaires that are related in content yielded some significant though modest correlation coefficients that corresponded to expectations [5, 11]. The Hostility-Directed-Inward Scale correlated at 0.35 with a standardized aggression questionnaire developed by Koch [16]. Correlations between corresponding scales of the Gottschalk-Gleser instrument and the Mood-Adjective Checklist by Hecheltjen and Mertesdorf [17] were surprisingly low.

Engel and von Rad [18] compared responses to the Holzmann Inkblot Technique and the Gottschalk-Gleser affect scores. Their findings suggested relatively high correlations between these techniques (r between 0.60 and 0.70), if both classification systems used the same material. If these techniques were employed independently of each other and one after the other, the correlations were low.

Our factor analysis of the Anxiety and Hostility Scales yielded four interesting factors: (1) the Overt-Hostility-Outward Scale (HDO$_o$) and guilt, (2) the Covert-Hostility-Outward (Scale (HDO$_c$) and death anxiety, (3) the Hostility-Directed-Inward Scale (HDI) and shame, and (4) the Ambivalent-Hostility-Scale (AH) and death and separation anxiety. The factorial structure has proven to have a time and situational stability [6].

4.2 Clinical Research

The clinical studies are only indirectly concerned with testing the validity of the Gottschalk-Gleser technique. These studies are primarily designed to test certain psychosomatic hypotheses. Schofer, Muller, and Kerekjarto [19] compared three patient groups suffering from allergies with control groups (a group of surgery patients and a group of healthy subjects). Their findings suggested that the asthmatics significantly differed from controls on a number of scales (HDO$_c$, AH, Death, HDI, Shame, Mutilation). Patients suffering from neurodermatitis showed differences on the Death Anxiety and Mutilation Scales, whereas surgery patients and patients with urticaria showed no differences when compared with controls. Ahrens and Henskes [20] found no significant differences between patients with ulcer and hypertension and patients with regular somatic disease using standard instructions.

Von Rad et al. [21] tested the validity of the alexithymia hypothesis by comparing a group of neurotics with psychosomatic patients. Speech samples collected with standard instructions showed no differences between groups on the Affect Scales. After employing the first 1000 words of the initial psychosomatic interview as a basis considerable differences were evident (psychoneurotics showing higher scores on a number of Affect Scales). These authors attempted to explain these findings by suggesting that the alexithymia phenomenon is only revealed in the interaction of the interview setting.

Reimer and Koch [22] recently conducted a study on attempted suicide cases. Independent variables were sex as well as the manner of the suicide. Men who used more violent methods showed higher scores on the Hostility-Directed-Inward Scale. The same scale has proven, in another study of Glasenapp, to be a good predictor for complications during invasive cardiologic diagnostic measures [23].

The Gottschalk-Gleser technique has also been used in some investigations of psychotherapeutic courses. Koch and Schofer [9] reported findings of a pre- and posttherapeutic comparison in patients with sexual disturbances. Substantial decreases in anxiety and hostility were evident. Muhs [24] investigated schizophrenics at admission and upon discharge from inpatient care. The anxiety and hostility scores were much higher compared with normal subjects at admission but decreased down to a normal range at the time of discharge.

Wirsching et al. [25] employed the Gottschalk-Gleser Scales to predict the occurrence of benign versus malignant tumors in patients suspected of having cancer. The scores were calculated from the first 1000 words of a psychodiagnostic interview. The findings of these group comparisons revealed that the patients in whom a excision showed breast cancer were significantly more talkative during the interview and exhibited, according to their hypothesis, more suppression of stressful feelings (low scores on HDO_o and diffuse anxiety) than women who had benign tumors.

Since the Gottschalk–Gleser technique may be employed for all shorts of texts and dialogues, and not only with use of the standardized instructions, it appears to be appropriate for the analysis of clinical interviews and recordings from psychotherapeutic sessions. Some of the studies mentioned earlier, for example, von Rad and Lolas [21] and Wirsching et al. [25], used text taken from interviews. The advantage of using interview material is that no specialized methods of data collection are needed. The standard artificial sampling procedure represents a considerable stressor for the patients, as shown in a psychophysiological investigation by Stemmler, Thom, and Koch [10]. In natural settings, the Gottschalk–Gleser technique may be referred to as nonreactive measurement. The disadvantage of such a procedure is that possible effects from the client–therapist interaction are not easily controlled for.

Such client–therapist interaction can be controlled to some extent using a standardized form of the interview as, for example, the fully structured interview method for the classification of type A coronary prone behavior. Koch and Schmidt [26] investigated the differences between type A and type B on the Gottschalk–Gleser Anxiety and Hostility Scales. The only difference found between types A and B was the amount of words spoken in the interview. Type A subjects spoke more than type B. No differences were evident, however, in the anxiety and hostility scores.

Koch et al. [27] used the Gottschalk–Gleser technique to analyze the verbal behavior in patient–physician dialogue during inpatient care. A normal ward for internal medicine was compared with a psychosomatically oriented ward where doctors placed more emphasis on emotional aspects of the patient communication. Sodemann and Kohle [28] also investigated the verbal behavior between patient and doctor during the ward visit. Some of the Anxiety Scales were able to differentiate between the dialogues with the mortally ill and those who would recover from their illness. Several authors have used the Gottschalk–Gleser technique in the analysis of recorded dialogue from psychotherapeutic sessions.

The research group in Hamburg has applied the Gottschalk–Gleser methods most intensively. The numerous findings cannot be reported here. I should be mentioned, however, that the technique proved *not* to be effective in supporting those hypotheses tested if only isolated utterances of single persons in the dialogue were used in the analysis. If entire therapeutic sessions or larger segments were used, the Gottschalk–Gleser method revealed interesting information with respect to the client–therapist interaction. For example, the development of anxious and hostile emotions could be depicted over the course of psychotherapy, and differences between therapeutic techniques were quite evident.

Tschuschke, Volk and Ehlers [29] have employed the scales for analyzing transcripts from psychoanalytic group sessions. Angermeyer and Hecker [30] used the same scales for the analysis of family therapeutic sessions in families with schizophrenic children.

4.3 Conclusions

Although there has been considerable effort invested to establish the validity of the Gottschalk-Gleser technique in German-speaking countries, more work needs to be done. In establishing construct validity, final validations cannot be expected even after 10 years. Since the affects of anxiety and hostility are considered to be fluctuating states and since we lack adequate criteria for the validity of such measures, substantiating the validity of the Gottschalk-Gleser technique is difficult.

The failure to support some clinical hypothesis involving the affects of anxiety and hostility in no way repudiates the construct validity of these Gottschalk-Gleser Content Analysis Scales. Rather, such an outcome has more bearing on the lack of validity of the clinical hypothesis. At the same time, it can be said to thereby contribute to the construct validation of these Anxiety and Hostility Scales. Viewed in a more positive way, the recent findings reviewed here concerning the German form of Gottschalk's Scales give evidence to suggest that the Gottschalk-Gleser method exhibits validity in several research areas.

4.4 Summary

Since 1973 a German team has been investigating the applicability and validity of the Gottschalk-Gleser Anxiety and Hostility Scales in German-speaking countries. Twenty basic and clinical studies are reported. After 10 years of research experience with the German version of the Gottschalk-Gleser Scales, it can be stated that though the process of construct validation is not completed, clear indications of the construct validity of the Anxiety and Hostility Scales have been found.

References

1. Gottschalk LA, Gleser GC (1969) The measurement of psychological states through the content analysis of verbal behavior. University of California Press, Berkeley
2. Gottschalk LA, Winget CN, Gleser GC (1969) Manual of instructions for using the Gottschalk-Gleser content analysis scales: anxiety, hostility, and social alienation-personal disorganization. University of California Press, Berkeley
3. Gottschalk LA (ed) The content analysis of verbal behavior: further studies. Spectrum, New York
4. Gottschalk LA (1982) Manual of uses and applications of the Gottschalk-Gleser verbal behavior scales. Res Commun Psychol Psychiatry Behav 7: 273
5. Schofer G, Koch U, Balck F (1979) The Gottschalk-Gleser content analysis of speech: a normative study (The relationships of hostile and anxious affects to sex, sex of the interviewer, socioeconomic class, and age). In: Gottschalk LA (ed) The content analysis of verbal behavior: further studies. Spectrum, New York, p 95

6. Schofer G, Koch U, Balck F (1979) Test criteria of the Gottschalk–Gleser content analysis of speech: objectivity, reliability, validity in German studies. In: Gottschalk LA (ed) The content analysis of verbal behavior: further studies. Spectrum, New York, p 119

7. Kordy H, Lolas F, Wagner G (1986) Zur Stabilität der inhaltsanalytischen Erfassung von Affekten nach Gottschalk und Gleser. In: Koch U, Schofer G (eds) Sprachinhaltsanalyse in der psychosomatischen und psychiatrischen Forschung: Grundlagen und Anwendungsstudien mit den Affektskalen von Gottschalk und Gleser. Beltz, Weinheim

8. Bruhn M, Stemmler G, Koch U (1986) Die Abhängigkeit von Angst, Aggressivität und Hoffnungswerten von experimentell manipulierter Befindlichkeit und variierten Instruktionstypen. In: Koch U, Schofer G (eds) Sprachinhaltsanalyse in der psychosomatischen und psychiatrischen Forschung: Grundlagen und Anwendungsstudien mit den Affektskalen von Gottschalk und Gleser. Beltz, Weinheim

9. Koch U, Schofer G (1978) Abhängigkeit aggressiver und ängstlicher Affekte von klinischen settings – eine Untersuchung an Patientenpaaren mit dem Gottschalk-Gleser-Verfahren. Z Klin Psychol 7: 110

10. Stemmler G, Thom E, Koch U (1986) Psychologische Muster von indizierten Affekten von Gottschalk-Gleser-Sprachproben. In: Koch U, Schofer G (eds) Sprachinhaltsanalyse in der psychosomatischen und psychiatrischen Forschung: Grundlagen und Anwendungsstudien mit den Affektskalen von Gottschalk und Gleser. Beltz, Weinheim

11. Muthny FA (1986) Gottschalk-Gleser Auswertung von Probandenäußerungen im Rahmen psychophysiologischer Aktivierungsforschung. In: Koch U, Schofer G (eds) Sprachinhaltsanalyse in der psychosomatischen und psychiatrischen Forschung: Grundlagen und Anwendungsstudien mit den Affektskalen von Gottschalk und Gleser. Beltz, Weinheim

12. Gottschalk LA, Springer KJ, Gleser GC (1961) Experiments with a method of assessing the variations in intensity of certain psychological states occurring during two psychotherapeutic interviews. In: Gottschalk LA (eds) Comparative psycholinguistic analysis of two psychotherapeutic interviews. International Universities Press, New York

13. Gottlieb AA, Gleser GC, Gottschalk LA (1967) Verbal and physiological responses to hypnotic suggestion of attitudes. Psychosom Med 29: 172

14. Stegie R (1986) Zur Anwendung des Gottschalk-Gleser Verfahrens in einer psychophysiologischen Traumstudie. In: Koch U, Schofer G (eds) Sprachinhaltsanalyse in der psychosomatischen und psychiatrischen Forschung: Grundlagen und Anwendungsstudien mit den Affektskalen von Gottschalk und Gleser. Beltz, Weinheim

15. Gottschalk LA, Stone WN, Gleser GC, Iacano JM (1966) Anxiety levels in dreams: relation to changes in plasma free fatty acids. Science 153: 654

16. Koch U (1974) Der standardisierte Aggressionsfragebogen SAF. In: Koch U, Schofer G (eds) Arbeitsbericht, Sonderforschungsbereich 115, Projekt Cl, p 11

17. Hecheltjen G, Mertesdorf F (1973) Entwicklung eines mehrdimensionalen Stimmungsfragebogens (MSF). Gruppendynamik 2: 110

18. Engel K, von Rad M (1986) Zwei Verfahren zur Messung von Angst und Aggressivität. Ein empirischer Vergleich des Gottschalk-Gleser-Verfahrens und der Holtzman-Inkblot-Technik. In: Koch U, Schofer G (eds) Sprachinhaltsanalyse in der psychosomatischen und psychiatrischen Forschung: Grundlagen und Anwendungsstudien mit den Affektskalen von Gottschalk und Gleser. Beltz, Weinheim

19. Schofer G, Muller L, von Kerekjarto M (1979) Die Differenzierung psychosomatischer Krankheitsgruppen mit der Gottschalk-Gleser-Sprachinhaltsanalyse. Med Psychol 5: 24

20. Ahrens D, Henskes D (1986) Affektive Regulation bei psychosomatischen Erkrankungen. In: Koch U, Schofer G (eds) Sprachinhaltsanalyse in der psychosozialen und psychiatrischen Forschung: Grundlagen und Anwendungsstudien mit den Affektskalen von Gottschalk und Gleser. Beltz, Weinheim

21. von Rad M, Drucke M, Knauss W, Lolas F (1979) Alexithymia: anxiety and hostility in psychosomatic and psychoneurotic patients. Psychother Psychosom 31: 223

22. Reimer C, Koch U (1986) Untersuchung zur Aggressionsproblematik von Suizidenten. In: Koch U, Schofer G (eds) Sprachinhaltsanalyse in der psychosomatischen und psychiatrischen Forschung: Grundlagen und Anwendungsstudien mit den Affektskalen von Gottschalk und Gleser. Beltz, Weinheim

23. Glasenapp H (1980) Vorhersagen zur Angst und Aggressivität als mögliche Risikofaktoren der Herzkatheteruntersuchung mit Hilfe einer mehrdimensionalen Regressionsanalyse und der non-stochastischen additiven Verbundstruktur. Dissertation, Hamburg

24. Muhs A (1982) Veränderung ängstlicher und aggressiver Affekte schizophrener Patienten bei einer stationären psychiatrischen Behandlung. Eine Untersuchung mit dem Gottschalk-Gleser-Verfahren. Dissertation, Freiburg

25. Wirsching M, Hoffmann F, Stierlin H, Stummeyer D, Weber G, Wirsching B (1986) Angst, Harmonisierung und Opferbereitschaft – Affektäußerungen von Frauen, die sich wegen Brustkrebsverdacht einer Probebiopsie unterziehen mußten. In: Koch U, Schofer G (eds) Sprachinhaltsanalyse in der psychosomatischen und psychiatrischen Forschung: Grundlagen und Anwendungsstudien mit den Affektskalen von Gottschalk und Gleser. Beltz, Weinheim

26. Koch U, Schmidt T (1984) Verbalisierte Affekte im Typ A-Interview – Eine Analyse nach den Gottschalk-Gleser-Skalen. In: Koch U, Schofer G (eds) Sprachinhaltsanalyse in der psychosomatischen und psychiatrischen Forschung: Grundlagen und Anwendungsstudien mit den Affektskalen von Gottschalk und Gleser. Beltz, Weinheim

27. Koch U, Fauler T, Safian P, Jahrig C (1982) Affekte bei Ärzten und Patienten während der Visite: Eine Analyse verbalisierter Affekte mit dem Gottschalk-Gleser-Verfahren an Hamburger und Ulmer Visitengesprächen. In: Kohle K, Raspe H-H (eds) Das Gespräch während der ärztlichen Visite. Empirische Untersuchungen. Urban and Schwarzenberg, München, p 196

28. Sodemann U, Kohle K (1984) Anwendung des Gottschalk-Gleser-Verfahrens und eines Angstthemenwörterbuchs bei der Affektanalyse von Visitengesprächen. In: Koch U, Schofer G (eds) Sprachinhaltsanalyse in der psychosomatischen und psychiatrischen Forschung: Grundlagen und Anwendungsstudien mit den Affektskalen von Gottschalk und Gleser. Beltz, Weinheim

29. Tschuschke V, Volk W, Ehlers W (1980) Die Verwendbarkeit der Gottschalk-Gleser-Sprachinhaltsanalyse für Verlaufsuntersuchungen in der analytischen Gruppenpsychotherapie. Gruppendynamik 16: 257

30. Angermeyer MC, Hecker H (1979) Ausdruck psychischer Gestörtheit im Sprachverhalten von Eltern schizophrener Patienten: Eine quantitative inhaltsanalytische Studie. Soc Psychiatry 14: 85

5 Assessment of Psychological States Through Content Analysis of Verbal Communications*

Linda L. Viney

5.1 Introduction

The focus of many psychologists today is not so much on the traits and long-term characteristics of the people who participate in our research as on their reactions to events and situations. Psychologists are concerned with changing transitory psychological states, but have not yet developed fully effective techniques for their assessment. Content analysis of verbal communications can be helpful in assessing such states. Content analysis is based on the assumption that the language in which people choose to express themselves contains information about the nature of their psychological states. This assumption implies a representational or descriptive model of language, in contrast to the instrumental or functional model preferred, for example, by Mahl [1]. Content analysis can be applied only to verbal, not to nonverbal communications. However, although content analysis cannot be applied to nonverbal communications, inferences can be made about people's states through objective and systematic identification of specified characteristics of their verbal communications [2, 3]. Content analysis of verbal communications is a way of listening to and interpreting people's communicated accounts of events. When agreement between independent interpretations is achieved, the essential requirement of scientific endeavor (intersubjective agreement) is met [4].

The form of content analysis on which I intend to focus is, therefore, the content analysis scales which have been developed to measure psychological states through the application of the technique to a wide range of verbal communications to which content analysis is applicable. This will be followed by summaries of information about the reliability and validity of some major content analysis scales in current use. Attention will then be drawn to their theoretical and practical advantages, as well as their problems and limitations. I will give several examples from some of the existing research by psychologists using content analysis in the areas of personality, developmental psychology, and social psychology and others from the more applied areas of clinical psychology, community psychology, and health psychology to show the versatility of the technique of content analysis. Some of the possibilities which the application of computers to content analysis raise will next be explored. I will then consider the advantages of content analysis as an ethical technique for data analysis and the ethical model it assumes.

---

* Reprinted from the *Psychological Bulletin* (94: 542–563, 1983) with permission of the author and publisher.

5.2 A History of Content Analysis in Psychology

Content analysis has been used by multidisciplinary researchers in the field of communications. Berelson was one of the first to see its value as "an objective, systematic and quantitative description of the manifest content of communication" [5]. Only 15 years later Budd, Thorp and Donahew [6] were able to refer to over 300 content analysis studies of the print and radio media. The *Psychological Abstracts,* however, lists no entries for content analysis before 1978, although since then it has listed some 25–35 content analysis articles each year. That content analysis was not listed earlier in the *Abstracts* is strange since the technique had been in use for several decades. The two areas in which it had been most employed were of interest mainly to clinical psychologists: assessment based on projective techniques and investigations of the process of psychotherapy.

Content analysis of verbal responses has been employed with projective techniques since their inception. It has also been used with a wide variety of such techniques. Some examples follow. Elizur [7] in 1949 published a now classic study using content analysis of Rorschach responses to measure anxiety and hostility. Finney [8] identified content of Rorschach percepts associated with assaultive behavior. Holt [9] differentiated content representing primary and secondary process in the same material. Clinical interpretations of Rorschach responses are still based on such procedures [10], and researchers continue to develop new sets of inkblot-based content analysis categories. MacHove [11], for example, had devised a set of categories based on descriptions of percepts which are animate/inanimate and activated/deactivated to distinguish between affective and thought disorders.

Content analysis has been similarly important in the development of story-based projective techniques such as the Thematic Apperception Test. Eron [12] carried out the early classic content analyses with this technique. As for Rorschach interpretation, this type of analysis continues to be central to contemporary diagnostic use in apperception tests [13], and researchers are still developing new thematic content categories to measure concepts such as hostility [14]. Users of the Hand Test have also employed content analysis to some extent [15], as have psychologists who analyze early childhood memories [16, 17]. Much of this work has been for clinical purposes. However, it has also formed the bases from which measures have developed which have been much used in psychological research. Examples include the assessment of achievement motivation [18–21]. Horner's [22] concept of fear of failure, and the work of Winter [23] and McClelland [24] on power.

Content analysis has been and continues to be of importance for psychologists who employ projective techniques. It has not had the same continuing importance for investigators of psychotherapeutic process, although they have used a number of sets of content analysis categories with some success [25]. Content analysis was frequently employed in the 1950s, as the reviews of the work on psychotherapeutic process of that period show [26, 27]. Its use continued into the 1960s [28]. Then followed a period in which the researchers in this area turned elsewhere, chiefly to Rogers' [29] conceptualization of psychotherapeutic process. This conceptualization was not based solely on verbal communication [30]. Occasional content analysis studies of psychotherapy were carried out in the 1970s. Some of them [31, 32] applied computer technology to provide faster and more reliable content analyses. I will comment later on the impact of this technology on the use of content analysis by psychologists. Other studies of psycho-therapeutic process used rigorosly devised content analysis scales [33, 34].

5.3 Construction of Content Analysis Scales

The content analysis scales employed in these last-named studies were developed in the United States by Gottschalk and Gleser [35] for use in clinical psychology and psychiatry. Their scales assess disruptive and distressing states, such as anxiety and hostility. Their work has continued, with the development of new scales to assess clinical syndromes and the refinement of the old scales [36]. It has been added to by research in Australia by Viney and Westbrook, who have developed scales to tap agreeable as well as distressing states, such as sociability [37] and positive feelings [38], as well as states of greater homogeneity than clinical syndromes, such as cognitively based anxiety [39]. How these scales have been developed will now be described.

There are nine steps which must be taken in the construction of a content analysis scale before its reliability and validity can be established:

1. A precise description of the psychological state to be assessed must be made, with all its dimensions defined if it involves a multidimensional concept. Failure to clarify this description sufficiently can be the cause of later difficulties both in achieving interjudge reliability and in establishing the validity of the measure.
2. The unit of content to be analyzed must be defined. For all of the scales described in detail in this article, the unit selected for scoring purposes has been the clause, the language structure which includes an active verb.
3. The content of the verbal communications or cues from which the psychological state is to be inferred must be specified in detail.
4. Any cues such as those used to indicate the intensity of the state should be specified.
5. The differential scoring weights to be applied to these cues should also be specified. These two steps are not considered necessary if the intensity of the state is not considered to vary.
6. A correction factor taking into account the number of words in a communication is included because research participants who are communicating in response to relatively unstructured instructions will give communications of different lengths. Similarly, news reports will vary in length.
7. A score and, in the case of multidimensional concepts, a set of subscores can now be derived.
8. Its distributions for samples of different research participants and over different events are then examined so that if they are skewed they may be transformed to facilitate the use of relatively robust statistical techniques based on symmetrical distributions.
9. Normative data may then be collected from specified samples of people and situations.

A description of the development of two content analysis scales following this pattern should be useful here. The scales to be described are the Origin and Pawn Scales [40], which grew out of the conceptual work of de Charms [41]. He chose the term "origin" to describe the state in which people perceive their actions to be primarily determined by their own choice and "pawn" for the state in which they do not believe themselves to have this choice. The second step was to choose the clause as the unit of measurement. Heider's [42] descriptions of differences in the perception of action, together with reading of samples of verbalizations, led Westbrook and Viney to select five types of communication content from which origin-like and pawn-like content were to be inferred. For the Origin Scale the content types were: (a) expressions of intention (e.g., "We decided to go ahead with the party"), (b) expressions of exertion (e.g., "I am working hard"), (c) expressions of ability (e.g., "I can walk as far as the garden now"), (d) descriptions of oneself as overcoming or influencing others or the environment (e.g., "I went right on the spite of their criticisms"), and (e) descriptions of oneself as the cause or origin (e.g., "I made sure the place was clean when we left"). For the Pawn Scale the types of verbal content to be scored were: (a) indications that the speaker or writer did not intend the outcome described (e.g., "I didn't mean to hurt my mother"), (b) indications that the speaker or writer did not try to bring about such an outcome (e.g., "I didn't exert myself, but the job got done"), (c) expressions of lack of ability (e.g., "I'm no good at schoolwork"), (d) descriptions of oneself as being controlled by or at the mercy of external forces (e.g., "They won't let me wear any jewelry here"), and (e) descriptions of oneself as a pawn at the mercy of uncontrollable events (e.g., "I was a victim of circumstances").

Here is an example of a communication from a young unemployed man which has been scored for the Origin (O) and Pawn (P) Scales. These scales are referents for concepts akin to Rotter's [43] notion of perceived locus of control but have been devised in such a way as to avoid the assumption of unidimensionality which is built into the questionnaire measures of it:

> Being unemployed is pretty bad. / You don't know / what to do with yourself most of the time. / I try to get my days organized. / I am able to get up (O) / when the family does / for a few days ... but I soon get trapped into staying in bed longer and longer (P) / whether I want to or not. (P) / That's / what being unemployed does to me. (P)

Steps (4) and (5) relating to intensity cues and their weighting were not considered appropriate for the Origin and Pawn Scales. Westbrook and Viney did include, however, a correction factor (CF) to take into account the number of words in the scored communication. The Gottschalk-Winget-Gleser correction factor was used, that is, the number of words in the scored verbalization divided into 100 $\left(CF = \dfrac{100}{N}\right)$ [44]. The score was then defined in each case as: total raw score $\times$ CF. Further, some verbalizations contained no scorable content and would all have received the same score. Yet, they differed in length of verbalization, and longer verbalizations provided greater opportunity for such content. Half the correction factor was, therefore, added to each score: (total raw score $\times$ CF) $+ \frac{1}{2}$ CF. When these scores were plotted, their distributions were found to have a negative skew. The square root transformation provided the most symmetrical distribution of the transformations tested. The final O and P scores, then, were calculated as:

$$\sqrt{(\text{total raw score} \times \text{CF}) + \frac{1}{2}\,\text{CF}}$$

For some scales based on content analysis, it would now have been appropriate to collect normative data. For these scales, however, this step was considered to be inappropriate since it did not prove feasible to select samples of people in situations which could be said to be "normal" with respect to these psychological states. Even people in apparently normal situations have been found to be recovering from or anticipating life events which are known to affect these states [45]. Comparative data from specified people and situations have, however, been published [40].

The reliability and validity of the Origin and Pawn Scales are examined in detail later in this paper. Generally speaking, their interjudge reliability has been at a consistently acceptable level, but the Origin Scale is very unstable over time. No evidence is available on the internal consistency of the Origin and Pawn Scales. As to validity, there is some evidence (also examined later) that these scales measure the psychological states they were designed to measure. They have also made possible data collections which have cast doubt on the unidimensionality assumption of the questionnaire measures of perceived locus of control. If it is a unidimensional concept, its opposite poles should correlate negatively. Scores on these Origin and Pawn Scales have been found to be independent over many samples of people and situations [40].

5.4 Types of Verbal Communications to Which Content Analysis is Applicable

Data collection and data analysis are two separate phases of the process of assessment. Content analysis of verbal communications is a form of data analysis. As such it is applicable to verbal data which have been collected in a variety of ways. The communications to which it is applied may be written or spoken, spontaneous or planned, public or private. They may be isolated statements such as suicide notes [46] or parts of an ongoing interaction, as in psychotherapy [47]. Since this technique can transcend time, it may be applied to old communications (as in the written records of past civilizations) as well as to current communications. However, researchers must be able to understand the language in which they are expressed. Of course care must be taken to sample units of meaning in a representative manner, as in any form of data collection. Units of communication are usually sampled either by time taken to give the communication (as in a set of 5-min samples of verbal behavior) or a number of words (as in a set of 500-word samples of Churchill's speeches). The value of the results of any form of content analysis is limited by the representativeness of the data on which they are based.

If the communications to be analyzed have been made in response to specific instructions, those instructions can vary from highly structured to relatively unstructured, depending on the purpose of the research. Whatever the purpose of the research, instructions need to be sufficiently open-ended that the research participants have a range of choice in the meanings they communicate and the words they choose to communicate them. An example of such instructions follows [46]:

I'd like you to talk to me for a few minutes about your life at the moment – the good things and the bad – what it is like for you. Once you have started I shall be here listening to you; but I'd rather not reply to any questions you may have until a five-minute period is over. Do you have any questions you would like to ask now, before we start?

Responses to such intructions are usually transcribed from tape recordings for analysis.

Content analysis scales can, of course, be applied to communications given in response to the unstructured material or projective techniques [49], where they may provide solutions to what Cronbach and Gleser [50] have described as the "wide band width" problem of projective techniques. This problem can be described as follows. Compared with other psychological assessment devices, projective techniques provide a wide breadth of coverage but much "noise" in interpretation. Content analysis can do justice to that breadth while reducing the level of "noise".

There is also the question of the language of the verbal material to be analyzed. Content analysis has been used effectively with communications in Spanish [51], Italian [52], German [53], French [54], and Swedish [55], as well as in English. Some English-language content analysis scales have been translated and used by German researchers [56, 57]. It has also proved possible to use content analysis scales developed in one English-speaking culture in another English-speaking culture without changes in the scoring, although careful monitoring of the scoring and nuances of the local idiom and of the comparability of different samples of scores is necessary [58].

5.4.1 Reliability

An assessment technique is reliable to the extent that it is consistent in measurement. The technique cannot be consistent if errors occur when it is used [59]. One type of error which is of central importance for the measurement of transitory states by content analysis is interjudge error. Interjudge reliability indicates the consistency with which the technique can be used by different, independent raters, that is, the consistency with which interpretations of verbal communications can be made. Table 1 shows the arithmetic means and ranges of the interjudge reliability coefficients of a set of ten content analysis scales, which have been reported with some frequency in the literature. This set has been selected because more information is available by which to evaluate these applications of content analysis than has been provided for most of the other content analyses used by psychologists. For these ten scales, 18 published reports which refer to their interjudge reliability are currently available. They provide information from a total of 35 studies. Most of the average coefficients are acceptably high, although that for one scale, Hostility-Out Scale, falls somewhat below the general level. Their range shows that they are also consistently high, with that scale being less consistent and three other scales showing an occasional low estimate. For these content categories, it can be said that the concepts underlying them have meanings which can be communicated between research participant and researcher and so reliably scored. For many other content analysis scales, no evidence of interjudge reliability has been provided. Such scales are reported once or twice in the literature, then do appear again, probably because the definition of their content categories is not clear enough to permit their independent use by other researchers. When the scoring of content analysis scales is effectively programed for computers, checks on interjudge agreement will not be so important. Until that time, demonstrated interjudge reliability serves as a basis for that important transition from qualitative assessment with relatively simple scale categories to quantitative assessment with a wider range of complete scale categories.

Table 1. Reported interjudge reliability estimates for ten content analysis scales

	Average coefficient[a]	Range of coefficients	Literature source	Refs.
Positively toned scales				
Hope	–	0.85 +	Gottschalk (1974)	[94]
Origin	0.92	0.91–0.94	Westbrook and Viney (1980)	[40]
Positive Affect	0.93	–	Westbrook (1976)	[38]
Sociality	0.96	0.95–0.97	Viney and Westbrook (1979)	[37]
Negatively toned scales				
Cognitive Anxiety	0.96	0.71–0.99	Viney and Westbrook (1976)	[39]
Hostility In	0.94	0.76–0.98	Gottschalk and Gleser (1969)	[35]
			Viney and Manton (1973)	[58]
			Schofer et al. (1979)	[34]
Hostility Out	0.79	0.58–0.87	Gottschalk and Gleser (1969)	[35]
			Viney and Manton (1973)	[58]
			Schofer et al. (1979)	[34]
Pawn	0.90	0.87–0.93	Westbrook and Viney (1980)	[40]
Total Anxiety	0.90	0.76–0.94	Gottschalk and Gleser (1969)	[35]
			Viney and Manton (1973)	[58]
			Schofer et al. (1979)	[34]

[a] Arithmetic mean of several coefficients when more than one has been obtained in one or more studies.

The internal consistency of content analysis measures must also be considered. Table 2 shows that for the same set of ten commonly used content analysis scales, there is information available relating to the internal consistency of only four. The five reports of six studies in this area have dealt with intercorrelations of subcategories, that is, at the level of subscales but not descriptive categories, and with their contribution to total scores. For example, the subscales of the Sociality and Total Anxiety Scales have been judged to show sufficient statistical independence to be used individually to assess the relative importance of different sources of sociality or anxiety, but enough interrelationship to be summed together to provide a more global measure. No information is available about relationships between content categories, such as those two sets of five categories which have been defined for the scoring of the Origin and Pawn Scales. Such information about the internal consistency of content analysis scoring categories is much needed. The only internal consistency study I have found which employs a different paradigm to examine the split-half reliability of content analysis scales does so with a German version of the four negatively toned Gottschalk-Gleser Scales [60]. The average correlation coefficient achieved in this way was only 0.50. Further studies of this kind, as well as those intercorrelating categories, need to be carried out.

Table 2. Reports on the internal consistency of ten content analysis scales

	Evidence concerning internal consistency	Literature source	Refs.
Positively toned scales			
Hope		Gottschalk (1974)	[94]
Origin			
Positive Affect			
Sociality	Subscales not significantly intercorrelated and making separate contributions to the total score	Viney and Westbrook (1979)	[37]
Negatively toned scales			
Cognitive Anxiety			
Hostility In			
Hostility Out	Subscales significantly intercorrelated	Gottschalk and Gleser (1969)	[35]
Ambivalent Hostility			
Pawn			
Total Anxiety	Subscales intercorrelated differently for different samples and making separate contributions to the total score	Gottschalk and Gleser (1969)	[35]
		Westbrook and Viney (1977)	[89]

The other form of reliability which remains to be investigated is test-retest reliability. Stability over time is not a necessary requirement for measures of psychological states because such states should vary in response to situational change. It is however, important to have information about stability. Some psychological projects in which they might be employed, such as evaluation studies, require a certain level of stability. Table 3 provides a summary of the information available for the ten scales, all of which has been reported in the form of generalizability coefficients. They have been estimated over periods ranging from only 1 h to 5 months. For the ten scales, information is available concerning nine. This information is based on six publications reporting the results from 29 studies. They suggest that the scales vary considerably in their stability. They also suggest that estimates of the stability of any one content analysis scale may vary as a function of the population of research participants or events being considered. More information is needed about the consistency over time of these relatively well developed scales, as well as about their internal consistency.

Table 3. Reported stability estimates for ten content analysis scales

	Generalizability coefficient	Literature source	Refs.
Positively toned scales			
Hope		Gottschalk (1974)	[94]
Origin	Over 5 occasions: 0.22[a]	Westbrook and Viney (1980)	[40]
Positive Affect			
Sociality	Over 5 occasions: 0.67	Viney and Westbrook (1979)	[37]
Negatively toned scales			
Cognitive Anxiety	Over 5 occasions: 0.63	Viney and Westbrook (1976)	[39]
Hostility In	Over 2 occasions: 0.00[a], 0.00[a], 0.52	Gottschalk and Gleser (1969)	[35]
Hostility Out	Over 2 occasions: 0.15, 0.28[a], 0.39 Over 3 occasions: 0.30, 0.38, 0.59	Gottschalk and Gleser (1969)	[35]
Ambivalent Hostility	Over 2 occasions: 0.27[a], 0.37, 0.40 Over 3 occasions: 0.27[a], 0.46, 0.61	Gottschalk and Gleser (1969)	[35]
Pawn	Over 5 occasions: 0.51	Westbrook and Viney (1980)	[40]
Total Anxiety	Over 2 occasions: 0.19[a], 0.32, 0.38, 0.43 Over 3 occasions: 0.33 Over 5 occasions: 0.64	Gottschalk and Gleser (1969)	[35]

[a] For the associated F value for the occasion factor, $P < 0.01$.

5.4.2 Validity

Of content, criterion, and construct validities described by the A.P.A. [59] in its *Standards for Educational and Psychological Tests,* it is construct validity that best reflects whether a content analysis scale is achieving its aims. Since the content comes directly from the research participant, a content analysis scale seems likely to have inherent content validity. However, this is the case only if its categories adequately represent the intended content and do so consistently. Criterion validity procedures are used to provide information about what states the content analysis scales measure. A network of information about their relationships with other indices provides support for hypotheses generated by the constructs underlying the scales and so constitutes evidence of construct validity. Certain criteria are relevant for every scale. For example, any biases according to the sex, age, educational level, and occupational status of the research participants should be known for every scale. This information is provided in Table 4 for the ten content analysis scales under consideration, together with other empirical findings which contribute to their validity.

The other types of validational information include correlations with other measures of the same construct, for example, from self-reports and observations of behaviors scale. This information is provided in Table 4 for the ten content analysis scales under consideration, together with findings related to the construct, psychiatrists' ratings,

Table 4. Reported evidence of validity for ten content analysis scales

	Evidence of validity	Literature source	Refs.
Positively toned scales			
Hope	Independent of sex, age, educational level	Gottschalk (1974)	[94]
	Significantly negatively correlated with measures of negatively toned states	Gottschalk (1974)	[94]
	Significantly correlated with measures of other positively toned states	Gottschalk (1974)	[94]
	Discriminated medical patients leaving hospital from those staying	Gottschalk and Gleser (1969)	[35]
	Predicted medical patients' reaction to treatment	Gottschalk (1974)	[94]
Origin	Independent of sex, age, but correlated with occupational status	Westbrook and Viney (1980)	[40]
	Significantly correlated with measures of other positively toned states	Viney and Westbrook (1981)	[48]
	Significantly correlated with other measures of this state	Westbrook and Viney (1980)	[40]
	Significantly correlated with reported use of appropriate coping strategies	Westbrook and Viney (1980)	[40]
	Discriminated those who were experiencing controllable	Westbrook and Viney (1980)	[40]
	Discriminated youth workers from the clients they worked with	Viney (1981)	[126]
Positive Affect	Independent of sex, age, education, and occupational status	Westbrook (1976)	[38]
	Independent of measures of negatively toned states	Westbrook (1976)	[38]
	Discriminated women who were moving to a new home from those who were not	Viney and Bazeley (1977)	[130]
	Discriminated mothers reporting on childbearing from women reporting on other events	Viney (1980)	[45]
Sociality	Independent of sex, age, occupational status	Viney and Westbrook (1979)	[37]
	Significantly negatively correlated with negatively toned states	Viney and Westbrook (1979)	[37]
	Discriminated informants who were maintaining good relationships from those who were not	Viney and Westbrook (1979)	[37]
	Discriminated youth workers from the clients they worked with	Viney (1981)	[131]
	Predicted good rehabilitation of medical patients	Viney and Westbrook (1982)	[135]
	Responded as predicted to experimental manipulation	Viney (1981)	[131]

Table 4. (continued)

	Evidence of validity	Literature source	Refs.
Negatively toned scales			
Cognitive Anxiety	Independent of sex, age, but correlated with occupational status	Viney and Westbrook (1976)	[38]
	Significantly correlated with measures of other negatively toned states	Viney and Westbrook (1976)	[38]
	Significantly correlated with measures of state anxiety, not trait anxiety	Viney and Westbrook (1976)	[38]
	Discriminated people in situations which were new to them from those who were not in new situations	Viney (1980)	[45]
	Discriminated peoples' accounts of situations which were unpredictable from those which were not	Viney and Westbrook (1976)	[38]
	Discriminated relatives' accounts when waiting for emergency medical patients from those who were not	Bunn and Clarke (1979)	[123]
Hostility In	Independent of sex, age, educational level	Gottschalk and Gleser (1969)	[35]
	Significantly correlated with self-reports of depression	Gottschalk and Gleser (1969)	[35]
	Significantly correlated with ratings of depression-related behaviors by observers	Gottschalk and Gleser (1969)	[35]
	Significantly correlated with psychiatrists' ratings of depression	Gottschalk (1979)	[36]
	Discriminated psychiatric admissions from others	Viney and Manton (1973)	[58]
	Discriminated chronically ill from others	Westbrook and Viney (1982)	[90]
	Predicted good rehabilitation of medical patients	Viney and Westbrook (1982)	[135]
Hostility Out	Independent of sex, age, educational level	Gottschalk and Gleser (1969)	[35]
	Significantly correlated with self-reports of anger	Gottschalk (1979)	[36]
	Significantly correlated with ratings of angry behaviors by observers	Gottschalk (1979)	[36]
	Discriminated "empty nest" mothers from other women	Viney (1980)	[40]
	Predicted good rehabilitation for medical patients	Viney and Westbrook (1982)	[135]
	Responded as predicted to experimental (psychological and drug) manipulation	Gottschalk and Gleser (1969)	[35]
Ambivalent Hostility	Independent of sex, age, educational level	Gottschalk and Gleser (1969)	[35]
	Significantly correlated with measures of indirectly expressed anger, negativism, and suspicion	Gottschalk and Gleser (1969)	[35]

Table 4. (continued)

	Evidence of validity	Literature source	Refs.
	Discriminated psychiatric admissions from others	Viney and Manton (1973)	[58]
	Discriminated unemployed youth from others	Viney (1983)	[129]
	Predicted poor rehabilitation of medical patients	Viney and Westbrook (1983)	[135]
	Responded as predicted to experimental (drug) manipulation	Gottschalk and Gleser (1969)	[35]
Pawn	Independent of sex, age, but correlated with occupational status	Westbrook and Viney (1980)	[40]
	Significantly correlated with measures of other negatively toned states	Westbrook and Viney (1980)	[40]
	Significantly correlated with other measures of this state	Westbrook and Viney (1980)	[40]
	Significantly correlated with appropriate use of coping strategies	Westbrook and Viney (1980)	[40]
	Discriminated chronically ill from others	Westbrook and Viney (1982)	[40]
	Discriminated unemployed youth from others	Viney (1983)	[129]
	Predicted poor rehabilitation for medical patients	Viney and Westbrook (1982)	[135]
Total Anxiety	Independent of sex, age, educational level	Viney and Westbrook (1982)	[135]
	Significantly correlated with self-reports of anxiety	Gottschalk (1979)	[36]
	Significantly correlated with ratings of anxiety-related behaviors by observers	Gottschalk (1979)	[36]
	Significantly correlated with psychiatrists' ratings of anxiety	Gottschalk and Gleser (1969)	[35]
	Significantly correlated with physiological measures of anxiety	Gottschalk and Gleser (1969)	[35]
	Discriminated chronically ill from others	Westbrook and Viney (1982)	[90]
	Discriminated relatives' accounts when waiting for emergency medical patients from those who were not	Bunn and Clarke (1979)	[123]
	Predicted good rehabilitation for medical patients	Viney and Westbrook (1982)	[135]
	Responded as predicted to experimental (psychological and drug) manipulations	Gottschalk and Gleser (1969)	[35]

and physiological measures. Relationships with certain types of content analysis scales rather than others, in accordance with the nature of the construct, are also relevant. For example, positive correlations with positively rather than negatively toned scales have been predicted for the Origin Scale but with negatively rather than positively toned scales for the Pawn Scale. Both of these procedures provide estimates of criterion-based validity, using concurrent criteria. Successful discrimination by the scales, either of appropriate groups of research participants or of situations experienced by them, is another form of concurrent criterion validity which has been considered. Some validational studies using criteria assessed later have also been reported. An even more difficult test than predictive validity is that concerning whether the scales respond in a manner appropriate to their underlying constructs when they are used to assess the effects of an experimental manipulation. These manipulations have consisted of both psychological and drug treatments [35, 36].

Table 4 shows that more of these types of information are currently available for some content analysis scales than others. The Total Anxiety Scale is the best validated to date, with evidence bearing on its independence from demographic factors, correlations with ratings by self and others of the psychological state in question, correlations with other measures of anxiety, discrimination of both people and situations, effective prediction, and responsivity to experimental manipulation. The Hostility-In and Pawn Scales are the next best supported. These are followed by a cluster of scales with roughly equivalent validational information: the Origin, Sociality, Hostility-In, and Ambivalent-Hostility Scales. Those with the least support are the Hope, Positive-Affect, and Cognitive Anxiety Scales. It should also be noted that three of the scales which have been discussed in detail – the Origin, Pawn, and Cognitive Anxiety Scales – have been influenced by socioeconomic variables. This does not invalidate their use but indicates the likely effects of such variables which should be taken into account when these scales are employed. Two factors seem to have influenced the amount of validational evidence available. One factor is the tone of the psychological state measured by the scale: negatively toned scales have been better validated than positively toned scales. This is probably because psychological conceptualizations and methodologies in relation to distressing psychological states have generally received more attention than the more agreeable states. The other factor is the time which has elapsed since the original construction of the scales. The Total Anxiety Scale was the first of its type and has had some 20 years in which to acquire validation. Most of the other scales were constructed more recently. If time since construction is an influential factor, then more extensive validational networks can be expected to develop for the later group. The short time since conception may also be the reason so few negative findings relating to validity have been reported. All of the content analysis scales described in detail will benefit from the development of their validational networks. However, it is for those applications of content analysis in which the categories are used only once or twice and then apparently discarded that validity must most be questioned.

5.5 Some Theoretical Advantages of Content Analysis

One major theoretical advantage of the technique of content analysis is that it may be applied by researchers of different theoretical perspectives. The propositions which each psychologist holds to be true may be built into the content analysis scales he or she develops. This applicability of the technique of content analysis with different theoretical approaches is important because the Zeitgeist of psychology is constantly changing. Psychologists who have engaged in longitudinal research know how "out-of-date" their carefully developed concepts can look 20 or even 10 years later. Of course, content analysis scales based on "old" concepts may look out-of-date too. Yet, because as methods of data analysis they are independent of the method of data collection, new content analysis scales which have the benefit of new psychological insights may be developed and applied to the old data. Developing these scales also has other theoretical advantages. The process of defining content analysis categories to represent the construct of interest is a heuristic one which, at the least, forces the researcher toward a greater clarity of conceptualization. The heuristic value of content analysis may also be greater if the psychologist approached interpersonal communications, insofar as is possible, free of presuppositions [61, 62]. As the Sedelows [63] have observed, content analysis in which the categories arise from the observed phenomena rather than from the researcher's prior conceptions can lead to new theories about these phenomena.

The content analysis scales which have been devised so far have been based on at least three different sets of internally consistent assumptions: a psychophysiological set, a psychoanalytic set, and a sociophenomenological set. First, content analysis scales have been viewed as a means of access to the physiological processes underlying the communications that are analyzed [64]. Working from this assumption, the words are seen as indicators of physiological activity [65]. The criteria against which the scales are validated within this framework are psychophysiological [66] and psychopharmacological [67]. Second, content analysis scales have been viewed, psychoanalytically, as a way of tapping emotions that are suppressed or repressed [68], in which case relationships of the scales' scored to behaviors of which the psychotherapy patient is unaware become of interest [69]. Third, they have also been used by those who take a sociophenomenological perspective of psychology. This approach implies a concern with the meanings people use to interpret their experiences, especially their interpersonal experiences, and personal construct theory [70] is one form of this approach. Its predominant methodology involves enlisting the cooperation of research participants [71, 72], asking them to talk freely about their experiences, and listening to their responses [73]. The content analysis scales provide a form of listening to and interpreting such responses [74].

Content analyses of peoples' communications about events can provide a valid subjective perspective to add to the objective perspective that psychologists generally prefer. Many techniques are available for appraising the observable behavior of others but few for tapping into their less accessible experience. The assessments that have been made of quality of life is a case in point. This is a topic currently of importance to psychologists because through it they can influence health and welfare policy and its practice [75]. No one would deny that the subjective aspects of quality of life are as important as the objectively observable aspects. Yet, most indices of quality of life have been based on observation [76–78]. Psychologists are now wanting to redress this balance [79], to advocate in-depth studies of the perceived quality of life of individuals [80], and to examine differences among people in terms of which aspect of quality of life is important to them [81]. Content analysis scales, because they can be used to represent a subjective perspective on quality of life [48], are appropriate for these purposes.

5.6 Practical Advantages of Content Analysis

There are some practical advantages to the use of content analysis scales. No expensive or cumbersome equipment is needed. A small cassette recorder is required. (It should be noted, however, that employing research assistance to apply the scales may be expensive.) Data collection is not time-consuming and demands minimal expertise or training. (It should also be noted that data analysis by applying the scales does require considerable time and training.) Of more importance is the general suitability of the method. While questionnaires and interviews must contain questions relating specifically to the situation or event of interest, the content analysis technique has no such predetermined specificity and so may be just as applicable in one situation as in the next. Also important is the absence of practice effects with this technique. Assessments may be made from the same people over time without introducing this kind of error, which helps to make them useful techniques for estimating change of psychological state. For most of the content analysis scales developed to date, the effects of different instructions and different interviewers have been minimal. They may, however, occur [35] and should be monitored.

A less tangible but nevertheless significant advantage, which I have already touched on in relation to projective techniques, is the richness of the data which may be represented by content analysis. Much of the complexity and true-to-life nature of data are lost with techniques such as questionnaires and rating scales. This is because content analysis may be used to tap into the flow of peoples' experience without interfering with it. It may be nonobtrusive, in the sense spelled out by Webb, Campbell and Schwartz [82], that is, it may avoid many of the errors introduced through peoples' awareness of being observed. Their perceptions of their own role as respondent, response stereotypes such as "nay-saying", interviewer interaction effects, and even the measurement process itself may all influence their responses. Content analysis should be a better technique than simple self-report techniques, such as self-rating scales, for assessing certain kinds of psychological states because it should be less susceptible to socially desirable responding [83]. It should also avoid the problem of responses intended to meet the expectations of the psychologist [84], as well as of faking or providing misleading information. There is some empirical evidence available in relation to the lesser susceptibility of content analysis to social desirability [37, 40]. There is, however, no such evidence yet available for the other claims. Content analysis may be used so as to overcome the problem that arises when research participants are ambivalent about an event they have experienced. Ambivalence cannot be tapped by "yes" or "no" or "true" or "false" responses. Content analysis is also, as Gottschalk [85] has noted, a more effective technique for many purposes than reports from observers, such as behavior rating scales, because external observers not only have their own biases but also do not have direct access to the same data which the people they observe have within their own experience. Of course, the two techniques can be effectively combined.

Psychologists are becoming more concerned with accounts from research participants of the events they are studying, whether their work is carried out in the laboratory or in the field [86–88]. Such accounts will not be readily interpreted until we have built up a body of knowledge about how people experience events. We need normative data of this kind [89]. It can be provided by the application of content analysis scales. This is also the case for our understanding of a complex event, such as the onset of chronic illness. With content analysis scales, it has been possible to identify common patterns of reaction to this event [90] and to check to see whether these patterns differ according to the nature of the disease process [91] or according to the severity of the resulting disability [92]. Such a program of research has been possible because the first step of identifying patterns of reaction could be taken using content analysis scales. Similar work may also be carried out with less complete and more readily controlled psychological phenomena.

5.7 Problems and Limitations of Content Analysis

Content analysis scales of the type examined here are limited in their application to verbal communications only. They ignore all information not presented in words. They do not deal with the functional aspects of language as Mahl [1] does with his "ums" and stutters, nor do they make use of the complex nonverbal sources of information which are combined with the verbal sources by Truax and Carkhuff [30] to measure, for example, respect. This is not to say that content analysis of extralinguistic data is not possible. Russell and Stiles [25] have reviewed a number of content analysis systems designed for this purpose. Psychologists seeking to measure psychological states which they believe may be better expressed in extralinguistic or a combination of linguistic and extralinguistic forms will not find the content analysis scales reviewed here useful.

Their viability, then, is partially determined by the nature of the observational referents of the definition of the psychological state. The clarity of this definition is also relevant. Content analysis cannot be applied if the concept the psychologist intends to assess is not precisely defined. (This limitation may work as an advantage since it may be said that no assessment would be preferable under such circumstances.) The technique cannot be used if language referents for the concept cannot be identified. Also, the results of content analysis can only be as meaningful as the verbalized data on which they are based are representative of their source. Interpretations of those research participants of many types and in many different situations are available. This is one reason why established content analysis scales with relevant bodies of empirical data are of more use than sets of content analysis categories developed only on the basis of specific data and limited in purpose to one specific research project.

The source of the data raises other problems as well. This content analysis technique should not be applied to data from research participants for whom it cannot be assumed that the language in which they express themselves may not provide viable data for content analysis. This may be because they are intellectually retarded, poorly educated, or using a language other than their native one which has not yet been mastered. Similarly, those research participants, the quality of whose psychological states seems neither marked nor varied, form another group for whom this assumption may not validly be made. Patients exhibiting the clinical syndrome of alexithymia, which is characterized by apparent lack of emotion and imagination, for example, are unlikely to score highly on content analysis scales, as has been reported by von Rad and his colleagues [93].

5.8 Some Psychological Applications of Content Analysis

Content analysis has been effectively applied by psychologists in a number of areas. Much of this work has involved the application of content analysis scales. An overview of these scales will first be supplied. Then, samples of research in the areas of personality, developmental, and social psychology will be examined. This examination will be followed by a discussion of some examples from the applied fields of clinical, community, and health psychology.

The research teams most active in developing content analysis scales based on adequate samples of research participants have been led by Gottschalk in the United States and Viney in Australia. Many of the applications of content analysis discussed here have employed their scales, although some applications of other, once or twice used content analyses are also considered. The research teams have developed scales to measure negatively toned emotional states, such as uncertainty [39], anxiety, anger, and depression [44, 68]. There are also scales to measure the more positive emotions, both generally [38] and in the more specific form of hope [94]. There are the Origin and Pawn Scales, which have been described [40]. There is also an alternative measure of achievement strivings [35]. Scales have been developed which tap people's perceptions of interpersonal interactions, for example, the Sociality Scale [37], which assesses the extent to which people are experiencing satisfying relationships. Similar scales have been devised which focus on less homogeneous or multidimensional states. These are the Social Alienation and Personal Disorganization Scale [35], which assesses the withdrawal and disruption of the schizophrenic state, and the Cognitive Impairment Scale [95], which measures the transitory intellectual dysfunctions that can occur in people concurrently with physiological and emotional changes. All of these scales assess complex psychological phenomena and so take time to learn to score to criterion.

This time and effort may be warranted because other information is also available from these scales. For example, the independent subscales of the Total Anxiety Scale [35], make possible the assessment of the relative contributions of different sources of anxiety to the total score for any person at any point in time. Similarly, the scales dealing with anger permit differentiation between different ways of expressing anger: whether it is expressed directly or whether it is experienced ambivalently and thus in a more indirect way. The Sociality Scale subscales [37] can be used to identify which types of satisfying relationships are being experienced by people. It is also possible to use the scales in combination. Westbrook and Viney have developed, for example, a ratio score which measures the psychological cost of an event to people. Cost estimates are based on the relative proportion of the positive and negative emotions of the research participants [48].

Samples of research using content analysis in the area of personality are the first to be examined. Epstein [96] has called for personality psychologists to study individuals in depth and over time. Content analysis scales are well suited to these tasks. Questions like "How are psychological states linked with behavioral states?" and "How do such psychological states come about?" fall within the boundaries of the field of personality. Content analysis has been used to find some preliminary answers to these questions. In relation to the first question, for example, Freedman and his colleagues [97] have used some Gottschalk-Gleser Content Analysis Scales to differentiate between anger which is directed out from oneself to the world and anger directed in on oneself and have looked for body movements associated with each of these states. They found anger directed out to be associated with object-focused movements. Hermann [98] developed his own content analysis procedure to assess the needs for control, power and affiliation, conceptual complexity, distrust of others, and task orientation of Soviet Politburo members. Similarly, some preliminary answers to the second question have become available with the aid of content analysis scales. Thus, one study has related different types of evaluative feedback to increases in anxiety [99]. Another has examined the impact of coping strategies on anxiety and hostility [100]. Yet another content analysis-based study has focused on the media messages associated with the extent to which individuals feel controlled by situations and events [101].

Content analysis scales have been successfully applied to communications from people during all stages of development after the preverbal state. They have been used to measure anxiety and hostility with school-age children [102, 103] and with adolescents [104, 105] through to retired and elderly people [45]. The patterns of their uncertainty, anxiety, frustration, anger, depression, positive feelings, origin and pawn percepts, and sociability have been examined. Some research has been carried out with womens' accounts of their major transitions. Different patterns of women's psychological states have been observed for life changes, such as moving from primary to high school, going to work, finding a life partner, becoming a mother, creating a home in a new community, and being left by young adult offspring in the "empty nest" [45]. More intensive study of one of these life changes – childbearing – has also been conducted using this range of content analysis scales [106]. Westbrook has been concerned with identifying socioeconomic differences in the childbearing experience [107] as well with the relation of such differences to the birth order of the child [108] and to the quality of the mother's relationship with the father of the child [109].

Social psychologists, as well as developmental psychologists, have used content analysis [110]. Buckmorse [111] has recently suggested that Adorno's F Scale, a questionnaire measure of authoritarianism, should not be considered to be his greatest contribution to psychology. She argues that the content analysis which Adorno developed to decipher texts, believing language to represent a form of social reality, will ultimately be recognized to be of greater value. Attitudes are one interest of social psychologists; roles are another. Sex roles determine the focus of much social interaction in our culture. Their dimensions can be gleaned through content analysis, for example, of popular novels [112]. Group interactions, too, are an interest of social psychologists. A content analysis scale based on social influence theory has been developed to evaluate group process [113]. Similarly, balance theory has been used as a basis for another type of content analysis to test hypotheses about the nature of international conflict [114]. For this research, the content to be analyzed was not spontaneous verbal communications, but news items about a specific conflict.

Of the more applied fields of psychology it is, as I foreshadowed, that of clinical psychology which has seen the most work with content analysis. Analyses of the content of the delusions of patients diagnosed as reactive and process schizophrenics have been related to ratings of their integration and autism, for example, to differentiate the two groups [115]. Standardized scales were not used here. Standardized procedures have been used to provide new assessment tools, as well as being applied to old techniques, such as the Rorschach or Thematic Apperception Test. Content analysis scales have proved effective for clinical work with both children [116] and adults [36]. The work with children has focused on assessing emotional states, such as anxiety and hostility, an area which, compared with intellectual functioning, has been largely neglected. The work with adults has concentrated on intellectual impairment, with the aim of providing some information about impairment more quickly than the more complex and time-consuming tools which are available [117]. Content analysis has also been used to assess the effects on anxiety levels of physical disaster, through analysis of the dreams reported by the survivors [118]. It has proved valuable, too, in psychotherapy research. The process of psychotherapy, insofar as it involves changing psychological states, is being reexamined through the use of content analysis scales, for example, by Grunzig, Holzscheck and Kächele [119], Schofer [120], and Brunink and Shroeder [121]. Gottschalk [64] has also pointed to the value of his content analysis scales as predictors of psychotherapy outcome. Perley, Winget and Placci [122] have tested the long-accepted belief that patients' experience of hope is an important factor in their choice to continue treatment. They found support for their hypothesis. Content analysis scales have also been used to evaluate the immediate outcomes of different forms of treatment, for example, crisis interventions on anxiety and uncertainty [123] and the effects of outpatient treatment on the anxiety and hostility of adolescent clients [124]. They have also been employed to evaluate the immediate outcomes of treatments using psychoactive drugs [125].

I have discussed elsewhere the appropriateness of the Gottschalk-Gleser and Viney-Westbrook Content Analysis Scales for research in community psychology [126]. They may be used in this context to gain understanding of communities, societies, and cultures [127, 128]. They have provided information about how the members of a community experience their lives, how they experience community change, and how they are affected by community-oriented intervention programs. Here are some examples of such work. Using the content analysis scales, it has been possible to gain greater understanding of how unemployed people view their role in their community in terms of alienation (or low sociality) but many pawn percepts [129]. The loneliness and frustration of the experience of relocation from one community to another have also been explored [130]. It has been possible, too, to demonstrate some of the more immediate outcomes of a youth work program in terms of less loneliness and increased sociability [131]. Two training programs for lay counselors based on opposed theoretical perspectives have also been evaluated to reveal different types of emotions elicited by and attributed to their clients by the counselors [132].

In health psychology, content analysis scales have been used to assess the psychological states which are associated with certain types of illness [133], treatment [134], and rehabilitation programs [135]. The scales are useful techniques for researchers in the field of psychosomatic medicine [64, 136]. The anxiety levels of patients with chronic illness have, for example, been traced over time. This in turn has enabled the identification of some aspects of their illness which are more anxiety arousing than others [137] and of the types of anxiety aroused as well as of some anxiety-based reactions to rehabilitation programs [135]. The experiences of coronary patients have been studied using some of the scales [91, 138], as have those of hypertensive patients [139]. Patients' emotional reactions to treatment have been assessed in this way, for example, those of mastectomy patients to radiotherapy [140]. The meanings patients ascribe to illness have also been explored using a combination of the Gottschalk-Gleser and Viney-Westbrook Scales [73, 141].

5.9 Is Computerization of Content Analysis Scales Possible?

Considerable training is necessary for the effective use of content analysis scales. They also can be time-consuming to apply since scoring must be checked and rechecked. Many psychologists may therefore consider them too expensive for use in their present form. Computer programs for scoring the scales could, however, alter the balance of such cost-benefit considerations. Researchers using content analysis are now looking to computer technology to achieve this objective [142]. There are some software programs available for content analysis, but they tend to deal only with frequencies of single words or sentences or with some of the instrumental aspects of speech on which Mahl has focused and not with meaning [143]. The clauses which are currently scored on content analysis scales by hand are complex, multimeaning units and so have not yet yielded to such an analysis. The two main approaches to content analysis by computer have been through dictionaries stored in the computer memory or through the use of models of artificial intelligence [3].

The dictionary approach seems attractive. The Harvard III Psychosociological Dictionary [144] was constructed over 20 years ago, employing the theories and concepts relevant to psychologists and sociologists, and is still in use [145]. The Harvard Need-Achievement Dictionary [144], designed to perform McClelland's need achievement content analysis, is another example of this approach. However, there are problems to be considered. Decisions about which word from the available verbal communications to use and how to store and gain access to the dictionary are difficult to make. The size of a vocabulary of words is another problem in need of rapid access store of a computer so that this work is often more time-consuming than it should be. There is also the problem raised by the different vocabularies of different populations of research participants. Heroin addicts may have different vocabularies from those of seminarians. Applying a dictionary with both populations would require revision of the dictionary with both populations would require revision of the dictionary. This approach may therefore imply constant revision. Such revision may also be needed for other populations also because of cultural changes in language usage over time. Revision of the constantly changing and more extensive vocabulary of human scorers is likely to be less necessary but, if necessary, more readily accomplished.

While a finite dictionary of words is possible, a finite dictionary of sentences, with the endless variety of word combinations available, would not be. It should, however, be possible for the finite number of rules which govern sentence structure of the categorization of linguistic information to be defined. The General Enquirer, which is used in conjunction with the two dictionaries which have been mentioned, is an example of this artificial intelligence approach [144]. There is current work in Japan on parsing algorithms which are developed by starting with the available verbal communication and working up to identification of its governing rules [146, 147]. This work may provide a sounder basis for the computerized content analysis of language. The problems with this parsing approach include those raised by research participants who do not follow such rules. People do not always speak grammatically although they may be able to write grammatically. Other people can understand them, but computers cannot yet be effectively programmed to do so. Also, meaning is often partly determined by context which is also difficult to represent in software programs for computer scoring. The result is that the necessary preediting and large array of rules currently make this approach also time-consuming and expensive. This is why the most common solution has been the combine the dictionary and artificial intelligence approaches, and advocated by Stone and his colleagues. This has been the solution adopted by the Bierschenks in their attempts to develop computer-based content analysis of interview texts in Swedish [55, 148–150].

Three attempts to develop computer-based scoring programs for the Gottschalk-Gleser Scales have been reported to date. Gottschalk, Hausmann and Brown [151] have used a parser to deal with the rules governing sentence structure. With a content analysis scale measuring anger, they were able to achieve 60% correct scoring. When scores from the computer program were compared with those from experienced scorers, a rank correlation coefficient of 0.80 was achieved. Results from more robust indices of correlation and from comparisons of score sizes, however, were not so encouraging. The program was missing too many scorable clauses. In Germany, Grunzig, Holzscheck and Kächele [119] have dealt with only four subcategories of the Total Anxiety Scale (castration and separation anxiety, and guilt and shame) when comparing computer and human scoring. The level of agreement they were able to achieve was only 40%. In a more recent attempt, Gottschalk and Bechtel [152] have developed a three-stage program. First, each clause is converted into an internal representation which contains information about the scoring categories present in the clause and its syntactic structure. Then the information about scoring and structure is combined to assign a score in each clause, and these scores are combined to assign a score in each clause, and these scores are combined to produce a total score. Gottschalk and Bechtel have been able to achieve Pearson product moment correlation coefficients of 0.85 between computer scoring and hand scoring, but still find unacceptable differences in score sizes as determined by the two methods. Computerization, then, seems feasible and probably cost beneficial in the long term.

5.10 Is Content Analysis an Ethical Technique?

Insofar as content analysis is a technique for analyzing data and not for collecting it, it raises no ethical issues. Yet, because it can be applied to data collected in ethically appropriate ways, it has value. It provides a means of making sense of and rendering useful the information from a simple question posed to research participants such as "I am interested in X. I'd like you to tell me about your experience of X." Research participants then become responsible for their own account of the events they have experienced. They also are able to work with the researcher in the kind of open and honest relationship which the APA Code of Ethics [153] recommends, avoiding the coercion and deception that concern many psychologists today [154]. Baumrind [155] has criticized psychologists for not taking more seriously the informed consent of research participants. With the content analysis technique, this consent can develop into the even more active and responsible role of cooperating co-researcher or co-assessor, as Fischer [156] has shown. This role is appropriate for a model of the person as active and aware, constructing his or her psychological world, and influencing and being influenced by his or her environment [157]. Participants in this kind of research become responsible for guarding their own privacy [158]. If they choose to retain total privacy, by not communicating, then content analysis cannot be applied effectively. As Kelman [159] observed, psychologists must leave to their "subject" decisions about the extent to which they share themselves with us. They are as entitled to self-determination in research as they are in other areas of their lives.

Kelman has also viewed as an ethical issue the debate between rigor and vigor which has split psychology, as well as other social sciences, into two opposing camps. Research which favors rigor he has described as "scientific," quantitative, and precise. Research which favors vigor he has described as humanistic, qualitative, and relying on clinical intuition. Content analysis, because it can represent an accurate quantification of clinical intuition, can bridge the gap between these two camps. Content analysis is a way of listening to people talk (or reading what people write) and arriving at consistent interpretations of their reports. It allows for the combining of hypothesis testing with description, verification with discovery, accuracy with empathy. Most importantly, it combines reproducibility with human relevance. It may be said to combine rigor with vigor.

5.11 Content Analysis: An Evaluation

Many different measures of psychological states based on content analysis have been identified in this review. Examples of work employing content analysis have been cited in the areas of personality, developmental, and social psychology. I have also described content analysis research in the applied areas of clinical, community, and health psychology. However, relatively few psychologists are using this technique in their research.

Psychologists should be able to make better use of this technique as it becomes better known and is more fully developed. Unlike many of the more theoretically bound techniques which are available, content analysis requires the acceptance of only one major assumption: that the language in which people choose to express themselves contains information about the nature of their psychological states. It is useful for the range of verbal communications, which have been elicited in different ways and at different times. It can be employed nonobtrusively and is not situation specific. It can be applied to already recorded data as well as to new. It can take account of the richness and complexity of the material with which it deals and provide a valid subjective perspective to add to the objective perspective which has come to dominate psychology. It can be used in such a way as to promote an open and honest relationship between researchers and research participants.

Content analysis does not, however, provide answers to all the problems psychologists have encountered in their attempts to assess psychological states. There are, as I have noted, limitations on its application. Also, many sets of content analysis categories have been developed by psychologists and psychiatrists, reported once with inadequate information about their reliability and validity, and then never discussed in the literature again. Such applications of content analysis do not accurately indicate the potential of the technique. The major exceptions to this pattern have been the Gottschalk-Gleser and Viney-Westbrook Content Analysis Scales for which some of this information has been summarized in this article. Yet even with these scales, some reservations have been expressed concering their reliability. Evidence for the consistency of interjudge agreement of their categories is available, but more information is needed concerning their internal consistency and, where appropriate, the stability of their scores over time. Also, some of the evidence of their validity provides inferred rather than direct support. This problem, which is a result of the lack of available criterion measures, content analysis shares with many other methods of psychological assessment. The lack of information about stability is likely to be the most serious problem because it calls into question the use of existing content analysis scales to evaluate change over time. However, they can be used to evaluate the process of change when information about the amount and direction of change is made available through designs employing matched control groups or research participants as their own controls. It is possible that the cost of their application and development may outweigh their usefulness. The extent to which software programs can be developed to perform content analysis using computer technology may determine the extent to which the technique is used by psychologists in the future.

Content analysis can range in form from simple coding of verbal data into one of two mutually exclusive categories to complex scales based on multidimensional concepts. It can be used with the aim of describing phenomena in a new field or for testing hypotheses in a more developed area. The value of this technique for psychologists lies in its capacity to provide accurate and consistent interpretations of people's accounts of events without depriving these accounts of their power or eloquence.

5.12 Summary

Content analysis of verbal communications is a technique by which psychologists can assess the transitory psychological states of their research participants. A history of the use of this technique in psychology is given. The development of content analysis scales is then described, together with an example of a scale in construction. The variety of verbal communications to which content analysis is applicable is also considered. Issues of reliability and validity are considered in a survey of the literature concerned with a sample of ten relatively well-developed content analysis scales. Some of the theoretical and practical advantages of the technique over other methods of assessment of psychological states are also examined, as are some of its problems and limitations. Information about available content analysis scales is provided. Applications of content analysis in personality, developmental, and social psychology are considered, together with others in clinical, community, and health psychology. The scoring of content analysis scales by computer is also discussed, as is their contribution to an ethical relationship between researcher and research participant. This review concludes with an evaluation of the viability of content analysis as an aid in psychological research.

Acknowledgment. The author would like to acknowledge the contributions of Goldine C. Gleser, Louis A. Gottschalk, and Mary T. Westbrook to this work.

References

1. Mahl GF (1959) Exploring emotional states by content analysis. In: Pool I (ed) Trends in content analysis. University of Illinois Press, Urbana
2. Holsti O (1969) Content analysis for the social science and humanities. Addison-Wesley, Reading
3. Krippendorf K (1980) Content analysis. Sage, Beverly Hills
4. Popper KR (1959) The logic of scientific discovery. Basic Books, New York
5. Berelson B (1952) Content analysis in communication research. Glencoe, New York, p 31
6. Budd RW, Thorp RK, Donehew L (1967) Content analysis of communications. MacMillan, New York
7. Elizur A (1949) Content analysis of the Rorschach with regard to anxiety and hostility. Res Ex J Proj Tech 13: 247–284
8. Finney BC (1955) Rorschach test correlates of assaultive behaviour. J Proj Tech 19: 6–16
9. Holt RR (1956) Gauging primary and secondary processes in Rorschach responses. J Proj Tech 20: 14–25
10. Aronson E, Rezinoff M (1958) Rorschach content interpretation. Van Nostrand, New York
11. MacHove FJ (1982) Differentiating affective from thought disorders by semantic analysis of Rorschach responses. J Pers Assess 46: 12–17
12. Eron LD (1950) A normative study of the thematic apperception test. Psychol Monog 64 (9)
13. Bellak L (1970) The TAT and CAT in clinical use. Grune and Stratton, New York
14. Henry RM (1981) Validation of a projective measure of aggression – anxiety for five-year-old boys. J Pers Assess 45: 359–369
15. Hoover TO (1978) The hand test fifteen years later. J Pers Assess 42: 128–138
16. Mayman M, Garis M (1960) Early memories of expressions of relationship paradigm. Am J Orthopsychiatry 30: 507–520
17. Bruhn AR, Schiffman H (1982) Prediction of control stance from earliest childhood memory. J Pers Assess 46: 380–390
18. Atkinson JW (ed) (1958) Motives in fantasy, action and society. Van Nostrand, New York
19. Atkinson JW, Raynor JO (eds) (1974) Motivation and achievement. Hemisphere, Washington DC
20. McClelland DC, Atkinson JW, Clark RA, Lowell EL (1953) The achievement motive. Appleton-Century-Crofts. New York
21. McClelland DC (1961) The achieving society. Free Press, New York

22. Horner MS (1968) Sex differences in achievement and performance in competitive and non-competitive conditions. Doctoral dissertation. University of Michigan
23. Winter D (1973) The power motive. Free Press, New York
24. McClelland DC (1961) Power the inner experience. Free Press, New York
25. Russell RL, Stiles WB (1979) Categories for classifying language in psychotherapy. Psychol Bull 86: 404–419
26. Auld F, Murray EJ (1955) Content analysis studies of psychotherapy. Psychol Bull 52: 377–395
27. Frank GH (1961) On the history of the objective investigation of the process of psychotherapy. J Psychol 51: 89–95
28. Frank GH, Sweetland A (1962) A study of the process of psychotherapy. The verbal interaction. J Consult Psychol 26: 135–138
29. Rogers CR (1967) The therapeutic relationship and its impact. University of Wisconsin Press, Madison
30. Truax CB, Carkhuff RR (1967) Toward effective counseling and psychotherapy. Aldine, Chicago
31. Zimmer JM, Cowles KH (1972) Content analysis using fortran: applied to interviews conducted by Rogers C, Perls F and Ellis A. J Counsel Psychol 19: 161–166
32. O'Dell JW, Bahmer AJ (1981) Rogers, Lazarus and Shostrum in content analysis. J Clin Psychol 37: 507–510
33. Lewis HB (1971) Shame and guilt in neurosis. International Universities Press, New York
34. Schofer G, Balck F, Koch U (1979) Possible applications of the Gottschalk-Gleser content analysis of speech in psychotherapy research. In: Gottschalk LA (ed) Content analysis of verbal behavior: further studies. Wiley, New York
35. Gottschalk LA, Gleser GC (1969) The measurement of psychological states through the content analysis of verbal behavior. University of California Press, Berkeley
36. Gottschalk LA (ed) (1979) The content analysis of verbal behavior: further studies. Spectrum, New York
37. Viney LL, Westbrook MT (1979) Sociality: a content analysis scale for verbalizations. Soc Behav Personal 7: 129–137
38. Westbrook MT (1976) Positive affect: a method of content analysis for verbal samples. J Consult Clin Psychol 44: 715–719
39. Viney LL, Westbrook MT (1976) Cognitive anxiety. A method of content analysis for verbal samples. J Pers Assess 40: 140–150
40. Westbrook MT, Viney LL (1980) Scales of origin and pawn perception using content analysis of speech. J Pers Assess 44: 157–166
41. De Charms R (1968) Personal causation. Academic, New York
42. Heider JB (1958) The psychology of interpersonal relations. Wiley, New York
43. Rotter JB (1966) Generalized expectancies for internal versus external control of reinforcement. Psychol Monog 80: 1–28
44. Gottschalk LA, Winget CN, Gleser CG (1969) Manual of instructions for using the Gottschalk-Gleser content analysis scales: anxiety hostility and social alienation-personal disorganization. University of California Press, Berkeley
45. Viney LL (1980) Transitions. Cassell, Sydney
46. Gottschalk LA, Gleser GC (1960) An analysis of the verbal content of suicide notes. Br J Med Psychol 33: 195–204
47. Gottschalk LA (1961) Comparative psycholinguistic analysis of two psychotherapeutic interviews. International Universities Press, New York
48. Viney LL, Westbrook MT (1981) Measuring patient's experienced quality of life: the application of content analysis scales in health care. Community Health Stud 5: 45–52

49. Hafner AJ, Kaplan AM (1960) Hostility content analysis of the Rorschach and TAT. J Proj Tech 24: 137–143
50. Cronbach LJ, Gleser GC (1957) Psychological tests and personnel decisions. University of Illinois Press, Urbana
51. Lolas F, Von Rad M (1977) Anxiety and hostility in psychosomatic and psychoneurotic patients: content analysis of verbal expressions. Acta Psiquiatr Psicol Am Lat 23: 184–193
52. Daini S, Solano L, Antonioli M, Torre A (1978) Affective resonance in hypogogic reveries: A content analysis evaluation. Arch Psicol Neurol Psichiatr 39: 249–262
53. Scobel WA (1979) Speech and client-centred therapy: a content analysis research. Psychother Med Psychol 29: 66–72
54. Thirard J (1976) Survey of a system of content analysis. Bull Psychol 30: 65–73
55. Bierschenk BA (1976) Theoretical and psychometrical problems of a computer-based analysis of interview. Pedagogist-Psykologiska, Problem no 287
56. Schofer G (1977) The Gottschalk-Gleser method: a content analysis of speech to measure hostile and anxious affects. Z Psychosom Med Psychoanal 23: 86–102
57. Koch U, Schofer G (1978) Relationships of anxious and angry affects to clinical conditions: An example of married couples with the Gottschalk-Gleser method. Z Klin Psychol 7: 110–125
58. Viney LL, Manton M (1973) Sampling verbal behavior in Australia: the Gottschalk-Gleser content analysis scales. Aust J Psychol 25: 45–55
59. American Psychological Association (1974) Standards for educational and psychological tests. APA, Washington DC
60. Schofer G, Koch U, Balck F (1979) Test criteria of the Gottschalk-Gleser content analysis of speech: Objectivity, reliability, validity in German studies. In: Gottschalk LD (ed) The content of verbal behavior: further studies. Spectrum, New York
61. Horner W (1968) Sex differences in achievement and performance in competitive and non-competitive conditions. Doctoral dissertation. University of Michigan
62. Speigelberg H (1969) The relevance of phenomenological philosophy for psychology. In: Lee EN, Nandelbaum M (eds) Phenomenology and existensialism. Nijhoff, The Hague
63. Sedelow WA, Sedelow SY (1978) Formalized historiography, the structure of scientific and literary texts. Some issues posed by computational methodology. J Hist Behav Sci 14: 247–263
64. Gottschalk LA (1977) Recent advances in the content analysis of speech and the application of this measurement approach to psychosomatic research. Psychother Psychosom 28: 73–82
65. Gottschalk LA (1974) The application of a method of content analysis to psychotherapy research. Am J Psychother 28: 488–499
66. Gottschalk LA, Cleghorn JM, Gleser GC, Iacono JM (1965) Studies of relationships of emotions to plasma lipids. Psychosom Med 27: 102–111
67. Stone WW, Gleser GC, Gottschalk LA (1973) Anxiety and beta adrenergic blockage. Arch Gen Psychiatry 29: 620–622
68. Gottschalk LA (1971) Some psychoanalytic research into the communication of meaning through language: the quality and magnitude of psychological states. Br J Med Psychol 44: 131–148
69. Gottschalk LA, Uliana RL (1977) Further studies on the relationship of nonverbal to verbal behavior. In: Freedman N, Grand S (eds) Communicative structures. Plenum, New York
70. Kelly G (1955) A theory of personality, Norton, New York
71. Kelly G (1965) The strategy of psychological research. Bull Br Psychol Soc 18: 1–15
72. Kelly G (1969) Humanistic methodology in psychological research. J Human Psychol 9: 53–65
73. Viney LL (1983) Images of illness. Krieger, Malabar, Florida

74. Keen E (1975) A primer in phenomenological psychology. Holt, Rinehart and Winston, New York
75. Katzner DW (1979) Choice and quality of life. Sage, Beverly Hills
76. Grogono AM, Woodgate DJ (1971) Index of measuring health. Lancet 102: 1024–1028
77. Lui BC (1975) Quality of life indicators in US metropolitan areas. US Environmental Protection Agency, Washington DC
78. Pliskin N, Taylor AK (1977) General principles: Cost benefit and decision analysis. In: Bunker IK (ed) Costs, risks and benefits of surgery. Oxford University Press, Oxford
79. George LK, Bearon LB (1980) Quality of life in order persons: Measuring and measurement. Human Sciences, New York
80. Flanagan JC (1978) A research approach to improving our quality of life. Am Psychol 33: 138–147
81. Hoods DL, Raymond JS (1981) Quality of life and the competent community. Am J Community Psychol 9: 293–301
82. Webb EN, Campbell DT, Schwartz RD (1966) Unobtrusive measures: nonreactive research in the social sciences. Rand McNally, Chicago
83. Edwards A (1957) The social desirability variable. Dryden, New York
84. Rosenthal RR (1976) Experimenter effects in behavioral research. Appleton-Century-Crofts, New York
85. Gottschalk LA (1974) Quantification and psychological indicators of emotions: the content analysis of speech and other objective measures of psychological states. Int J Psychiatry Med 5: 587–610
86. Abelson RP (1981) Psychological status of the script concept. Am Psychol 36: 715–729
87. Peele S (1981) Reductionism in the psychology of the eighties: can bio-chemistry eliminate addiction, mental illness and pain? Am Psychol 36: 807–818
88. Thompson SC (1981) Will it hurt less if I can control it? A complex answer to a simple question. Psychol Bull 90: 89–101
89. Westbrook MT, Viney LL (1977) The application of content analysis scales to life stress research. Aust Psychol 12: 157–166
90. Westbrook MT, Viney LL (1982) Psychological reactions to the onset of chronic illness. Soc Sci Med 16: 220–230
91. Viney LL, Westbrook MT (1980) Psychosocial reactions to heart disease: an application of content analysis methodology. Proceedings of the Geigy symposium on behavioral medicine, Melbourne
92. Viney LL, Westbrook MT (1981) Psychological reactions to chronic illness-related disability as a function of its severity and type. J Psychosom Res 25: 513–523
93. Von Rad M, Drucke M, Knauss W, Lolas F: Alexithymia a comparative study of verbal behavior in psychosomatic and psychoneurotic analysis of verbal behavior: further studies. Spectrum, New York
94. Gottschalk LA (1974) A hope scale applicable to verbal samples. Arch Gen Psychiatry 30: 779–785
95. Gottschalk LA (1979) Cognitive impairment associated with acute or chronic diseases. Gen Hosp Psychiatry 6: 344–346
96. Epstein S (1979) Explorations in personality today and tomorrow. Am Psychol 34: 649–653
97. Freedman N, Blass T, Rifkin A, Quitkin F (1973) Body movements and the verbal encoding of aggressive affect. J Pers Soc Psychol 26: 72–85
98. Hermann MG (1980) Assessing the personalities of Soviet Politburo members. Pers Soc Psychol Bull 6: 332–352
99. Viney LL (1971) Anxiety as a function of self-evaluation and related feedback. Personality 2: 205–217

100. Viney LL, Manton M (1974) Preference for defense mechanisms and expression of anxiety. Pers Soc Behav 2: 50–55
101. Levine GF (1977) Learned helplessness and the TV news. J Commun 27: 100–105
102. Gottschalk LA (1976) Children's speech as a source of data toward the measurement of psychological states. J Youth Adolesc 5: 11–36
103. Gottschalk LA, Uliana RL (1979) Profiles of children's psychological states derived from the Gottschalk-Gleser content analysis of speech. J Youth Adolesc 8: 269–282
104. Gleser GC, Winget C, Seligman R (1979) Content scaling of affect in adolescent speech samples. J Youth Adolesc 8 (3): 283–297
105. Winget C, Seligman R, Rauh JL, Gleser GC (1979) Social alienation-personal disorganization assessment in disturbed and normal adolescents. J Nerv Ment Dis 167(5): 282–287
106. Westbrook MT (1978) Analysing affective responses to past events: women's reactions to a childbearing year. J Clin Psychol 34: 967–971
107. Westbrook MT (1979) Socioeconomic differences in coping with childbearing. Am J Commun Psychol 7: 397–412
108. Westbrook MT (1978) The effect of the order of birth on women's experience of childbearing. Journal of Marriage and the Family 40: 165–172
109. Westbrook MT (1978) The reaction to childbearing and early maternal experience of women with different marital relationships. Br J Med Psychol 51: 191–199
110. Holsti O (1968) Content analysis. In: Lindzey G, Aronsen E (eds) The handbook of social psychology, Vol 2. Addison-Wesley, Reading
111. Bucksmorse S (1977) The Adorno legacy. Pers Soc Psychol Bull 3: 707–713
112. Weston LC, Ruggiero JA (1978) Male-female relationships in best selling "modern gothic" novels. Sex Roles 4: 647–655
113. Bonoma TC, Rosenberg H (1978) Theory based content analysis: a social influence perspective for evaluative group process. Soc Sci Rev 7: 213–256
114. Moore M (1978) An international application of Heider's balance theory. Eur J Soc Psychol 8: 401–405
115. Heilbrun AB, Heilbrun KS (1977) Content analysis of delusions in reactive and process schizophrenics. J Abnorm Psychol 86: 597–608
116. Gottschalk LA, Uliana RL, Hoigaard JC (1979) Preliminary validation of a set of content analysis scales applicable to verbal samples for measuring the magnitude of psychological states in children. Psychiatry Res 1: 71–82
117. Gottschalk LA, Eckardt MJ, Pautler CP, Wolf RJ, Terman SA (1983) Cognitive impairment scales derived from verbal samples. Compr Psychiatry 24: 6–19
118. Gleser GC, Green BL, Winget CN (1981) Prolonged psychosocial effects of disaster: a study of Buffalo Creek. Academic, New York
119. Grunzig HJ, Holzscheck K, Kachele H (1976) EVA – Ein Programm-System zur maschinellen Inhaltsanalyse. Med Psychol 2: 208–217
120. Schofer G (1977) Assessment of affective changes in the course of psychotherapy using the Gottschalk-Gleser content analysis. Z Klin Psychol 25: 203–218
121. Brunik SA, Shroeder HE (1979) Verbal therapeutic behaviour of expert psychoanalytically orientated, gestalt and behavior therapists. J Consult Clin Psychol 47: 567–574
122. Perley J, Winget C, Placci C (1971) Hope and discomfort as factors which influence treatment continuance. Compr Psychiatry 12: 557–563
123. Bunn TA, Clarke AM (1979) Crisis intervention: an experimental study of the effects of a brief period of conselling on the anxiety of relatives of seriously injured or ill hospital patients. Br J Med Psychol 52: 191–195
124. Gleser GC, Winget C, Seligman R, Rauh JL (1979) Evaluation of psychotherapy with adolescents using content analysis of verbal samples. In: Gottschalk LA (ed) Content analysis of verbal behavior: Further studies. Spectrum, New York

125. Gottschalk LA (1978) Content analysis of speech in psychiatric research. Compr Psychiatry 19: 387–392
126. Viney LL (1981) Content analysis: a research tool for community psychologists. Am J Commun Psychol 9: 269–281
127. Rapoport A (1969) A system theoretic view of content analysis. In: Gerbner G, Holsti O, Krippendorff K, Paisley WS, Stone PJ (eds) The analysis of communication content. Wiley, New York
128. Pool I (1970) The prestige press: a comparative study of political symbols. MIT Press, Cambridge
129. Viney LL (1983) Psychological reactions of young people to unemployment. Youth Soc 14: 457–474
130. Viney LL, Bazeley P (1977) The affective responses of housewives to community relocation. J Commun Psychol 5: 37–45
131. Viney LL (1981) An evaluation of an Australian youthwork programme. Aust Psychol 16: 37–47
132. Viney LL (1983) Experiences of volunteer counselors: a comparison of pofessionally-orientated approaches to their training. J Commun Psychol 11: 259–268
133. Viney LL, Westbrook MT (1982) Patterns of anxiety in the chronically ill. Br J Med Psychol 55: 87–95
134. Viney LL, Benjamin YM (1985) Evaluation of a hospital-based counselling programme. Adv Behav Med (to be published)
135. Viney LL, Westbrook MT (1982) Patients' psychological reactions to chronic illness: do they predict rehabilitation? J Appl Rehab Counseling 13: 38–44
136. Gottschalk LA (1977) Quantification and psychological indicators of emotions: the content analysis of speech and other objective measures of psychological states. In: Lipowski ZJ, Lipsitt DR, Whybrow P (eds) Psychosomatic medicine: current trends and clinical applications. Oxford University Press, New York
137. Viney LL (1984) Loss of life and loss of bodily integrity: two different sources of threat for people who are ill. Omega 15: 207–222
138. Miller CK (1965) Psychological correlates of coronary artery disease. Psychosom Med 27: 257–265
139. Kaplan SM, Gottschalk LA, Magliocco EB, Rohovit DD, Ross WD (1961) Hostility in verbal productions and hypnotic dreams of hypertensive patients: Studies of groups and individuals. Psychosom Med 23: 311–322
140. Holland CJ, Rowland J, Lebowitz A, Ruselen R (1979) Reactions to cancer treatment. Psychiatr Clin North Am 2: 347–350
141. Viney LL (1983) Experiencing chronic illness: a personal construct commentary. In: Adams Webber J, Mancuso JC (eds) Applications of personal construct theory. Academic, London
142. Bierschenk BA (1978) Content analysis as a research method. Kompendieserien 25: 1–93
143. Wildgrube W (1979) A Fortran IV program for quantitative content analysis. Educ Psychol Meas 39: 695–696
144. Stone PJ, Dunphy DC, Smith MS, Ogilvie DM (1966) The general enquirer: a computer approach to content analysis. MIT Press, London
145. Oxman TE, Rosenberg SD, Tucker GJ (1982) The language of paranoia. Am J Psychiatry 139: 275–282
146. Sekimoto S (1980) A characterization of lookahead stateless DPDAs of a bottom-up type. Trans Inst Elect Comput Eng Jpn E63: 490–491
147. Tanaka E (1980) A bottom-up parsing algorithm for content-sensitive language. Trans Inst Elect Comput Eng Jpn E63: 483–489
148. Bierschenk BA (1977) Computer-based analysis of interview texts. Numeric description and multivariate analysis. Didakometry No 53

149. Bierschenk I (1975) Computer-based content analysis: Theoretical and practical considerations. Pedagogisk-Psykologiska, problem no 283
150. Bierschenk I (1977) Computer-based content analysis: coding manual. Pedagogisk dokumentatin no 52
151. Gottschalk LA, Hausmann C, Brown JS (1975) A computerized scoring system for use with content analysis scales. Compr Psychiatry 16: 77–90
152. Gottschalk LA, Bechtel RJ (1982) Developing a computer system to perform content analysis of verbalizations. Compr Psychiatry 23: 364–369
153. American Psychological Association (1973) Ethical principles for the conduct of research with human subjects. APA, Washington DC
154. Diener E, Crandall R (1978) Ethics in social and behavioral research. University of Chicago Press, Chicago
155. Baumrind D (1975) Metaethical and normative considerations covering the treatment of human subjects in the behavioral sciences. In: Kennedy EC (ed) Human rights and psychological research. Crowell, New York
156. Fischer CT (1971) The testee as co-evaluator. In: Giorgi A, Fischer WF, Von Eckartsberg R (eds) Duquesne studies in phenomenological psychology, vol 1. Duquesne University Press, Pittsburg
157. Mischel W (1977) On the future of personality measurement. Am Psychol 32: 246–254
158. Vineey LL (1973) Toward a more relevant Code of Professional Conduct. Aust Psychol 8: 100–108
159. Kelman HC (1968) A time to speak. Jossey-Bass, San Francisco

Recent Procedural and Technical Contributions

6 An Interpersonal Measure of Hostility Based on Speech Context*

Thomas Gift, Robert Cole, and Lyman Wynne

6.1 Introduction

While the importance of family and social factors in the prognosis of schizophrenia has long been recognized, the work of Brown, Birley and Wing [1] and Vaughn and Leff [8] on criticism and emotional overinvolvement in families of discharged schizophrenic patients is at present a major research focus. In their replicated studies, the Expressed Emotion (EE) ratings of key relatives (e. g., a spouse or parent) predicted with high accuracy the relapse or acute exacerbation of symptoms within the 9 months after discharge of schizophrenic patients who have returned to live with these relatives. The informant's EE was measured on three primary scales: Critical Comments, Hostility, and Emotional Overinvolvement [7, 8]. The Critical Comments and Emotional Overinvolvement Scales depend partly on the contents of the informant's speech and partly on tone of voice. The ratings were made from audiotape recordings of interviews and have yielded high interrater reliability.

These EE findings from the United Kingdom were dramatic and clearly of great practical significance for prevention and treatment programs. A replication carried out in the United States [9] using similar methods produced closely parallel findings, underscoring the importance of attempts to advance understanding of these phenomena.

A major concern, however, is that the methods employed in assessing EE involve the use of highly trained raters and require an interview usually lasting about 1.5 h. If for training purposes it is desirable that the interview be transcribed, the time investment is increased further. In an attempt to assess hostility expressed by family members toward the patient, but avoid the cumbersome features of the Brown-Vaughn-Leff approach, Wynne and Gift [10] devised a modification of the Gottschalk Five-Minute Speech Sample [4] for use with family members.

6.1.1 Wynne-Gift Speech Sample Procedure

In the context of a series of assessment interviews and procedures, the subject is seated so that a tape recorder will pick up his speech. He is told that a tape recorder will be used so that important points will not be missed. Further inquiry about tape recording may lead to appropriate reassurances (such as "No one except the research group will hear the tape"). We have found in work with several samples of families that subjects of great di-

---

* Reprinted from *Psychiatry Research* (in press) with permission of the authors and publisher.

versity can become comfortable with this modification of the Five-Minute Speech Sample technique by introducing this procedure in a context in which rapport is first established. This can be accomplished by use of simple social amenities, rather than by having a stranger suddenly introduce an unfamiliar procedure set apart as "research." One can begin by asking the subject about basic facts, such as the duration of the marriage and the names and ages of members of the current household. The subject then does not feel obliged to give such information during the Five-Minute Speech Sample and avoids using up variable portions of the task time before starting (if ever) to express feelings about the person who is the "object". The subject is then given a standard, verbal introduction to the task:

> When I ask you to begin I'd like you to speak for five minutes, telling me what kind of a person (patient's first name) is and how you get along together. After you've begun to speak, I'd prefer not to answer any questions until the five minutes are over. Do you have any questions you'd like to ask before we begin?

The subject's inquiries are dealt with, whenever possible, by repeating relevant portions of the instructions. For example, if the subject asks what he or she should talk about, the interviewer replies, "I'd like you to talk about your son, Jack, and how you get along together." The focus, as in the Brown-Vaughn-Leff procedure, is on the respondent's view of the patient rather than on the generalized expression of the subject's emotional status that is elicited with the standard Gottschalk instructions, in which the subject is asked to describe an interesting or dramatic life experience.

We here report preliminary results pointing to the validity of the Wynne-Gift modification of the Gottschalk-Five-Minute Speech Sample technique in assessing group differences in interindividual hostility in marital couples.

6.2 Methods

As part of a larger investigation, parents of 4-year-old children were solicited for participation in the study. Data were collected from ten separated or divorced mothers of such children and 11 married subjects. Subjects were matched on race (all were white) and on socioeconomic status employing the Hollingshead Four-Factor Index of Social Status [6]. Using the Wynne-Gift instructions, the wives or ex-wives in the marital pairs were asked to describe their husbands or former husbands. Their verbal productions were tape-recorded and transcribed. The protocols then were scored (by Gift) using the usual Gottschalk rating of hostility outward, which involves, in essence, assigning a score for expression of anger, dislike, criticism, and rejection, and assigning a weight to reflect the intensity of the feeling expressed [5]. In the Gottschalk approach to hostility expressed outward, there is a scaling of "direct" statements (in which the speaker is the agent) and "indirect" statements (in which someone other than the speaker is the agent). Gift and Gottschalk have achieved an interrater reliability of $r = 0.92$ with this scale using a set of transcripts obtained from subjects responding to standard Gottschalk-Gleser instructions. This set of transcripts has proven useful in the past in assuring that a trainee's scorings are sufficiently close to an expert's; scoring issues in the training set and in the transcripts obtained in the course of the present study are the same.

Four ratings were differentiated: (1) overall "direct" hostility as described by Gottschalk, regardless of the target or object; (2) overall "indirect" hostility, regardless of target; (3) the individual items reflecting expressions of hostility by the key informant *toward the spouse or ex-spouse* were summed separately; this will be referred to as the *key set;* (4) Gottschalk items from the key set that indicated expression of personal criticism, denigration, and the low worth of the object (*personal criticism* rating) were summed separately, while the other two constituents of the key set, Gottschalk scores that reflect anger and rejection but do not necessarily imply that the object is depreciated as a person, were omitted. The personal criticism rating parallels the content-based aspect of the rating of critical comments and criticism in the Camberwell Family Interview (CFI) procedure. A second aspect of the CFI rating of critical comments and hostility depends on tone of voice. Gottschalk and Frank [3] have demonstrated elsewhere the vocal qualities heard from the tape recording of interviews while reading the typescripts of speech provided only negligible information with respect to assessing magnitude of affect from the typescripts of speech alone using the Gottschalk-Gleser Scales. These authors concluded that semantic and vocal qualities of speech serve to amplify one another and tend to be redundant in terms of the communication of affects. Therefore, the additional assessment of tone of voice in such studies may or may not be superfluous. The Gottschalk content-based scoring system, hence, omits listening to the tone of voice. Both key set and personal criticism ratings reflect and are based on Gottschalk scorings for direct hostility outward.

Table 1. Hostility measures based on the Gottschalk Hostility-Outward Scale[a]

Score	Derivation[b]
Total hostility	Sum of all clauses positive for hostility, weighted for intensity of expression
Direct hostility	Sum of all clauses positive for hostility, in which speaker is grammatical subject, weighted for intensity of expression
Indirect hostility	Sum of all clauses positive for hostility, in which agent other than speaker is grammatical subject, weighted for intensity of expression
Key set	Sum of all clauses positive for hostility in which speaker is grammatical subject, individual identified in instructions (in this study spouse or ex-spouse) is grammatical object, weighted for intensity of expression
Personal criticism	Sum of all clauses in which speaker is grammatical subject, individual identified in instructions (in this study, spouse or ex-spouse is grammatical object), positive for hostility on the basis of expression of personal criticism, denigration, or low worth of the object, weighted for intensity of expression

[a] Descriptions are presented in simplified fashion to illustrate basic concepts; readers are referred to Gottschalk et al. [4] for more complete understanding of scoring system.
[b] All scores are corrected for amount of speech by dividing by total word count, as per standard Gottschalk procedure.

It was hypothesized that on all measures the separated or divorced women would express more hostility toward their ex-spouses than married women reported toward their present spouses.

6.3 Results

As hypothesized, the overall level of hostility was greater for the divorced or separated women than for married women, as shown in Table 2. When direct and indirect hostility were analyzed separately, the indirect hostility was significantly greater for the divorced or separated group than for the married women, although the measure of direct hostility fell just short of statistical significance in the hypothesized direction. These scores involved a correction for total number of words spoken, following Gottschalk's standard method [4].

Table 2. Hostility by marital status

Hostility measure	Married ($n=11$) $\bar{x}$	Separated/divorced ($n=10$) $\bar{x}$	F	P
Total hostility	1.4	1.9	6.7	0.018
Direct hostility	1.41	2.27	3.6	NS
Indirect hostility	0.88	1.11	5.6	0.029
Key set	0.0034	0.0076	4.8	0.041
Personal criticism	0.0011	0.0050	9.5	0.006

When the key set, representing items in which the woman was the subject and the spouse or ex-spouse the object, was examined (controlling for word count), the divorced women showed more hostility than the married women ($P<0.4$). When the personal criticism score was examined, controlling for word count, the divorced women again showed more hostility than the married women ($P<0.006$).

When individual protocols were reviewed, it seemed evident that the Gottschalk scorings represented expressions of hostility toward spouse or ex-spouse that would be recognizable by clinically untrained readers, based on the literal meaning of the text. Additionally, the married women were more likely to make positive comments about their husbands, although this is not reflected in the Gottschalk scores discussed above. At the same time, other subtle expressions of hostility or criticism that could apparently be discerned on a clinical basis were not picked up by the application of the Gottschalk scoring rules.

6.4 Discussion

The results presented above point to the validity of the Gottschalk scoring of hostility of family members through the use of the Wynne-Gift instructions. These findings have important implications for research. The existence of a short method of measuring interpersonal hostility makes feasible research designs that examine this component of EE with a variety of family types (e.g., marital, parental, extended families, etc.) and across different types of pathology in the identified patient. At the same time, its ease of administration makes it possible to measure changes in hostility at several points over time. In particular, the effects of therapeutic intervention, as in family therapy or treatment, can be monitored using repeat assessments of hostility. While these issues have been discussed particularly in the context of the family, it seems reasonable to assume that similar phenomena may exist in other social contexts, such as on an inpatient ward, among college dormitory residents, or among military personnel. Not only is the ease of administration important, but since the one probe in the Five-Minute Speech Sample technique is quite general, it can be used in contexts other than the family, while the CFI has many aspects that do not translate well into nonfamily contexts.

The ease of administration of the technique permits serial recording at a number of sampling points. This, in turn, will permit use of a variety of statistical techniques, such as analysis of variance with repeated measures and reciprocal modeling, which cannot be carried out so well with cross-sectional data or two-point, before-and-after assessments.

A great number of clinical applications seem evident. The use of serial Five-Minute Speech Samples to measure treatment effectiveness has been noted above. Logically prior to this would be the use use of the Five-Minute Speech Sample technique to assess dimensions of family emotional atmosphere in a way that would aid in the selection of appropriate treatment. Feelings of other social network members toward the identified patient also might be explored with the technique and appropriate therapy begun in instances where there are high levels of hostility or emotional overinvolvement. While the impetus for our work was provided by interest in the EE investigations noted, clearly the measurement of hostility between spouses and ex-spouses is itself an important topic. In a recent review, Emery [2] described the important negative consequences for children of hostility expressed between parents and the problem posed in this field by lack of appropriate measures for such hostility.

An important practical issue with the use of the Wynne-Gift procedure is that of maintaining rapport with the subject. As noted, eliciting the Five-Minute Speech Sample invariably results in some anxiety for the subject. In our experience, the degree of anxiety varies with the level of education and verbal ability of the subject. Those who are educated and verbal can get into the task fairly easily, whereas those who are less educated and whose verbal skills are less developed may respond by saying relatively little, while becoming relatively more anxious.

An important aspect of dealing with the anxiety that may be generated with research subjects is to "debrief" the subject after the 5-min-period is over. This is often best done by saying something like, "The five minutes are up. How was it to talk for five minutes at a stretch?" If the patient was obviously quite anxious, it is often helpful to say something like, "Most people find it makes them pretty nervous to have to talk for five minutes at a time." This debriefing, in our experience, has been remarkably effective in turning a situation which might result in diminution of rapport into one which seems to enhance the relationship between subject and interviewer.

The fact that almost all subjects set some time limits regarding their participation in research confers an important advantage upon the Wynne-Gift technique in contexts in which the researcher is interested in an extensive data collection since the technique requires only 5 min of the subjects' time. On the other hand, the total time required of the researchers is significantly greater. Transcribing the tapes requires 5–20 min, depending on number of words spoken, the speaker's style, and the quality of the recording. The person doing the transcription need not be clinically trained, but should have above-average verbal ability and some experience with verbatim transcriptions. After the transcript is prepared, approximately 20 min per transcript are required of the rater. A rater can by anyone who has learned the scoring of the Gottschalk Hostility-Outward Scale; appropriate training requires approximately 20 h.

Many closely similar issues arise regarding the use of both the Wynne-Gift modification and the original Gottschalk method; interested readers are referred to the basic instruction manual [4] as well as a recent compendium of reports utilizing the Gottschalk Five-Minute-Speech Sample approach [5].

In evaluating the findings presented here, it must be noted that this sample differs considerably from that in the CFI studies. In the CFI work, the family member being described, either the offspring or spouse of the informant, was hospitalized for a psychiatric illness of major proportions, while in this study the spouse or ex-spouse had never been identified as having a psychiatric illness of any sort. The CFI work involved eliciting expression of affect toward a family member who had been residing with the informant until the index hospitalization or rehospitalization and who was expected to return to the informant's home after hospital discharge. In contrast, in the present study the married informants were living with the family member (husband) being described, while the divorced or separated informants had not been living with the family member being described (husband or ex-husband) for months or years and had expressed no plan to resume living with them.

Thus, the present report is not a replication of the British or more recent California CFI work. Rather, it is an attempt to facilitate further research in this area by providing a more efficient alternative and more widely applicable means of examining expression of interpersonal hostility.

References

1. Brown GW, Birley JLT, Wing JK (1972) Influence of family life on the course of schizophrenic disorders: a replication. Br J Psychiatry 121: 241–258
2. Emery RE (1982) Interparental conflict and the children of discord and divorce. Psychol Bull 92: 310–330
3. Gottschalk LA, Frank EC (1967) Estimating the magnitude of anxiety from speech. Behav Sci 12: 289–295
4. Gottschalk LA, Winget CN, Gleser GC (1969) Manual of instructions for using the Gott-

schalk-Gleser content analysis scales: anxiety, hostility, and social alienation – personal disorganization. University of California Press, Berkeley

5. Gottschalk LA (ed) (1979) The content analysis of verbal behavior: further studies. Spectrum, New York
6. Hollingshead AS (1977) Four factor index of social status. Yale University Press, New Haven
7. Leff JP, Wing JK (1971) Trial of maintenance therapy in schizophrenia. Brit Med J 3: 599–604
8. Vaughn CE, Leff JP (1976) The influence of family and social factors on the course of psychiatric illness: a comparison of schizophrenic and depressed neurotic patients. Br J Psychiatry 129: 125–137
9. Vaughn CE, Snyder KS, Jones S, Freeman MA, Falloon IR (1984) Family factors in schizophrenia relapse: replication in california of british research on expressed emotion. Arch Gen Psychiatry 41: 1169–1178
10. Wynne LC, Gift TE (1979) A five-minute speech sample technique for assessing family emotional atmosphere, presented at the NIMH conference on expressed emotion, Washington DC, april 17–18

7 Microcomputers as Aids to Avoid Error in Gottschalk–Gleser Rating[*]

Gerhard Deffner

7.1 Introduction

The use of the Gottschalk–Gleser technique of content analysis [1] in empirical studies involves a large amount of work. The different steps in this kind of analysis of verbal data are: transcription of audio recordings, selection of coding units, rating of units, addition of raw scores, compilation of raw scores, counting of words, and punching of cards. The amount of work and the large number of different steps can lead to serious impairment to the Gottschalk–Gleser technique's precision. The main problem is that each step in this procedure may contribute cumulative error to the content analysis of speech samples. In this paper, various sources of error are discussed, and a small microcomputer system and its use is described which was designed to help avoid or at least reduce these errors.

7.2 Random Error

One type of error is common to all empirical procedures – unsystematic mistakes without relation to content. Such random error may result in an overall loss of clearness in the effects under study, but it will not change the outcome of a study in any other way. Random errors can in Gottschalk–Gleser analysis be expected to happen during: addition of raw scores, compilation of tables, counting of words, and punching of cards. The persons who are performing these tasks can be expected to make mistakes, but there is no reason to assume that these mistakes are in any systematic way related to the content of the speech samples. They thus can be considered random errors.

---

[*] Reprinted from *Psychiatry Research* (in press) with permission of the author and publisher.

7.3 Systematic Error (Bias)

One potential source of nonrandom error involves the transcription of audio recordings. Very often, audio recordings of speech samples are of poor quality. Even if care is taken to ensure good technical quality, there frequently are utterances that are spoken in such a way (low voice, very fast, etc.) that they are very difficult to understand. Unfortunately, this mostly happens in the case of utterances with strong emotional or affective content and which therefore are of special importance for Gottschalk–Gleser scoring. If such utterances are hard to understand, then consequently they easily lend themselves to misunderstanding, omissions, etc. This in turn could be a potential source of systematic error, if the person who performs the transcriptions were biased toward a certain kind of misunderstanding. (If, for instance, this person chooses to overhear utterances of aggressive tone.)

The second and most important source of bias involves the actual scoring. There are two ways in which errors may occur at this stage: one is that rating decisions can vary between different persons who perform such rating, and the other is that raters may not be stable in their decisions over time. Both possibilities describe different aspects of reliability, which can be measured as a correlation across raters or over time. As this has long been acknowledged to be crucial for the objectivity of content analysis, high coefficients of reliability are desired in these techniques. In the manual for Gottschalk–Gleser content analysis, it is recommended that the scores from all different raters employed in a study should be correlated as highly as 0.80 [2]. If this high degree of correspondence is not achieved, then raters have to receive further training. In practice, this means that after an initial stage of thorough training during which the same material is scored by several persons, the rest of the material in the study will be split up, and individual speech samples will be scored by only one particular person. If such is the case (and it seems to be so in most studies), then there is no possibility to even make a statement about the quality of this person's scoring because there are no other scores on the basis of which reliability coefficients could be computed. At this point, one can only speculate on the possible effects that this knowledge may have on raters!

The possibility of errors has been a problem ever since techniques of content analysis were used. The main concern has been about reliability, a problem for which no clear and easy to follow remedy could be found other than thorough training of raters. It therefore is no surprise that there is a long tradition of attempts to mechanize the rating procedure. If rating could be performed by computer programs, then the question of reliability would finally be solved: interrater reliability and reliability over time will be 1.0 for any same versions of the particular program run at various times. Still there is an important trade off to pay attention to: in many cases an increase in reliability is achieved at the cost of low validity. In the current context this could mean that although a particular computer program will assign the same ratings anytime it is run, it nevertheless may not achieve a very good representation of content by the scores it assigns. However, before this issue can be discussed in any detail, a short description of such approaches shall be given.

7.4 Description of Three Different Approaches to Computerized Content Analysis

1. Systems in the tradition of the "General Inquirer" [3] or the German system "EVA" [4] detect the occurrence of critical words which have previously been compiled into a lexicon. For further data analysis, such systems give information on the frequency with which words from different categories were present in the text analyzed. One important aspect of all such systems is that they do not "understand" any of a text's meaning. The only possibility to improve the performance of such systems is by improving the lexicon and by adding mechanisms to identify different syntactic occurrences of the same word. An example of such extensions is Grünzig and Mergenthaler's system "ATD" [5], which is designed to detect words that express anxiety.

2. The next possible line of approach is that of concentrating on words that are of special importance in determining the meaning of sentences (i.e., the main verb); if such words can be identified, it should then be possible to obtain some degree of information about a sentence's meaning. For this, a syntactic analysis of the input text is required. To do so by means of a computer program, new developments in computer science have to be used. The field of "artificial intelligence" offers special types of computer programs – "parsers" – which have been developed for this kind of analysis (cf. Winston [6]). Gottschalk and his co-workers have presented a system based on these principles [7]. They used Wood's ATN-parser [8] to identify the "action verb" in each sentence together with the corresponding noun phrases describing the actor and the recipient person. In the next step, semantic features were assigned to these words or phrases on the basis of a special lexicon. The program then performs Gottschalk-Gleser scoring on the semantic features which have been assigned to each sentence; the rules for this have also been built into the program. It is hard to say whether this program "understands" the input texts, but it is certain that this approach makes it possible to capture much more of a text's content than the first approach, which is based on the categorization of individual words. Still, Gottschalk et al.'s program does not perform as well as human raters: in tests of the program's performance, only 60 of 100 sentences were scored correctly [7].

3. The third kind of approach makes even more advanced use of techniques developed in artificial intelligence, those of "natural language understanding" (see Shank and Riesbeck [9]). In contrast to the two approaches described above, an attempt is made to go beyond the level of categorizing features of the text according to an inflexible lexicon; such systems try to combine previous knowledge stored in the program with the results of syntactic and semantic analyses of the verbal input material. This very closely resembles the hermeneutic method of human "language understanders" (cf. Schnotz [10] who also use their background knowledge in the act of understanding. This possibility has been explored by Gottschalk and Bechtel [11]. They tried to incorporate artificial intelligence programs of language understanding into a computer program for Gottschalk-Gleser scoring. Their system has sofar been put into operation for the six Gottschalk-Gleser Anxiety Scales, and it has achieved ratings which are highly correlated with the scoring done by human raters ($r = 0.58–0.92$ for individual scales; $r = 0.85$ for the total anxiety score). One thing needs to be pointed out though: all scores arrived at by the computer program were lower than scores as-

signed to the verbal material by human raters. This means that the computer program does not understand all of the anxiety-related contents in a text.

The evaluation of these approaches to computerized content analysis should be related to the three different sources of error which were mentioned at the beginning of this paper. It needs to be pointed out that all three approaches do very well in avoiding random error during counting of words, addition of raw scores, etc. because all of these tasks are performed by the computer. Also, reliability of scoring is optimal. Only two difficulties remain: the possibility of bias during transcription and the possibility of a reliability/validity trade off. "Validity" in this context can be understood as "full understanding of a text's meaning." As has already been mentioned, there is a clear rank order within the three approaches, and the third one which is based on computerized language understanding clearly is the most promising. On the other hand, it could be argued that even Gottschalk and Bechtel's system does not perform at the same level as human raters and that therefore computer programs are not really useful for a deep understanding of content, but perhaps the scope of further developments in the field of artificial intelligence should not be underestimated. Statements about "what computers can't do" (cf. Dreyfus [12]) have very often become outdated before very long. One difficulty with the use of artificial intelligence approaches also is that those programs have mainly been designed for simple language with fairly simple syntactic structure. Speech samples from clinical studies on the other hand tend to contain idiomatic expressions, unfinished sentences, etc., which pose additional problems for such programs and which would require more complicated mechanisms of language understanding.

Instead of speculating upon the fundamental impossibility of thorough understanding by computer programs, it is safe to say that a lot of work will have to be invested to make such sophisticated systems perform at the same level as human raters, that is, high validity will only be achieved at the price of many more man-hours of complex programming. For this reason, it seems justified to look for other possibilities of using computers to reduce error in Gottschalk-Gleser scoring.

As an alternative to the attempt of substituting human raters (language understanders) by computer programs, I suggest using a small-scale computer system which relies on conventional means to reduce bias in language understanding (during transcription and scoring) and which can be used interactively to perform all those steps where random error can easily be avoided (i. e., counting words, etc.). This is a somewhat different philosophy of computer use since no attempt is made to substitute human intelligence. Computers are used for tasks which hardly require intelligence but still should be done error-free, and secondly they are used in a fashion which makes it easier for humans to exercise their intelligence. In this way, one advantage of computerized scoring – elimination of random error – can be retained whereas the problem of validity would again be exchanged for that of reliability as in any traditional procedure of content analysis. Nevertheless, it has been possible to facilitate conventional means of avoiding bias and improving reliability by working with this system. This approach is based on a program by Deffner, Heydemann and v. Borstel [13], which was developed for the analysis of verbal protocols. The original program was extended for the purposes of Gottschalk-Gleser scoring [14] and was adapted to run on small-scale computers, which today can be found in almost any research environment: eight-bit microcomputers.

7.5 Eight–Bit Microcomputer System

7.5.1 Transcription

Audio recordings are typed in at the computer terminal using the regular editor program of the particular machine. The ease with which corrections can be made to the text makes transcriptions more exact because corrections can be inserted repeatedly without regard to readability as in the case of writing on paper. At the same time, the ease of changing the layout of text on the screen is used to break up speech samples into coding units in such a way that there is one unit per line. Finally, texts can be stored on floppy disks for further processing.

This mode of producing transcriptions has an important advantage: the person who produces transcriptions need not be a skilled typist. In the case of many audio recordings of speech samples, most of the time is taken up by the attempt to understand what the particular person said. It often is necessary to replay the recording several times, and when that is finished, the transcription has to be checked against the recording. Typing speed therefore is of minor importance because unskilled users can rely on the ease of making corrections and changes of layout that the computer offers. For this reason, it is possible to have this task performed by someone who is well informed about the Gottschalk-Gleser technique and, what is more, someone who understands the danger of letting his or her own personality bias the transcription process. Ideally, transcription should be performed by persons who have been sensitized to issues of a psychodynamic nature.

7.5.2 Interactive Scoring

Gottschalk-Gleser scoring is performed with the help of a program that allows interactive processing of speech samples. The main characteristic of this program is that it is written to be "user friendly", that is, the user needs to have no programing experience, is safe from accidentally causing errors or breaks in the run of the program, and the program will in most cases also detect mistakes in typing. Scoring a text proceeds as follows: first, the user is asked for his or her name and then the program searches for the next text on the disk which has not yet been scored by that particular user. After that, the text is presented on the screen so that the user can read the complete speech sample. The program will then print individual coding units and ask the user to assign a Gottschalk-Gleser score and its appropriate weight according to the German adaptation developed by Schöfer [15]. If no score should be assigned to the coding unit, then the user can just type n. All input which is not n or a legal combination of a Gottschalk-Gleser Scale and a weight will cause the program to print "Du hast Dich vertippt" (you made a typing error), and the cycle will be repeated for that coding unit. When all coding units have been gone through, the text is printed again. This time scores are displayed along with the text. Should the user want to make any changes to the scoring, he or she can do so by typing the required line number, and the program will then go back to the scoring routine for that coding unit. Display and alteration can be performed until the user is satisfied with his or her scoring decisions and wants to proceed to the next speech sample; scores in their final form will then be stored on a disk. The main advantages of this system (for an example see Table 1) are:

1. No coding units can be overlooked because each is called by the program. One kind of bias – systematic overlooking of certain statements – can thus be avoided.
2. The user need not know more about using a computer than the basic layout of keys on the terminal's keyboard. All that is required is typing one's own name and the few symbols used for denoting Gottschalk-Gleser scores.
3. All scores are stored on a disk. There can be no mistakes during the recording of scores (random error) because no additional tables have to be compiled.
4. All scoring which has been done sofar with the use of this program (over 150 speech samples) has been shown to be much faster than traditional paper and pencil scoring.

Table 1. Scoring session[a]

① *The movie was quite obvious*	
That's what I feel about most physicians, too	
The young man was treated as though he were a number	
He was simply brushed aside	
Something I also miss from the physician	
is warm and open behavior toward the patient	
Yes – taken together it is a very cold atmosphere	

Next, you will be prompted for a score that you want to assign to each segment:

Segment 1:
② *The movie was quite obvious*
What score do you want to assign? n

Segment 2:
③ *That's what I feel about most physicians, too*
What score do you want to assign?   Ic2
    You made a typo
    Correction: Ic2

Segment 3:
    The young man was treated as though he were a number
What score do you want to assign?   IIb2/4b

Segment 4:
    He was simply brushed aside
What score do you want to assign?   IIb2/3b

Segment 5:
    Something I also miss from the physician
What score do you want to assign?   Ic3

Segment 6:
    is warm and open behavior toward the patient
What score do you want to assign?   IIb2/3b

Segment 7:
    Yes – taken together it is a very cold atmosphere
What score do you want to assign?   Ic1

Table 1. (continued)

That was all. Here is an overview of the speech sample together
with your scoring:

(4)   1. *The movie was quite obvious:*   n
         2. *That's what I feel about most physicians, too:*   *Ic2*
         3. *The young man was treated as though he were a number:*   *IIb2/4b*
         4. *He was simply brushed aside:*   *IIb2/3b*
         5. *Something I also miss from the physician:*   *Ic3*
         6. *is warm and open behavior toward the patient*   *IIb2/3b*
         7. *Yes – taken together it is a very cold atmosphere:*   *Ic1*
Do you want to make any changes (yes/no)?   Yes
In which line?   23
(5)   There is no line of this number.
         Which is the line number you want?   3
         3: *The young man was treated as though he were a number*
What score do you want to assign?   *IIb2/5b*
Do you want to make further changes? (yes/no)?   No
Your work on this speech sample is now finished.

Results
         Number of words: 53
(6)   Gottschalk–Gleser raw scores:

I	II	III	IV	A1	A2	A3	A4	A5	A6
6	6	0	0	0	0	4	0	2	0

[a] Explanations for the sample dialogue:
   (1) Initial display of the complete text.
   (2) Beginning of the unit-by-unit query for a score (*n*, "no score").
   (3) Example of internal typechecking and error handling interaction with the user.
   (4) Display of text and scores.
   (5) Attempt to call a line that does not exist, subsequent correction of score (to "IIb2/5b").
   (6) Display of results: word count and Gottschalk–Gleser raw scores.

7.5.3 Checking for Reliability and Improving It

The ease and speed of interacitve scoring can be turned to advantage concerning reliability: it will be possible to have two persons score all material in about the same time as
would normally have been required for just one person to perform this task. The program for interactive scoring has been extended accordingly and now offers additional
routines for the comparison of scores from two raters. In the case that a text has been
scored before, the program will then compute coefficients of reliability. Also, it can give
feedback to the user if his or her scores do not agree with the ones that were assigned in
the previous run of the program. This feature can either be used during training of raters, or it can be used to single out difficult coding units which need to be discussed before a score can finally be assigned.

    There are two advantages of this: 1. it is possible to compute coefficients of reliabil-
ity and thus give feedback on interrater correspondence, and 2. it is possible to use the
system for efficient training of raters or for achieving consensus on difficult scoring decisions.

7.5.4 Computation of Scores

After all scores have been assigned, a second program can be run, which counts words, computes scores from raw scores, and writes them onto disks in a format which is suitable for further statistical analysis. Random error during this stage is thereby avoided.

7.6 Conclusion

The experience in using this microcomputer-based system has been most encouraging so far. It has been used on over 150 speech samples from a study of descriptions of experimental stimuli (friendly vs unfriendly interaction in a short film) involving depressive and psychosomatic patients (Ahrens and Deffner [16]). Some speech samples were not only transcribed by a nontypist trained in the procedure as described earlier in this paper, but by a regular typist as well. The former transcriptions proved to be more accurate and also to contain less omissions.

Interactive scoring was done successfully, and the comments from raters (who had had experience in traditional paper and pencil scoring) were that they felt comfortable working with the interactive program and that they felt the quality of their scoring to be much better because they could get feedback and also single out difficult coding units for discussion. In general, this approach seems to be a good alternative to more advanced approaches of content analysis by computer.

7.7 Summary

In this article, different types of error during the various steps of Gottschalk-Gleser content analysis of speech samples are discussed. Several attempts have in the past been made to avoid error by using computer programs to categorize verbal material. Although these systems offer the great advantage of increasing reliability to a maximum, validity is a problem. More recent approaches which utilize artificial intelligence methods of language understanding by computer nevertheless do show promising results. However, these computer systems will have to be developed even further before they can perform at the same level as human raters. For this reason, an alternative approach is presented which only relies on computers in a limited way. All steps of Gottschalk-Gleser content analysis are performed with a collection of programs on a small eight-bit microcomputer: transcription, scoring, storage and computation of scores.

References

1. Gottschalk LA, Gleser GC (1969) The measurement of psychological states through the content analysis of verbal behavior. University of California Press, Berkeley
2. Gottschalk LA, Winget CN, Gleser GC (1969) Manual of instructions for using the Gottschalk-Gleser content analysis scales: anxiety, hostility, and social alienation – peronal disorganization. University of California Press, Berkeley
3. Stone PJ, Dunphy DC, Smith MS, Ogilvie DM (1966) The general inquirer: computer approach to content analysis. MIT, Cambridge
4. Grünzig H-J, Holzscheck K, Kächele H (1976) EVA – Ein Programmsystem zur maschinellen Inhaltsanalyse von Psychotherapieprotokollen. Med Psychol 2: 208–217
5. Grünzig, H-J, Mergenthaler E (1986) Computerunterstützte Ansätze. In: Koch U, Schöfer G (eds) Sprachinhaltsanalyse in der psychiatrischen und psychosomatischen Forschung. Beltz, Weinheim
6. Winston PH (1977) Artificial intelligence. Addison-Wesley, Reading
7. Gottschalk LA, Hausmann C, Brown JS (1975) A computerized scoring system for use with content analysis scales. Compr Psychiatry 16: 77–9O
8. Woods W (1973) An experimental parsing system for transition network grammars. Natural Language Processing Algorithmics Press, New York
9. Shank RC, Riesbeck CK (1981) Inside computer understanding. Erlbaum, Hillsdale
10. Schnotz W (1982) Rekonstruktion von individuellen Wissensstrukturen. In: Huber GL, Mandl H (eds) Verbale Daten. Beltz, Weinheim
11. Gottschalk LA, Bechtel RJ (1982) The measurement of anxiety through the computer analysis of verbal samples. Compr Psychiatry 22: 364–369
12. Dreyfus HL (1972) What computers can't do. Harper and Row, New York
13. Deffner G, Heydemann M, v. Borstel G (1984) Ein Kategoriensystem und interaktives Ratingverfahren für die Vorverarbeitung von Protokollen des Lauten Denkens. Arch Psychol 136: 147–162
14. Deffner G (1986) Durchführen des Gottschalk-Gleser Ratings auf Kleincomputern. In: Koch U, Schöfer G (eds) Sprachinhaltsanalyse in der psychiatrischen und psychosomatischen Forschung. Beltz, Weinheim (to be published)
15. Schöfer G (1980) Gottschalk-Gleser Sprachinhaltsanalyse. Beltz, Weinheim
16. Ahrens S, Deffner G (1985) Affektive Reaktion bei Crohn-, Colitis- und depressiven Patienten. (to be published)

8 A Depression Scale Applicable to Verbal Samples*

Louis A. Gottschalk and Julia Hoigaard

8.1 Introduction

Many measures of psychological dimensions have been developed, and these measures can be broadly classified into three categories: self-report scales, rating scales, and content analysis scales. The strengths and weaknesses, in terms of measurement errors, inherent in these three kinds of assessment approaches have been described by others [1, 2]. For the purposes of this paper, it is sufficient to say, by way of an overview of these methods, that the content analysis approach combines the personal and subjective strengths of self-report measures and the objective and impartial strengths of the rating of the magnitude of psychological dimensions by independent observers.

No validated content analysis measure of depression has been developed, though the use of the content analysis of verbal behavior has been applied to the measurement of many psychological dimensions, for example, anxiety [3], hostility [4], social alienation-personal disorganization [5], cognitive impairment [6–9], hope [19], pawn and origin – locus of control [11], and positive emotions [12, 13]. This paper will describe a Depression Scale we have developed which is applicable to verbal samples.

8.2 Definition of Depression

Some of the problems in measuring depression involve how to identify it, at what point in a scale magnitude is it pathological, and what does a score in a pathological range tell us about its etiology?

Though this paper is concerned with a verbal behavioral measure of depression, other presumptive measures or so-called markers of depression have to deal with similar issues. These include *physiological measures,* for example, rapid-eye-movement (REM) sleep latency, REM distribution throughout the night [14] or enlarged cerebral ventricles [15], and *biochemical measures,* for example, the dexamethasone test [16], decreased platelet histamine uptake [17], decreased platelet imipramine binding [18], or cerebrospinal fluid 5-HIAA [19].

---

* Previously published in modified form in Psychiatry Research (1986) 17: 213–227 with permission of the authors and publisher.

These various issues on how to identify depression and what its signs mean with respect to cause cannot be taken separately. If the underlying basis for the phenomena of depression is an unitary disease versus multiple diseases or disorders, the phenomena to pay attention to and measure could well be different. For example, simple behavioral dimensions could, perhaps, suffice for an investigator espousing a unitary disease concept of depression. Such an investigator might, also, comfortably arrive at an arbitrary cutoff score on a linear scale to distinguish a pathological from a nonpathological depression, whereas the concept of multiple underlying causes for depression would exact more demands on the variety of phenomena to include within the construct classified as "depression." An investigator holding this multiple etiological point of view of depression would want to consider and record many details of the phenomena of depression to try to discern and describe pertinent phenomenological subtypes, possibly with different natural history courses, prognoses, and preferred treatments. Furthermore, determining what constitutes a pathological degree of any one of these subtypes of depression would become more complex. For example, at what point on a Depression Scale would the symptoms and signs of acute grief after a relative's death or the manifestations of depression triggered by a sudden serious illness, for example, myocardial infarction, be considered pathological?

Convincing data have not been obtained to support a unitary disease concept of depression. Hence, a behavioral measure of depression should provide measurement categories compatible with the concept that there are a number of potentially relevant subdimensions of the construct of depression which have significant statistical relationships with different underlying pathogenic processes. If the subdimensions of depression do not covary significantly with different premorbid personality traits, precipitating circumstances, responsiveness to different pharmacological agents or psychological therapeutic approaches, or physiological or biochemical markers, then the detection and assessment of these dimensions may not prove necessary. In the absence of such empirical data, the content analysis measure of depression described here has a broad range of phenomenological subscales (see Table 1).

Table 1. Depression Scale

Weights	I. Hopelessness[a]
−1	1. References to not being or not wanting to be or not seeking to be the recipient of good fortune, good luck, God's favor, or blessing
−1	2. References to self or others not getting or receiving help, advice, support, sustenance, confidence, esteem from: (a) others, (b) self
−1	3. References to feelings of hopelessness, losing hope, despair, lack of confidence, lack of ambition, lack of interest; feelings of pessimism, discouragement experienced by: (a) others, (b) self

II. Self-Accusation

A) Guilt Depression:[b] References to adverse criticism, abuse; condemnation, moral disapproval, guilt, or threat of such experienced by:

−3	a) Self (3)
−2	b) Others (2)
−1	c) Denial (1)

Table 1 (continued)

Weights

	B) *Shame Depression:*[c] References to ridicule, inadequacy, shame, embarrassment, humiliation, overexposure of deficiencies or private details or threat of such experienced by:
−3	a) Self (3)
−2	b) Others (2)
−1	c) Denial (1)

C) *Hostility Directed Inward*[d]

−4	a) References to self, attempting or threatening to kill self, with or without conscious intent
−4	b) References to self, wanting to die, needing or deserving to die
−3	a) References to self, injuring, mutilating, disfiguring self, or threats to do so, with or without conscious intent
−3	b) Self-blaming, expressing anger or hatred to self, considering self worthless or of no value, causing oneself grief or trouble, or threatening to do so [similar to guilt Depression (IIA) and Shame Depression (IIB)]
−2	a) References to self needing or deserving punishment, paying for one's sins, needing to atone or do penance
−2	b) Self adversely criticizing, depreciating self; references to regretting, being sorry or ashamed for what one says or does; references to self mistaken or in error
−2	c) References to feelings of deprivation, disappointment, lonesomeness
−1	a) References to feeling disappointed in self; unable to meet expectations of self or others
−1	b) Denial of anger, dislike, hatred, blame, destructive impulses from self to self
−1	c) References to feeling painfully driven or obliged to meet one's own expectations and standards

III Psychomotor Retardation

−1	References to general retardation and slowing down in thinking, feeling, or action

IV Somatic Concerns

−1	A) *Hypochondriacal Component* References to bodily malfunctioning or physical problems in total body or any parts or systems
−1	B) *Sleep Disturbances* References to any disturbances in sleeping
−1	C) *Sexual Disturbances* References to sexual malfunctioning of any kind, including menstrual disturbances or complaints
−1	D) *Gastrointestinal Disturbances* References to appetite disturbances, changes in bowel habits, abdominal discomforts
−1	E) *General Somatic Symptoms* Including heaviness in limbs back or head, backaches, headaches, muscle aches, loss of energy, fatiguability, and loss of weight

V. Death and Mutilation Depression[e]

A) *Death Depression*
References to death, dying, threat of death, or anxiety about death experienced by or occurring to:

Table 1 (continued)

−3	a) Self (3)
−2	b) Animate others (2)
−1	c) Inanimate objects (1)
−1	d) Denial of death anxiety (1)

B) Mutilation Depression
References to injury, tissue or physical damage, or anxiety about injury or threat of such experienced by or occurring to:

−3	a) Self (3)
−2	b) Animate others (2)
−1	c) Inanimate objects destroyed (1)
−1	d) Denial (1)

VI. Separation Depression[f]

References to desertion, abandonment, ostracism, loss of support, falling, loss of love or love object, or threat of such experienced by or occurring to:

−3	a) Self (3)
−2	b) Animate others (2)
−1	c) Inanimate objects (1)
−1	d) Denial (1)

VII. Hostility Outward[g]

A) Hostility Outward-Overt

−3	a) Self-killing, fighting, injuring other individuals or threatening to do so
−3	b) Self-robbing or abandoning other individuals, causing suffering or anguish to others, or threatening to do so
−3	c) Self adversely criticizing, depreciating, blaming, expressing anger, dislike of other human beings
−2	a) Self-killing, injuring, or destroying domestic animals, pets, or threatening to do so
−2	b) Self-abandoning, robbing, domestic animals, pets, or threatening to do so
−2	c) Self-criticizing or depreciating others in a vague or mild manner
−2	d) Self-depriving or disappointing other human beings
−1	a) Self-killings, injuring, destroying, robbing wildlife, flora, inanimate objects, or threatening to do so
−1	b) Self adversely criticizing, depreciating, blaming, expressing anger or dislike of subhuman, inanimate objects, places, situations
−1	c) Self-using hostile words, cursing, mention of anger or rage without referent

B) Hostility Outward-Covert

−3	a) Others (human) killing, fighting, injuring other individuals or threatening to do so
−3	b) Others (human) robbing, abandoning, causing suffering or anguish to other individuals, or threatening to do so
−3	c) Others adversely criticizing, depreciating, blaming, expressing anger, dislike of other human beings
−2	a) Others (human) killing, injuring, or destroying domestic animals, pets, or threatening to do so
−2	b) Others (human) abandoning, robbing, domestic animals, pets, or threatening to do so

Table 1 (continued)

Weights	
−2	c) Others (human) criticizing or depreciating other individuals in a vague or mild manner
−2	d) Others (human) depriving or disappointing other human beings
−2	e) Others (human or domestic animals) dying or killed violently in death-dealing situations or threatened with such
−2	f) Bodies (human or domestic animals) mutilated, depreciated, defiled
−1	a) Wildlife, flora, inanimate objects, injured, broken, robbed, destroyed, or threatened with such (with or without mention of agent)
−1	b) Others (human) adversely criticizing, depreciating, expressing anger or dislike of subhuman, inanimate objectsm, places, situations
−1	c) Others angry, cursing without reference to cause or direction of anger, also instruments of destruction not used threateningly
−1	d) Others (human, domestic animals) injured, robbed, dead, abandoned, or threatened with such from any source including subhuman and inanimate objects, situations (storms, floods, etc.)
−1	e) Subhumans killing, fighting, injuring, robbing, destroying each other, or threatening to do so
−1	f) Denial of anger, dislike, hatred, cruelty, and intent to harm

[a] Derived from negative portion of Hope Scale [10].
[b] Same as guilt anxiety of Anxiety Scale [5].
[c] Same as shame anxiety of Anxiety Scale [5].
[d] Same as Hostility-Directed-Inward Scale [5].
[e] Same as death and mutilation anxiety of Anxiety Scale [5].
[f] Same as separation anxiety of Anxiety Scale [5].
[g] Same as Hostility-Directed-Outward Scale [5].

Table 1 lists and describes seven Depression Subscales. The sum of the scores obtained from these seven subscales constitutes the total depression score.

8.3 Theories of Content Analysis

There are a number of different ways of classifying content analysis [5, 20–22]. One useful classification system includes classical, pragmatic, and linguistic analysis.

Classical content analysis does not limit content analysis to lexical content but may include investigation of the musical, pictorial, plastic, and gestural systems of communication [23]. In the classical model, the units are coded to categories descriptive of the content itself. With the classical model, once the units are coded, further inferences may be made about the internal state of the communicator, and these inferences are subject to validation only by other procedures. Following the classical model, the statement "she is fearful" would be coded to the category she (other) afraid, and only subsequently could one hypothesize that such a statement might indicate some anxiety in the speaker. The classical model places a premium on objectivity, but such precision often leads to superficiality of results.

In the so-called *pragmatic* model [21], content units are coded into categories descriptive of some condition of the communicator or of the relationship between the communicator and his verbal behavior itself. Inference is used at the time of coding and is the basis of coding relevant semantic and syntactic content units to the categories of the content analysis system. For example, to code the statement "she is fearful" to signify that the speaker is fearful follows the pragmatic model. The pragmatic model aims to realize psychological meaningfulness by working with complex clinical constructs. It uses the skills and knowledge of the clinician while formalizing the conditions under which these skills are used to insure procedural rigor. In brief, the pragmatic model promotes research with psychodynamic constructs, such as anxiety and depression, for which behavioral cues cannot always be easily specified.

Linguistic analysis looks for behavioral cues in syntactic, grammatical, and paralinguistic variables through a nonquantitative approach or with appropriate statistical techniques. Dittmann and Wynne [24] explored the relationship between linguistic phenomena and affect. They found that linguistic features could be identified reliably but were not related to affect and that paralinguistic features could not be identified within acceptable standards of statistical reliability.

The approach presented here to the content analysis of depression, as well as to other psychological and behavioral dimensions we have developed [5], follows to a large extent the pragmatic model. Clinical inferences have been used in the categories to be coded. However, nonprofessional technicians and even the computer [25] can be trained to do the coding with approximately the same level of reliability that can be coded from "manifest" lexical content categories. Moreover, the system presented here is unusual from a theoretical point of view in that it borrows from several different bodies of theory – learning theory, linguistic theory, and psychodynamic theory are all involved. The theoretical approach being used is, hence, an *eclectic* one.

The problem of quantification has been dealt with by including both frequency and nonfrequency aspects of specific types of statements to assess intensity. The frequency of occurrence per 100 words of various themes considered to signify some aspect of depression and communicated in each grammatical clause is one method of assaying the magnitude of depression. Another method of indicating the magnitude of a psychological dimension, not based on frequency of occurrence of a verbal category but based on a linguistic or semantic cue, occurrs in language through the use of adjective or adverb modifiers or through the conotation of a word itself. For example, the use of a comparative adverb, such as "very" *depressed,* would augment the assigned weight for *depressed* by one point.

8.4 Methods of Obtaining and Scoring Verbal Samples

A variety of methods and material can be used to obtain verbal samples for scoring content [5]. The materials include personal letters, autobiographical reports, literature in general, projective test responses, recorded speeches, such as political speeches, psychotherapeutic interviews, and speech obtained in response to standardized instructions.

The method used in the present study was to elicit 5-min verbal samples from subjects by using standard, purposely ambiguous instructions to simulate a projective test procedure. The instructions which each subject received were:

> This is a study of speaking and conversational habits. Upon a signal from me, I would like you to speak for five minutes about any interesting or dramatic personal life experience you have had. Once you have started, I will be here listening to you, but I would prefer not to reply to any questions you may feel like asking until the five-minute period is over. Do you have any questions you would like to ask me now before we start? If not, then, you may start talking.

Some of the Depression Subscales are content analysis scales whose reliability and validity have been intensively studied and reported elsewhere, namely, anxiety [3, 5, 12], hostility [4, 5], and hope [5, 10].

To correct for skewness of the frequency distribution of affect scores and to obtain scores that approximate an interval scale when using the Gottschalk-Gleser Anxiety and Hostility Scales, already established mathematical transformation methods are used [5, 26]. The sum of the products is obtained for the frequency of use of relevant verbal categories and the numerical weights assigned to each thematic category. To this sum is added 0.5 to avoid the discontinuity occurring whenever no scorable items have occurred in some verbal samples. The resulting sum is multipled by 100 and divided by the number of words spoken, giving a corrected score. A further transformation, namely, the square root of the corrected score, is made to obtain the final score. The mathematical formula used to derive the anxiety and hostility scored and the respective subscale scores of these affects per 100 words =

$$\sqrt{\frac{100 \ (f_1 w_1 + f_2 w_2 + f_3 w_3 \ldots f_n w_n + 0.5)}{N}}$$

where f_n is the frequency per unit of time of any relevant type of thematic verbal reference, w_n is the weight applied to such verbal statements, and N is the number of words per unit time.

All of the Depression Subscales use the above procedure for obtaining a score, namely: (I) Hopelessness, (II) Self-Accusation, (III) Psychomotor Retardation, (IV) Somatic Concerns, (V) Death and Mutilation Depression, (VI) Separation Depression, and (VII) Total Hostility Out.

Several of these seven major Depression Subscale scores have their own minor subscales. II: Self-Accusation is comprised of three subscales: (IIA) Guilt Depression, (IIB) Shame Depression, and (IIC) Hostility Inward. V: Death and Mutilation Depression is comprised of two subscales: (VA) Death Depression and (VB) Mutilation Depression. VII: Total Hostility Out is composed of two subscales: (VIIA) Overt Hostility Out and (VIIB). Covert Hostility Out. These minor subscale scores are also obtained by summing the products of the frequency of use of the relevant verbal categories and the numerical weights assigned to each thematic category, adding 0.5, multiplying by 100, and dividing by the number of words spoken, and the square root of this number is obtained giving a corrected score (per 100 words spoken). The scores on the (II). Self-Accusation Scale, (V) Death and Mutilation Depression Scale, and (VII) Total Hostility-Outward Scale are not obtained by simple addition of their respective subscales. Rather, the sum of the relevant verbal categories multiplied by the weights of the verbal categories is added only once to 0.5, multiplied by 100, and divided by the number of words spoken in the verbal sample and then square-rooted.

The total depression score is obtained by summing all seven depression major subscale scores.

8.5 Normative Depression Scores for Adults and Children

Normative depression scores, derived from the content analysis of speech for non-psychiatric populations, provide a measure of the typical or average for a group of people in some situations. The methods of eliciting verbal behavior, for example, a request to the

Table 2. Comparison of depression scores obtained from speech samples from three groups of adults

	Groups				
	Normative adults			Detoxified chronic alcoholics	Depressed outpatients
	Males	Females	Total	Males	Males Females
Number of subjects	29	29	58	50	4 6
Age range (yrs)	32.4 ± 10.2	28.8 ± 9.8	30.6 ± 10.1	43.3 ± 9.2	40.2 ± 9.3
Depression Scales					
I. Hopelessness	0.90 ± 0.31	1.05 ± 0.38	0.95 ± 0.35	1.03 ± 0.42	1.66 ± 0.51
II. Self-Accusation	1.03 ± 0.58	1.41 ± 0.76	1.22 ± 0.70	1.52 ± 0.91	2.42 ± 1.06
II.A) Guilt Depression	0.37 ± 0.21	0.41 ± 0.18	0.39 ± 0.20	0.65 ± 0.49	1.00 ± 0.81
II.B) Shame Depression	0.79 ± 0.53	1.18 ± 0.78	0.99 ± 0.69	0.78 ± 0.56	1.69 ± 0.64
II.C) Hostility Inward	0.64 ± 0.38	0.75 ± 0.33	0.70 ± 0.35	1.13 ± 0.71	1.36 ± 0.72
III. Psychomotor Retardation	0.35 ± 0.10	0.41 ± 0.19	0.38 ± 0.15	0.38 ± 0.15	0.46 ± 0.25
IV. Somatic Concerns	0.34 ± 0.10	0.46 ± 0.17	0.40 ± 0.16	0.56 ± 0.34	0.46 ± 0.22
V. Death and Mutilation	0.93 ± 0.65	0.57 ± 0.40	0.75 ± 0.57	0.65 ± 0.43	0.87 ± 0.80
V.A) Death Depression	0.65 ± 0.50	0.48 ± 0.28	0.56 ± 0.41	0.56 ± 0.34	0.63 ± 0.40
V.B) Mutilation Depression	0.70 ± 0.50	0.46 ± 0.35	0.58 ± 0.44	0.46 ± 0.28	0.72 ± 0.67
VI. Separation Depression	0.86 ± 0.63	0.71 ± 0.35	0.79 ± 0.51	0.76 ± 0.44	1.22 ± 0.70
VII. Hostility Outward	1.06 ± 0.56	0.77 ± 0.33	0.91 ± 0.48	1.04 ± 0.42	1.44 ± 0.93
VII.A) Overt Hostility Out	0.72 ± 0.36	0.69 ± 0.31	0.70 ± 0.34	0.87 ± 0.42	1.24 ± 0.79
VII.B) Covert Hostility Out	0.81 ± 0.51	0.50 ± 0.19	0.65 ± 0.41	0.58 ± 0.31	0.75 ± 0.62
Total Depression	5.48 ± 1.87	5.39 ± 1.53	5.43 ± 1.70	5.94 ± 1.67	8.53 ± 3.51
Mean words/5-min speech samples	561	473	517	526	516

prospective speaker to free-associate versus to talk about all the sad or catastrophic events one has experienced, result in speech samples that, on the average, differ in the amount of depressive content. Similar effects of changing the instructions for eliciting speech on other affect scores have been observed by others [5, 27, 28]. Likewise, the milieu or context in which the verbal behavior is brought forth can influence the content of speech, for example, speech from a patient in a hospital bed versus speech from the same patient talking in an office or residence [5]. Considerable evidence has been accumulated, however, that 5-min speech samples elicited from normative groups of individuals located in widely distributed geographical areas in the United States by a standardized procedure, namely, to "talk about any interesting or dramatic personal life experiences" (see standardized instructions) [5, 26], have mean scores across groups that are not significantly different from one group to another for anxiety, hostility outward, hostility inward, and ambivalent hostility [5, 9]. More surprising, perhaps, is the fact that mean anxiety and hostility scores, derived by the Gottschalk-Gleser method from 5-min speech samples elicited by the same standardized procedure from normative groups from the United States, are not significantly different from comparable scores obtained from a normative group ($n = 355$) in Hamburg, Germany [29] or from a normative group ($n = 140$) in Australia [30]. This relative stability of mean affect scores obtained from the content analysis of verbal behavior elicited by standardized instructions from large groups of normative individuals from diverse national geographical areas and from individuals whose native language is English or German provides base-line scores which can be used to answer the question of what is a high or low score for this or that psychological dimension using these content analysis scales.

Psychological measurements are usually interpreted in a relative rather than abso-

Table 3. Normative depression scores for children derived from speech samples

Sex	Group Normative Children		
	Males	Females	Total
Number of subjects	16	16	32
Age range (yrs)	11.6 ± 3.4	12.2 ± 3.2	11.9 ± 3.3
Depression Scales			
I. Hopelessness	0.98 ± 0.54	1.15 ± 0.53	1.06 ± 0.53
II. Self-Accusation	1.11 ± 0.86	1.25 ± 0.75	1.18 ± 0.80
II.A) Guilt Depression	0.47 ± 0.18	0.50 ± 0.53	0.48 ± 0.27
II.B) Shame Depression	0.83 ± 0.80	0.85 ± 0.83	0.84 ± 0.80
II.C) Hostility Inward	0.77 ± 0.45	0.72 ± 0.30	0.74 ± 0.38
III. Psychomotor Retardation	0.41 ± 0.16	0.42 ± 0.28	0.42 ± 0.22
IV. Somatic Concerns	0.54 ± 0.32	0.51 ± 0.33	0.52 ± 0.32
V. Death and Mutilation	0.88 ± 0.78	0.86 ± 0.79	0.87 ± 0.77
V.A) Death Depression	0.52 ± 0.33	0.56 ± 0.35	0.54 ± 0.34
V.B) Mutilation Depression	0.84 ± 0.70	0.75 ± 0.70	0.79 ± 0.69
VI. Separation Depression	1.02 ± 0.75	0.94 ± 0.43	0.98 ± 0.60
VII. Hostility Outward	1.23 ± 0.62	1.19 ± 0.46	1.21 ± 0.54
VII.A) Overt Hostility Out	0.89 ± 0.49	0.88 ± 0.45	0.80 ± 0.46
VII.B) Covert Hostility Out	0.84 ± 0.60	0.80 ± 0.39	0.82 ± 0.50
Total depression	6.16 ± 2.82	6.37 ± 2.37	6.24 ± 2.56
Mean words/5-min speech samples	440	473	456

lute manner. The choice of populations for which separate standardization data are needed is not simple or obvious. Any factor that can influence the central tendency or range of scores can provide a basis for classification and differential interpretation. For example, the distribution of scores might vary as a function of the subject's age, sex, race, socioeconomic status, medical or psychiatric condition, the type of relationship to the examiner, or any combination of these factors [5, 31]. The normative depression scores we offer here, which were derived from 5-min speech samples elicited in response to standardized instructions [26], can hence be used to begin to ascertain the extent to which other factors affect the magnitude of these depression scores.

Table 2 gives the depression scores obtained from a sample of 29 white adult males and 29 white adult females, employees of the Kroger Company in Cincinnati, Ohio, who were adjudged free of medical illnesses and psychiatric disorders.

Table 3 gives the distribution of depression scores on a sample of 16 white boys and 16 white girls. Table 4 gives the distribution of depression scores by school grades.

Table 4. Mean scores on total Depression Scale for normative children by school grade

Grade	n	Males	n	Females
K – 3	4	5.88	4	5.00
4 – 6	4	7.75	4	6.74
7 – 9	4	5.57	4	8.36
10 – 12	4	5.81	4	5.01

8.6 Construct Validation Studies

Validation of this content-analysis-based Depression Scale requires enlistment of the many steps involved in the process of construction validation. The construct validity of a test is the extent to which the test may be said to measure a theoretical construct or trait [32]. Construct validation requires the gradual accumulation of information from a variety of sources. Any data throwing light on the nature of the psychological dimension under consideration and the conditions affecting its development and manifestations are relevant to construct validity. A first step in the preparation of a predictive (criterion-related) instrument may be to consider what *constructs* are most likely to provide a basis of discrimination and thus an effective assessment tool.

Depression is a construct, an abstraction, a name for a variously defined syndrome or collection of symptoms and signs. As such, the criteria for supporting what this measure assesses and what it does not assess need to be many and should involve some of the criteria employed in the commonly accepted usage of the term *depression*. On the other hand, there is no universal agreement among behavioral scientists and psychiatric clinicians on the subjective and objective psychological and behavioral cues required to identify *depression,* in spite of the efforts of the American Psychiatric Association (APA) to improve the reliability of diagnosing depressive phenomena, as exemplified by the DSM-III of the APA (1980) [33], or by the Schedule for Affective Disorders and Schizophrenia (SADS) [34] or the Research Diagnostic Criteria (RDC) [35]. There may well be some tests of depression in current usage which do not correlate highly with the phenomena measured by this content analysis scale. Such a measurement discrepancy has been observed in the assessment of the affects of anxiety and hostility [28, 36] using Anxiety and Hostility Scales of similar and different types, namely, self-report, rating, and content analysis measures.

Fully aware of these measurement problems in the fields of psychology and psychiatry, a systematic approach to construct validation will be applied to this content analysis measure of depression.

8.6.1 Face Validity

The simplest type of validation of a measure involves whether the instrument, on the face of it, appears to measure what it claims to measure. Many purported evaluative procedures or tests overlook this step in the process of construct validation. In our opinion, face validation is barely a beginning in construct validation, but it cannot be ignored.

Table 1 lists and briefly describes the scorable verbal categories of the seven Depression Subscales. In addition, the weights assigned to these verbal categories are given.

Some subscales [(II) Self-Accusation, (A) Guilt Depression, (B) Shame Depression, (C) Hostility Directed Inward; (V) Death and Mutilation Depression, (A) Death Depression, (B) Mutilation Depression; (VI) Separation Depression; (VII) Hostility Outward, (A) Overt and (B) Covert] assign weights of more than one to some verbal categories. These weights as well as the verbal categories have undergone construct validation studies reported in previous publications [5, 31]. Other Depression Subscales [(I) Hopelessness, (III) Psychomotor Retardation, and (IV) Somatic Concerns] have verbal category weights that are the same, namely, 1, because no empirical data have been yet obtained to give differential weights to these verbal categories.

A reader can peruse the verbal categories in Table 1 and decide – on the basis of face validity – whether the scorable categories, that is, the measurement items, include one's concept of the syndrome labeled "depression."

8.6.2 Comparisons Between Depression Scale Scores of Normative, Sober Chronic Alcoholic, and Depressed Individuals

Individuals who are classified as being depressed following the APA DSM-III classification (1980) should have significantly higher Depression Scale scores than nondepressed, psychiatrically normative individuals if this content analysis scale is valid. Likewise, some investigators [37, 38] have reported that sober chronic alcoholics come from families in which the prevalence of depression is higher than normative families, and these investigators have suggested that alcohol abuse may be a depressive equivalent.

Hence, a comparison of Depression Scale scores of normative, sober chronic alcoholic, and depressed individuals should show significantly higher depression scores for the chronic alcoholic and depressed subjects than for the normative subjects.

In this first validation study, ten male depressed outpatients, at the University of California, Irvine, Medical Center who were classified by the APA DSM-III system (1980) [33] as having depressive disorders, including such diagnoses as dysthymic disorder and major depressive disorder, gave 5-min speech samples elicited by the standard instructions to speak about any interesting or dramatic personal life experiences [5]. Also, a group of 50 detoxified alcoholic male patients in the Alcoholism Treatment Program, Veterans Administration Hospital, Long Beach, California gave 5-min speech samples in response to these standardized instructions. A group of nondepressed, normative adults (29 males and 29 females) also gave 5-min speech samples that were elicited by the same instructions. The typescripts of all speech samples were blindly scored on the Depression Scale by content analysis technicians capable of scoring on this content analysis scale with a reliability of 0.85 or better.

The mean depression scores obtained from these three groups of subjects are given in Table 2. The mean depression scores for the normative, alcoholic, and depressed subjects are, respectively, 5.43 ± 1.70, 5.94 ± 1.67, and 8.53 ± 3.51. The alcoholic group's mean depression score (5.94) is significantly higher ($P < 0.05$) than the normative group (5.43), and the depressed patient's mean depression score (8.53) is significantly higher than the normative group ($P < 0.01$) and the alcoholic group ($P < 0.01$) by the Scheffe test [39]. A more detailed presentation dealing with the psychological differences, as assessed by speech content analysis, between this group of 50 male detoxified chronic alcoholics and a normative nonalcoholic group of males has been published elsewhere [9].

8.6.3 Comparisons Between Depression Scale Scores from a Group of Normative Children and a Group of Hyperactive (Attention Deficit Disorder) Children

Depression scores on a group of normative, nondepressed children were compared with depression scores obtained from a group of hyperactive children. Speech samples, from which the depression scores were derived, were elicited by standard instructions [5].

Table 5. Psychological scores derived from content analysis of speech from boys with attention deficit disorder (hyperactive type) as compared with normative (nonhyperactive) boys

	Attention deficit disorder ($N = 13$)		Normative ($N = 16$)		t	P^a
	Mean scores	SEM	Mean scores	SEM		
Total depression	8.37	0.83	6.16	0.70	2.40	0.025
Hopelessness	1.66	0.15	0.98	0.13	2.32	0.025
Self-accusation	2.08	0.34	1.11	0.21	2.51	0.010
Psychomotor retardation	0.60	0.85	0.41	0.40	2.09	0.025
Cognitive impairment	4.04	0.32	2.75	0.32	2.86	0.005
Social alienation-personal disorganization	3.07	1.37	-0.78	1.50	1.86	0.040

[a] One-tail test

Mean depression scores from the group of hyperactive children were significantly higher ($P < 0.05$) than the depression scores from the group of normative children (see Table 5). The hyperactive children also showed elevated scores, derived by content analysis of the same verbal samples, on anxiety, social alienation-personal disorganization, and cognitive impairment [40].

8.6.4 Depression Scores, Using Different Criterion Measures from Depressed Patients

A group of 29 inpatients at the University of California, Irvine, Medical Center were diagnosed as having some type of depressive disorder based on DSM-III criteria. Five-minute speech samples were elicited by standard instructions and scored blindly by content analysis technicians. The Beck Depression Inventory [41], the Zung Depression Scale [42], and the Hamilton Depression Scale [43] were also administered to these depressed patients on the same day as the patient gave a 5-min speech sample for obtaining depression scores by content analysis.

The mean Depression Subscale scores obtained from the 5-min verbal samples given by this group of 29 depressed inpatients are reported in Table 6. The mean total depression score (8.31 ± 2.30) from this group of depressed inpatients is quite significantly higher than the mean total depression score (5.43 ± 1.70) obtained from the normative group of 58 adults (see Table 2) by the Scheffe test.

Both Pearson product moment correlations and Kendall nonparametric correlations were obtained between Gottschalk Depression Scale scores (total depression and major subscale scores) and scores from all criterion measures, that is, Zung, Beck, and Hamil-

Table 6. Depression scores from a group of depressed inpatients

Number of subjects	29	18	11
Age range (yrs)	36.5 ± 16.1		
Depression Scales	*Total*	*Females*	*Males*
I. Hopelessness	1.62 ± 0.49	1.76 ± 0.49	1.40 ± 0.43
II. Self-Accusation	2.26 ± 0.84	2.45 ± 0.86	1.95 ± 0.76
II.A) Guilt Depression	0.86 ± 0.68	0.90 ± 0.62	0.79 ± 0.80
II.B) Shame Depression	1.33 ± 0.73	1.46 ± 0.85	1.12 ± 0.45
II.C) Hostility Inward	1.47 ± 0.64	1.59 ± 0.67	1.27 ± 0.58
III. Psychomotor Retardation	0.49 ± 0.36	0.51 ± 0.41	0.45 ± 0.25
IV. Somatic Concerns	0.58 ± 0.29	0.65 ± 0.33	0.48 ± 0.18
V. Death and Mutilation	0.88 ± 0.68	0.95 ± 0.80	0.77 ± 0.46
V.A) Death Depression	0.68 ± 0.53	0.69 ± 0.61	0.66 ± 0.38
V.B) Mutilation Depression	0.65 ± 0.56	0.65 ± 0.61	0.65 ± 0.51
VI. Separation Depression	1.22 ± 0.76	1.28 ± 0.83	1.11 ± 0.65
VII. Hostility Outward	1.26 ± 0.66	1.29 ± 0.79	1.20 ± 0.41
VII.A) Overt Hostility Out	1.03 ± 0.61	1.11 ± 0.71	0.90 ± 0.37
VII.B) Covert Hostility Out	0.74 ± 0.39	0.69 ± 0.40	0.82 ± 0.37
Total depression	8.31 ± 2.30	8.89 ± 2.41	7.38 ± 1.85

ton. Since there were no essential differences in these correlations, only Pearson product moment correlations will be reported.

The correlations of the Gottschalk total depression scores with the total depression scores on the Zung, Beck, and Hamilton, from this group of 29 patients, were noted and reached a convincing level of significance ($P < 0.05$) with the Zung, Beck, and Hamilton total depression scores and, in addition, with highly relevant test items of all three concurrent criterion measures (see Table 7).

Table 7. Pearson correlations of Gottschalk total depression scores and total depression scores from the Zung, Beck, and Hamilton Scales ($n = 29$)

	Zung Scale	Beck Scale	Hamilton Scale
Gottschalk total depression scores	0.39	0.32	0.45

The semantic similarities in what is measured by the Gottschalk Depression Subscales with test items from the Beck, Zung, and Hamilton Scales can be estimated by examining the spectrum of Pearson product moment correlations of each Gottschalk Depression Subscale with these test items. It is realized that some of the intercorrelations might have occurred by chance because so many were run, and so one must consider that these findings are approximations. Careful examination of the intercorrelations of test items from the criterion measures and the seven Depression Subscales provides, nevertheless, a coherent, consistent, and plausible picture of the theoretical construct assessed by these subscales. Significant correlations ($P < 0.05$) occurred with many test items; many other test items had non-significant low correlations in the expected and predicted direction with the various Depression Subscales. Let us examine the significant intercorrelations ($P < 0.05$) between our seven Depression Subscale scores and various Zung, Beck, and Hamilton Depression Scale test items.

I Hopelessness
The higher subjects scored on this content analysis subscale, the higher they scored on the following test items: *Zung*–I do not enjoy, I do not feel useful, my heart beats faster; *Beck*–I look ugly; *Hamilton*–mental retardation, more psychic anxiety, more diurnal variation, more paranoid.

II Self-Accusation
The higher subjects scored on this content analysis subscale, the higher they scored on the following test items: *Zung*–wish I were dead, do not feel useful; *Beck*–feel I am a failure, feel disappointed, like to destroy self, believe I look ugly; *Hamilton* feel depressed, have more anxiety, feel paranoid.

III Psychomotor Retardation

The higher subjects scored on this content analysis subscale, the higher they scored on the following items: *Zung*—feel irritable, do not have weight loss; *Beck*—feel loss of interest in others, do not work well, feel too tired; *Hamilton*—feel depressed, think of suicide, do not feel agitated, do not have weight loss.

IV Somatic Concerns

The higher subjects scored on this content analysis subscale, the higher they scored on these test items: *Zung*—am constipated, things are not easy to do, do not enjoy life; *Beck*—feel disappointed, have trouble making decisions, feel tired; *Hamilton*—feel mental retardation, have somatic anxiety, have general symptoms.

V Death and Mutilation Depression

The higher subjects scored on this content analysis subscale, the higher they scored on the following test items: *Zung*—feel sad, do not have a clear mind, do not feel useful, wish I were dead; *Beck*—feel sad and blue, feel guilt, have trouble making decisions; *Hamilton*—have insomnia, have somatic anxiety, have weight loss, have diurnal variation, feel paranoid.

VI Separation Depression

The higher subjects scored on this content analysis subscale, the higher they scored on the following test items: *Zung*—have weight loss, feel restless, heart beats faster, do not feel useful; *Beck*—feel sad and blue, feel disappointed; *Hamilton*—do not feel agitation, do have weight loss.

VII Hostility Outward

The higher subjects scored on this content analysis subscale, the higher they scored on the following test items: *Zung*—do not cry, do not feel useful, do not enjoy a full life, wish I were dead; *Beck*—feel sad and blue, feel a failure, feel disappointed, feel ugly; *Hamilton*—feel agitated, have somatic anxiety, have weight loss.

8.7 Discussion and Conclusion

A description is provided of a measure of depression obtained by means of the content analysis of verbal behavior. Normative and construct validation studies give strong evidence that this measure assays major features of the depressive syndrome, which is subdivided into seven subscales or dimensions.

An earlier preliminary version of this Depression Scale included another subscale labeled Ambivalent Hostility, and papers have been published using this earlier version of this Depression Scale [9, 40]. Subsequent construct validation studies of a concurrent criterion measure type suggested that the Ambivalent Hostility Subscale was not uniformly correlated with other measures of the depressive syndrome and, hence, it was eliminated.

The content analysis approach to the measurement of psychological and behavioral measures embodies the characteristics and strengths of both self-report and independent observer rating methods. For this reason, it minimizes the measurement errors inherent in these methods when they are used independently [1]. This Depression Scale is now ready for broad applications to the assessment of the depressive syndrome in its many forms and manifestations.

References

1. Gottschalk LA (1984) Measurement of mood, affect, and anxiety in cancer patients. Cancer 53: 2236–2242
2. Lolas F (1986) Behavioral text and psychological context: On pragmatic verbal behavior analysis. In: Gottschalk LA, Lolas F, Viney U (eds) The content analysis of verbal behavior in clinical medicine and psychiatry. Springer, Berlin Heidelberg New York Tokyo
3. Gleser GC, Gottschalk LA, Springer KJ (1961) An anxiety scale applicable to verbal samples. Arch Gen Psychiatry 5: 593–605
4. Gottschalk LA, Gleser GC, Springer KJ (1963) Three hostility scales applicable to verbal samples. Arch Gen Psychiatry 9: 254–279
5. Gottschalk LA, Gleser GC (1969) The measurement of psychological states through the content analysis of verbal behavior. University of California Press, Los Angeles
6. Gottschalk LA, Eckardt MJ, Feldman DJ (1979) Further validation studies of a cognitive-intellectual impairment scale applicable to verbal samples. In: Gottschalk LA (ed) The content analysis of verbal behavior: further studies, Chapter 2. Spectrum, New York, pp 1–8
7. Gottschalk LA, Eckardt MJ, Pautler CR, Wolf RJ, Terman SA (1983) Cognitive impairment scales derived from verbal samples. Compr Psychiatry 24: 6–19
8. Gottschalk LA, Eckardt MJ, Hoigaard-Martin JC, Gilbert RL, Wolf RJ, Johnson W (1983) Neurophysiological deficit in chronic alcoholism: early detection and prediction by analysis of verbal samples. Subst Alcohol Actions Misuse 4: 45–58
9. Gottschalk LA, Hoigaard JC, Eckardt MJ, Gilbert RL, Wolf RJ (1983) Cognitive impairment and other psychological scores derived from content analysis of speech in detoxified male chronic alcoholics. Am J Drug Alcohol Abuse 9: 447–460
10. Gottschalk LA (1974) A hope scale applicable to verbal samples. Arch Gen Psychiatry 30: 779–785
11. Westbrook MT, Viney LL (1980) Scales of origin and pawn perception using content analysis of speech. J Pers Assess 44: 157–166
12. Gottschalk LA, Springer KJ, Gleser GC (1961) Experiments with a method of assessing the variations in intensity of certain psychological states occurring during two psychotherapeutic interviews. In: Gottschalk LA (ed) Comparative psycholinguistic analysis of two psychotherapeutic interviews. International Universities Press, New York
13. Westbrook MT (1976) Positive affect: a method of content analysis for verbal samples. J Consult Clin Psychol 44: 715–719
14. Knowles JB, MacLean AW, Cairns J (1982) Definition of REM latency: some comparisons with particular reference to depression. Biol Psychiatry 17: 993–1002
15. Jacoby RJ, Dolan RJ, Levy R, Baldy R (1983) Quantitative computed tomography in elderly depressed patients. Br J Psychiatry 143: 124–127
16. Kline MD, Beeber AR (1983) Weight loss and the dexamethasone suppression test. Arch Gen Psychiatry 40: 1034

17. Wood K, Harwood J, Cappen A (1983) Platelet accumulation of histamine in depression. Lancet 11: 519–520
18. Suranyi-Cadotte BE, Wood PL, Schwartz G, Vasian Nair NP (1983) Altered platelet ^{3}H-imipramine binding in schizo-affective and depressed disorders. Biol Psychiatry 18: 923–927
19. Banki CM, Arato M (1983) Amine metabolites and neuroendocrine responses related to depression and suicide. J Affectiv Disord 5: 223–232
20. Pool ID (1959) Trends in content analysis today: a summary. In: Pool ID (ed) Trends in content analysis. University of Illinois Press, Urbana
21. Marsden G (1965) Content analysis studies of therapeutic interviews: 1954 to 1964. Psychol Bull 68: 298–321
22. Viney LL (1983) The assessment of psychological states through content analysis of verbal communications. Psychol Bull 94: 542–563
23. Berelson B (1952) Content analysis in communication research. Free Press, Glencoe
24. Dittmann AT, Wynne LC (1961) Linguistic techniques and the analysis of emotionality in interviews. J Abnorm Soc Psychol 63: 201–204
25. Gottschalk LA, Bechtel RJ (1982) The measurement of anxiety through the computer analysis of verbal samples. Compr Psychiatry 23: 364–369
26. Gottschalk LA, Winget CN, Gleser GC (1969) Manual of instructions for using the Gottschalk-Gleser content analysis scales: anxiety, hostility, and social alienation-personal disorganization. University of California Press, Los Angeles
27. Gift T, Cole R, Wynne L (1986) A hostility measure for use in family contexts. In: Gottschalk LA, Lolas F, Viney U (eds) The content analysis of verbal behavior in clinical medicine and psychiatry. Springer, Berlin Heidelberg New York Tokyo
28. Koch U, Schofer G (eds) (1986) Sprachinhaltsanalyse in der psychosozialen und psychiatrischen Forschung: Grundlage und Anwendungsstudien mit den Affektskalen von Gottschalk and Gleser. Beltz, Weinheim
29. Schofer G, Koch U, Balck F (1979) The Gottschalk-Gleser content analysis of speech: a normative study. In: Gottschalk LA (ed) The content analysis of verbal behavior: further studies, Chapter 4. Spectrum, New York, pp 97–118
30. Viney LL, Manton M (1973) Sampling verbal behavior in Australia: Gottschalk-Gleser content analysis scales. Aust J Psychol 25: 45–55
31. Gottschalk LA (ed) (1979) The content analysis of verbal behavior: further studies. Spectrum, New York
32. Anastasi A (1968) Psychological testing, 3rd edn. MacMillan, New York
33. American Psychiatric Association (1980) Diagnostic and statistical manual of mental disorders, 3rd edn., American Psychiatric Ass'n, Washington, D.C.
34. Endicott J, Spitzer RL (1978) A diagnostic interview: the schedule for affective disorders and schizophrenia. Arch Gen Psychiatry 35: 837–844
35. Spitzer R, Endicott J, Robins E (1978) Research diagnostic criteria: Rationale and reliability. Arch Gen Psychiatry 35: 773–782
36. Gottschalk LA, Hoigaard JC, Birch H, Rickels K (1979) The measurement of psychological states: relationship between Gottschalk-Gleser content analysis scores and Hamilton anxiety rating scales scores, physician questionnaire rating scale scores, and Hopkins symptom checklist scores. In: Gottschalk LA (ed) Content analysis of verbal behavior: further studies, Chapter 3. Spectrum, New York, pp 41–94
37. Goodwin DW (1976) Psychiatric description and evaluation of the alcoholic. In: Tarter RE, Sugarman AA (eds) Alcoholism: interdisciplinary approaches to an enduring problem. Addison-Wesley, Reading
38. Winokur G, Reich T, Rimmer J, Pitts RN Jr (1970) Alcoholism III: diagnosis and familial psychiatric illness in 259 alcoholic probands. Arch Gen Psychiatry 23: 104–111

39. Nie NH, Hull CH, Jenkins JG, Steinbrenner K, Bendt DH (1975) Statistical package for the social sciences, 2nd edn. McGraw Hill, New York
40. Gottschalk LA, Swanson JM, Hoigaard-Martin JC, Gilbert RL, Fiore C (1984) Hyperactive children: a study of the content analysis of their speech. Psychother Psychosom 41: 125–135
41. Beck AT, Beamesderfer A (1974) Assessment of depression: the depression inventory in psychological measurements. In: Pichat P (ed) Psychopharmacology, Vol 7. Karger, Basel, pp 151–169
42. Zung WWK (1965) A self-rating depression scale. Arch Gen Psychiatry 12: 63–70
43. Hamilton M (1967) Development of a rating scale for primary depressive illness. Br J Soc Clin Psychol 6: 278–296

9 Content Analysis of Verbal Behavior in Psychotherapy Research: A Comparison Between Two Methods*

Fernando Lolas, Erhard Mergenthaler and Michael von Rad

9.1 Introduction

Content analysis of verbal behavior is a research technique for making inferences by systematically and objectively identifying specified characteristics in spoken or written language. By developing categories of speech units, content analytic procedures are designed to specify judgmental processes and transform intuitive evaluations into explicit rules (9, 16).

When applied to behavioral research, the process entails three steps: specification of the content characteristics to be measured, application of rules for identifying and recording the characteristics when they occur in the data, and establishment of relationships between the information so obtained and other aspects of the subject's behavior.

The present report is an outgrowth of previous work aimed at studying verbal behavior of patients during psychotherapeutic interviews. One of the basic tenets of this research has been the assumption that communicative styles and the way patients implement strategies for conveying emotional meaning could be construed as nosological principles of diagnostic, prognostic, and therapeutic value (10, 17, 18 Lolas F, unpublished observations). This investigation set out to compare two content analytical procedures applied to verbatim protocols from the same group of patients. These two types of verbal analysis involve different ways of specifying the characteristics to be measured, of defining the scoring units, and of implementing the process of identification and recording of the contents. Nevertheless, both procedures – the Gottschalk-Gleser method (4) and the "Anxiety Topics Dictionary" (ATD) developed at the University of Ulm (7, 14) – share a common body of theory and can be said to have pragmatic relevance. Their content categories are phrased, and can be interpreted, in "psychological" terms, thus linking verbal signs to the person who uses them and to the behavior within which they occur.

---

* Reprinted from *The British Journal of Medical Psychology* (55: 327–333, 1982) with permission of the authors and publisher.

9.2 Method

Verbatim protocols encompassing the patients' first 1000 words in psychotherapeutic interviews were obtained from 79 patients (50 women, 29 men) with a mean age of 28,5 years. They were interviewed by six therapists of comparable training to assess their suitability for psychotherapeutic treatment. The group included both subjects with predominantly psychic complaints and patients afflicted by a variety of somatic diseases (Table 1). The session was centered on self-description, complaints, and symptoms.

Transcripts of taped utterances were scored both by the method described by Gottschalk and Gleser (4) and by the ATD in its latest version. The latter is a computer-aided procedure, implemented as part of a comprehensive program for "electronic verbal analysis" (EVA) (7, 14).

The Gottschalk-Gleser method takes into consideration contextual aspects of the

Table 1. Survey of the sample ($n = 79$)

Diagnostic categories	
"Psychoneurotic" outpatient subgroup (n = 39)	
Narcissistic	6
Depressive	7
Depressive-narcissistic	5
Obsessional	4
Obsessional-depressive	2
Hysterical	3
Hysterical-depressive	10
Hysterical-obsessive	2
"Psychosomatic" outpatient subgroup (n = 40)	
Peptic ulcer	14
Ulcerative colitis	11
Neurodermitis	5
Asthma	3
Psoriasis	2
Others	5
Average age (years)	28.5
Sex	
Male	29
Female	50
Intelligence (Raven test)	
Within normal range	57
Above normal range	22
Socioeconomic class (without housewives, $n = 11$)	
Lower class	12
Middle class	56
Mode of referral	
Spontaneous	28
Physician/other persons	51

message, its coding unit being the grammatical clause as established by a coder. It relies on frequency counts of relevant categories modified by weighting. Weight depends upon "centrality" of the clause under examination (proximity to a predefined construct) and personal involvement of the speaker. For the scales included in the method, it has usually been established through an empirical validation process. Abundant information is available on the statistical features of Gottschalk-Gleser scores and on their relationships to psychometric data (2, 4, 6).

The EVA system is a computer-aided method relying on unweighted frequency counts of single words, grouped in accordance with preestablished dictionaries. Content categories are extensionally defined as lists of words (including different grammatical forms) related to psychologically meaningful constructs. The computer is employed both for the recognition and summary of coding units and tallies the occurrence of usage according to these categories of meaning (7, 13). See Appendix A for examples of entries.

Protocols were manually scored for the six forms of anxiety defined by the Gottschalk-Gleser method (death, mutilation, separation, guilt, shame, and diffuse anxiety) and the four hostility constructs considered by the same method (hostility directed outward overt and covert, hostility directed inward, and ambivalent hostility). After retyping the protocols in computer-readable form (IBM OCR-A Type), they were read into the data bank held at the Department of Psychotherapy, University of Ulm (12), and scored for four empirically derived and consensually validated anxiety "topics" from one of the EVA vocabularies (ATD) using the Telefunken TR440 computer facility. The four anxiety topics (shame, castration, guilt, and separation) were quantified in terms of content category frequency as a proportion of the analyzed text (1000 words). Gottschalk-Gleser scores were obtained according to a series of steps involving multiplication of frequency of use by weight, division by the number of words, and conversion to a standard score referred to 100 words. An additional step involved extraction of square root for normalizing the distribution. Gottschalk-Gleser Affect Scales do not form a set of exhaustive categories covering all themata so that cases of no codable content are possible (1, 4). Although the same holds true for the ATD, the probabilities for no scorable content are lower (single-word method). As a feature common to both methods, it may be said that they provide a measure of *relative* magnitude of the emotion or psychological state circumscribed by the constructs they employ.

9.3 Results

Raw mean scores and standard deviations for the variables studied in both methods are presented in Table 2. Although not directly comparable, these figures show different relative magnitudes of the anxiety subtypes common to both methods.

The statistical independence of Gottschalk-Gleser measures has been previously studied (11). Applying factor analytic techniques to the same data set as the one reported here, anxiety measures were shown to be uncorrelated. Guilt anxiety and ambivalent hostility (AH) loaded on the same factor. For the ATD, Table 3 shows that the four anxiety measures are independent.

Table 2. Raw mean scores and standard deviation

	ATD		GG	
	Mean	SD	Mean	SD
Shame	5.48	3.141	1.00	0.582
Castration	10.94	5.886	0.34	0.259
Guilt	7.56	3.986	0.62	0.495
Separation	12.51	6.177	0.69	0.444
Death			0.36	0.268
Diffuse			1.04	0.488
HDOo			0.74	0.498
HDOc			0.37	0.270
HDI			1.24	0.513
AH			0.80	0.411

HDOo, hostility directed outward overt; HDOc, hostility directed outward covert; HDI, hostility directed inward; AH, ambivalent hostility

Table 3. Intercorrelations between anxiety topics (ATD)

	Shame	Castration	Guilt	Separation
Shame	1.0			
Castration	−0.082	1.0		
Guilt	−0.046	−0.074	1.0	
Separation	0.008	−0.156	0.072	1.0

Table 4. Intercorrelations between the ATD and Gottschalk-Gleser content analytic categories in a mixed patient population ($n = 79$) (patients' initial 1000 words during interview)

Gottschalk-Gleser Scales	ATD			
	Shame	Castration	Guilt	Separation
Hostility				
HDOo	0.064	0.100	0.199	0.250[a]
HDOc	0.152	0.120	0.083	0.175
HDI	0.294[b]	−0.124	0.082	0.146
AH	0.189	−0.060	−0.005	0.030
Anxiety				
Death	−0.106	0.071	0.105	−0.021
Mutilation	−0.101	0.191	0.149	−0.291[b]
Separation	−0.030	−0.154	−0.044	0.462[b]
Guilt	0.221[a]	−0.193	0.229[a]	0.022
Shame	0.492[b]	−0.118	−0.124	0.077
Diffuse	−0.049	0.062	0.050	−0.004

[a] $P < 0.05$; [b] $P < 0.01$.

HDOo, hostility directed outward overt; HDOc, hostility directed outward covert; HDI, hostility directed inward; AH, ambivalent hostility

As shown in Table 4, positive product moment correlations were found between ATD and Gottschalk-Gleser content categories across the whole patient sample. Shame anxiety scores are linearly correlated, showing a significant positive correlation. The same holds true for separation anxiety at the 1% level of statistical significance. Although guilt anxiety scores also correlated positively, ATD shame showed also a relationship to Gottschalk-Gleser guilt scores. ATD separation anxiety correlated also with mutilation anxiety as measured by the Gottschalk-Gleser method. Hostility directed inward (HDI) showed a positive linear relationship to shame anxiety as assessed by the ATD in patients' utterances. Hostility directed outward overt (HDOo) correlated at the 5% level with ATD separation anxiety. Hostility directed outward covert (HDOc), ambivalent hostility (AH), death anxiety, and diffuse anxiety from the Gottschalk-Gleser method did not show any significant correlation with ATD scales.

9.4 Discussion

Aside from representing data reduction techniques, content analysis methods derive their usefulness for psychotherapy research from the fact that they help specify the speech features upon which intuitive evaluation rests. Biased associational contexts and connotational emphases related to the individual observer are replaced by explicit rules. Although language content is highly influenced by situational variables (8), a strong case can be made for the use of theory-related descriptive categories from a pragmatic point of view.

In the present study, the same material has been studied by means of two content analytic methods which share basic theoretical assumptions with regard to affect definition. In contrast to a purely physiological definition, their psychoanalytical frame of reference is based upon the notion that speech reflects feeling states and that these could be qualitatively and quantitatively operationalized in terms of textual markers. Language behavior would thus provide a relevant clue to a person's psychological organization. However, although both methods strive for inferential relevance in terms of psychologically sound categories and disregard somewhat the surface structure of the message (e.g., verbal tense), they differ in aspects that influence the scope and applicability of the permitted conclusions. In this sense, the "analysis program," that is, the series of steps from data collection to inference, may constitute by itself an added source of "noise" and should be taken into consideration. Both methods differ, for instance, in the way they operationalize the underlying constructs. Since the coding categories stem from the theory and not from the text, their relationship to textual features must be established or defined. However clear-cut meaning categories are, single-word methods such as the ATD require a judgmental fitting between the coding units (words) and the constructs they are supposed to reflect. Although the Gottschalk-Gleser method incorporates this feature in the coding process, observers' biases may play a role in the process of weighting and in assigning clauses to categories, where a decision has to be taken. On the other hand, the Gottschalk-Gleser method tends to be less sensitive to the speaker's vocabulary and word choice and incorporates contextual information embodied in word combinations. The ATD, as a representative of single-word based methods, can be greatly influenced by lexical choice. A case can be made for the predictive power of the isolated word (15), but the contention can be made that both methods, by their being sensitive to text units of different sizes, would emphasize different aspects of the underlying construct. The representativity of the textual markers (clause and word) in relation to the distal construct would then be critically dependent upon the operationalization process (dictionary construction and the like) despite an assumed common frame of reference. This is also relevant to the accurate depiction of intensity of psychological states.

From a practical point of view, both methods differ in ways that are not irrelevant to their clinical applications. Whereas the ATD can yield large amounts of data within a short time – provided appropriate computational facilities are available – implementation of the Gottschalk-Gleser method by computer has barely reached the stage of clinical application (3, 5). In German, the lack of reliable programms for syntactic analysis would demand a substantial precoding work to computerize a clause-based method.

Since the categories employed by the two methods do not exactly overlap, it is difficult to ascertain the extent to which they complement each other. By applying them both to the same extensive material (a practice seldom encountered in content analytic studies), the aim was to obtain suggestions for further inquiry. Since only correlational data have been presented, interpretation of the results can only be tentative. The fact that shame and separation anxiety are linearly related in both methods suggests that lexical choice (affecting predominantly ATD scores) might introduce less variability into these categories. Due to the heterogeneity of the sample, it appears unlikely that this is a sample-dependent phenomenon. A closer inspection at the operationalization process of these constructs would prove to be rewarding, particularly considering that the EVA system permits the reconstruction of the subject's vocabulary and examination of the frequency of specific words. Since different persons may convey the same emotional meaning through different words, this information – together with Gottschalk-Gleser scores – might be useful in constructing more discriminative "dictionaries" of content categories. Work now in progress is directed at identifying textual markers with a higher degree of specificity in relation to each category. The present results suggest that this process might be supported by information from the same text obtained by other methods. The fact that certain categories seem to be linearly related in their relative magnitudes may be useful in studies dealing with validation of constructs by external criteria.

In the present study, shame anxiety assessed by the ATD bears a positive linear relationship to hostility directed inward (HDI) of the Gottschalk-Gleser method. For this sample, the same relationship has been observed between Gottschalk-Gleser shame-anxiety scores and HDI scores (Lolas F, unpublished observations). This would further suggest a formal similarity between shame-anxiety constructs as operationalized by both methods.

The present results call for further investigation of analysis programs derived from similar bodies of theory and applied to the same samples of verbal behavior. Caution should be exercised in cross-comparisons between studies employing similar conceptualizations, irrespective of the validity of their categories. An analysis program and other aspects of the operationalization process are as decisive as the apparent theoretical allegiance a researcher may admit. Clinical verbal behavior analyses should be examined not only in relation to their predictive power, external validation, or ad hoc applicability, but also in terms of the consistency and comparability of their meaning categories.

Acknowledgment

This work was performed while the senior author was on a leave of absence from the University of Chile, aided by a fellowship from the Alexander von Humboldt Foundation, West Germany. Data processing and analysis were performed within the framework of the Sonderforschungsbereich 129, Projekt B 2, Deutsche Forschungsgemeinschaft. Thanks are expressed to Professor H. Kächele and to Miss U. Stöcklein for their help in conducting this study.

References

1. Gleser GC, Lubin A (1979) Response productivity in verbal content analysis: a critique of Marsden, Kalter, and Ericson. In: Gottschalk LA (ed) The content analysis of verbal behavior: further studies. Spectrum, New York
2. Gottschalk LA (1979) The content analysis of verbal behavior: further studies. Spectrum, New York
3. Gottschalk LA, Bechtel RJ (1982) The measurement of anxiety through the computer analysis of verbal samples. Compr Psychiatry 23: 364–369
4. Gottschalk LA, Gleser GC (1969) The measurement of psychological states through the content analysis of verbal behavior. University of California Press, Berkeley
5. Gottschalk LA, Hausman C, Brown JS (1975) A computerized scoring system for use with content analysis scales. Compr Psychiatry 16: 77–90
6. Gottschalk LA, Winget CN, Gleser GC (1969) Manual of instructions for using the Gottschalk-Gleser content analysis scales: anxiety, hostility, and social alienation-personal disorganization. University of California Press, Berkeley
7. Grünzig HJ, Holzscheck K, Kächele H (1976) EVA – Ein Programmsystem zur maschinellen Inhaltsanalyse von Psychotherapieprotokollen. Med Psychol 2: 208–217
8. Laffal J (1965) Pathological and normal language. Atherton, New York
9. Lisch R, Kriz J (1978) Grundlagen und Modelle der Inhaltsanalyse. Rowohlt, Reinbeck
10. Lolas F, von Rad M (1982) Communication of emotional meaning: a biopsychosocial dimension in psychosomatics. In: Day SB (ed) Life stress. Van Nostrand-Reinhold, New York
11. Lolas F, von Rad M, Scheibler D (1981) Situational influences on verbal affective expression of psychosomatic and psychoneurotic patients. J Nerv Ment Dis 169: 619–623
12. Mergenthaler E (1979) Das Textkorpus in der psychoanalytischen Forschung. In: Bergenholtz H, Schäder B (eds) Empirische Textwissenschaft. Scriptor, Kronberg
13. Mergenthaler E, Büscher U (1978) Elektronische Verbalanalyse (EVA-Textanalyse System). User's Handbook. Unpublished. Department of Psychotherapy, University of Ulm, Ulm
14. Speidel H (1979) Entwicklung und Validierung eines Wörterbuches zur maschinell-inhaltsanalytischen Erfassung psychoanalytischer Angstthemen. Unpublished MA thesis, University of Konstanz and University of Ulm, Konstanz
15. Spence DP (1980) Lawfulness in lexical choice: a natural experiment. J Am Psychoanal Assoc 28: 115–132
16. Stone PJ, Dunphy DC, Smith MS, Ogilvie DM (1966) The general inquirer: a computer approach to content analysis. MIT, Cambridge
17. Von Rad M, Drücke M, Knauss W, Lolas F (1979). Alexithymia: anxiety and hostility in psychosomatic and psychoneurotic patients. Psychother Psychosom 31: 223–234
18. Von Rad M, Lolas F (1978) Psychosomatische und psychoneurotische Patienten im Vergleich. Unterschiede des Sprechverhaltens. Psyche 32: 956–973

Appendix A. Examples of entries

Shame		*Guilt*	
Refusal	Ablehnung	Acquiescence	gewissenlos
	Zurückweisung		mißachten
	abweisen		obszön
Observe	anstarren		sündigen
	enthüllen	Punishment	ächten
	exhibitionistisch		bestrafen
Comparison	abnorm		entschuldigen
	erfolglos		sühnen
	mangelhaft	Jurisdiction	Anwalt
Humiliation	erröten		Eid
	ertappen		Zeuge
	genieren		gesetzlich
Insufficiency	falsch	Religiosity	Gott
	feige		entsagen
	häßlich		lossprechen
Safety	anerkennen		predigen
	erhaben	Innocence	Dankbarkeit
	furchtlos		erlauben
Hide	geheim		frei
	heimlich		legal

Castration		*Separation*	
Hostility	explosiv	Symbiosis	Abhängigkeit
	grausam		anbinden
	hacken		anklammern
Body	Zunge	Security	Haus
	anatomisch		Zuflucht
Sexuality	erotisch	Act of separation	abschieben
	erregend		fortziehen
	männlich		loslassen
Power	aktiv	Community	mitgehen
	fit		nahen
	mächtig		heim
Mutilation	giftig	Persons	Eltern
	quetschen		Familie
Female symbol	Loch		Mutter
	Spalte	Loss of love	Abneigung
Male symbol	Messer		Verlust
	bohren		entfremden
Inferiority	einschränken		hilflos
	passiv	Loneliness	allein
	schlaff		traurig

Some Applications of Verbal Behavior Analysis to the Clinical Sciences

10 Use of the Gottschalk–Gleser Verbal Content Analysis Scales with Medically Ill Patients*

Allen H. Lebovits, and Jimmie C. Holland

10.1 Introduction

The past several years have seen a dramatic upsurge in interest in the psychological aspects of medical illness [1–8]. Subdivisions of health psychology and behavioral medicine have developed within the field of psychology, paralleling the growth of the consultation liaison subspecialty within psychiatry. Such specialization is a result of greater interest among medical specialties in the psychological sequelae of technologically sophisticated therapies. Germ-free environments [9] and coronary care units [10] represent two types of environmentally stressful treatments. Radiotherapy [11–14] and chemotherapy [15] pose unique psychological stresses and psychiatric syndromes for patients with cancer.

The systematic study of patients with physical illness has been troubled by the absence of (a) psychological assessment methods developed for this population, (b) a sensitivity to the "normal" stresses of illnesses, recognizing the contribution of physical symptoms to symptom inventory of psychological morbidity, and (c) the ability to measure psychological states repeatedly over time as needed in physically ill patients.

One particularly sensitive evaluative instrument of mood state, the Gottschalk-Gleser Verbal Content Analysis Scales (G-G), has been used to assess several different populations of patients with different types of physical illness. This report reviews its efficacy in comparison with other report measures.

10.2 Assessment and Procedures

10.2.1 Self-Report Inventories

Most self-report inventories consist of a list of items or adjectives that the patient must rate. They have the distinct advantage of eliciting the patient's own subjective perceptions, and they require little professional time. The inventories do not require the presence of a skilled and trained interviewer and can usually be administered by a paraprofessional. In addition, the scoring may be accomplished quickly and easily, by computer or by hand.

---

* Reprinted from *Psychosomatic Medicine* (45: 305–320, 1983) with permission of the authors and publisher.

Self-report tests are limited in use, however, with a medical sample. Psychological defense mechanisms, such as denial or rationalization, mobilized by illness, may distort the patients' reports of their states. In addition, the patient may respond to self-report adjectives in terms of his general preillness state; he may be unable to refer to himself in relation to the present distressful situation. Furthermore, medical illnesses or treatments utilized may cause subtle subclinical changes in cognitive processes, including judgment and memory, that interfere with accurate reporting of psychological mood states. Self-report instruments are lengthy and therefore require long periods of concentration that may be frustrating to physically ill patients. In addition, single-affect scales also have the disadvantage of unidimensionality. Table 1 outlines some examples of usage of several self-report inventories with medically ill patients.

10.2.2 Observer-Report Rating Scales

Scales rated by an observer offer the advantage of objective observation of the patient. Such scales can take into account the possible role of psychological defenses, which can distort a self-report. They also eliminate the strain of writing, which may exist for a severely debilitated patient. These reports, however, require that the clinical raters be skilled and thoroughly familiar with the psychopathological complications of the particular disease process and its treatment (e.g., steroid effects), as well as able to rate psychological and psychiatric morbidity. The necessity for training of interviewers, establishment of interrater reliability, and carefully defined description of rating categories must be recognized. Table 2 outlines some examples of usage of observer-report rating scales with medically ill patients.

Table 2. Examples of observer-report rating scales used with medically ill patients

Instrument	Mood states	Scale format	Developers	Examples of use in medically ill	Problems of use in medically ill
Multidimensional					
Current and Past Psychopathology Scales	Depression, anxiety, hostility	18 rating scales of past, 8 of present psychological adjustment	Endicott, Spitzer [61]	Plumb, Holland [62]; Gorzynski et al. [63]	Some scales designed to measure more severe psychopathological symptoms than present in most medically ill samples
Symptom Checklist Analogue Scale	Depression, anxiety, hostility	Each symptom dimension represented on a 100-mm line extending from "not-at-all" to "extremely"	Derogatis [64]	Derogatis et al. [42]	Overly psychopathological symptom dimensions not appropriate with most medically ill patients
Single affect					
Hamilton Psychiatric Rating Scale for Depression	Depression	23 ratings	Hamilton [65]	Schwab [66]; Morris et al. [67]; Greer et al. [68]	Designed to assess primary depressive illness, seldom found in medically ill

10.3 Gottschalk–Gleser Verbal Content Analysis Scales

10.3.1 Introduction

Another method for measuring mood state in addition to self-report and observer-rated measures is a less well-known method, the content analysis of verbal behavior. Content analysis of an individual's speech has proved a useful alternative approach in evaluating the mood states of a medically ill patient. The G–G has been used with increasing frequency in the past several years among medically ill patients as a sensitive measure of immediate emotional states. It has been used with medical patients because of the ease of administration and the ability to repeat it frequently. The G–G was developed on the theory that psychological states are strongly influenced by biological roots. The definitions of each state and the selection of the specific verbal content items that are used in the assessment of each state are associated with the biological characteristics of the individual.

10.3.2 Method

The subject is instructed to speak into a tape recorder for 5 min. The instructions are general and are given to the subject as follows:

> This is a study of speaking and conversations habits. Upon a signal from me, I would like you to speak for five minutes about any interesting or dramatic personal life experiences you have had. Once you have started, I will be here listening to you, but I would prefer not to reply to any questions you might feel like asking me until the five minute period is over. Do you have any questions you would like to ask me now before we start? Well, then you may begin.

The instructions may be developed to suit the medical situation, as long as the same instructions are given to each patient at each assessment period. Holland et al. [12], for example, used the following instructions with mastectomy patients:

> I would like you to talk into the tape recorder for five minutes about anything that comes to your mind, such as interesting experiences you have had since your operation, or in the last months, or earlier in your life. During these five minutes, I won't speak to answer questions. You may begin now.

The 5-min verbal samples are transcribed verbatim, and the transcript is then scored by a trained technician for the presence and intensity of up to 16 psychological dimensions. A trained research technician follows a strictly empirical approach in the scoring of each grammatical clause of speech in the verbal sample, using well-delineated linguistic categories to define each of the separate verbal behavior scales. The technician then follows prescribed mathematic calculations to determine a final score for the magnitude of any one psychological state.

The speech analysis takes into account the syntax of the clause and the semantics of the words, phrases, and entire clause. Differential weights are assigned to semantic and linguistic cues that reflect magnitude of subjective experience. The number of words spoken per unit time is corrected so that intersubject and intrasubject comparisons can be made. Patients who speak less than 300 words are unscorable. Reliability increases with volume of words in the 5-min sample. A formal scale of weighted content categories is specified for each scale.

The most reliable and widely used scales are Anxiety, Hostility, and Depression. The Anxiety Scale yields a total anxiety score, which measures total manifest anxiety resultant from six Anxiety Subscales:

1. Death Anxiety – references to death, threat of death, or anxiety about death.
2. Mutilation (Castration) Anxiety – references to injury, tissue or physical damage, or anxiety about injury or threat of such.
3. Separation Anxiety – references to desertion, abandonment, ostracism, loss of support, falling, loss of love or love object, or threat of such.
4. Guilt Anxiety – references to adverse criticism, abuse, condemnation, moral disapproval, guilt, or threat of such.
5. Shame Anxiety – references to ridicule, inadequacy, shame, embarrassment, humiliation, overexposure of deficiencies or private details, or threat of such.
6. Diffuse or Nonspecific Anxiety – references to anxiety or fear without distinguishing type or source of anxiety.

There are three Hostility Scales:

1. Hostility Outward (which can be classified as overt or covert) focuses on destructive, injurious, or critical thoughts or actions directed at others.
2. Hostility Inward (which correlates strongly with depression [16]) measures immediate thoughts, actions, or feelings that are self-critical or self-destructive.
3. Ambivalent Hostility assesses destructive, injurious, or critical thoughts or actions of others (including situations) toward the person.

Other scales commonly scored include Hope, Cognitive-Intellectual Impairment, and Social Alienation-Personal Disorganization.

10.3.3 Scoring and Administration Issues

As with other projective tests, the procedures and instructions of the G-G must be adhered to strictly to achieve comparability with the norms of the scales and the findings of other investigators. This sensitivity to variability in procedure and instructions can be a serious drawback. The personality and sex of the interviewer have been shown to influence the content of the elicited speech [17]. Men, for example, may not verbalize hostility as readily with a female interviewer as with a male interviewer. Also, some interviewers may elicit greater emotional content in the verbal sample through such subtle means as nonvocal cues [17]. In addition to limiting comparability to other findings and normative data, this methodological problem may also be inherent in studies that employ more than one interviewer. Evaluation and control of interviewer differences should be an important part of any study using the G-G. In addition to interviewer variability, another important source of variability includes differences in instructions, which can elicit different verbal contents. The short administration time required (usually not more than 10 min) is an important consideration because medically ill patients are sometimes reluctant to agree to an extensive psychological assessment. The G-G Scale is easily administered. The evaluation requirements are a tape recorder and the reading of standardized instructions. The presence of a skilled evaluator is not necessary. The G-G test situation attempts to minimize the interviewer as a variable and maximize the internal psychological state of the subject. The instrument itself does not make any physical demands, such as writing, which can be a problem for physically ill patients. It requires only that the patient speak intelligible English and be willing to speak into a tape recorder.

Though administration of the G-G is relatively simple, scoring of the scales is not. Scoring of the G-G is much more complex and expensive than scoring standard self-report measures. Use of the G-G requires extensive training and practice for a scorer to reliably score the verbal content speech samples according to the scale developers' intent. If more than one scorer is used in a study, then extensive interrater reliability procedures must be used to ensure reliable agreement among the raters. Interscorer reliability must be .85 or higher to provide satisfactory reliability. Alternately, a scoring service is available through the scale's authors that, although costly, provides a greater assurance of reliable scoring.

The authors of the scale have achieved high interrater and test-retest reliability levels and have conducted many validation studies. The G-G has been used to study psychophysiological processes, such as the relationship of psychological state to phases of the menstrual cycle [18, 19], pharmacological studies [20–22], and psychotherapeutic processes and outcome [23]. For a more thorough description of the instrument and the many reliability and validity studies, see the reports of Gottschalk [24–27], Gottschalk and Gleser [17], and Gottschalk et al. [28].

10.3.4 Use with Medical Patients

The focus of this report is a review of studies that have used the G-G in evaluating medically ill patients: three studies of mood in cancer patients, three studies with coronary patients, and four studies evaluating patients with other medical diseases.

10.3.4.1 Use with Cancer Patients

Sholiton et al. [29] undertook a study to examine the possible etiological role of anxiety in adrenocortical hyperfunction in some patients with bronchogenic carcinoma. The G-G was one of three psychological measures administered to a group of 14 male patients with inoperable bronchogenic carcinoma and to a group of 14 male patients with chronic, moderately stabilized, nonneoplastic disease (such as heart disease or ulcer). There was no difference in levels of anxiety and hostility as measured by all of the instruments, including the G-G, between the two groups of patients. The G-G did reveal the only significant finding of the study: hostility outward and inward were positively correlated with overall plasma steroid levels in both groups. Anxiety failed to correlate.

Sixteen patients with metastatic carcinoma receiving total- or half-body irradiation as palliative treatment were evaluated before and after treatment and at six time intervals afterward with the Halstead Battery, the WAIS, the Reitan tests, and the G-G [30]. The battery of tests was given for assessment of cognitive and intellectual impairment and emotonal states such as anxiety, hostility, and hope. The G-G was the only instrument to yield a significant difference: Anxiety levels before treatment were significantly higher than those immediately after irradiation, reflecting apprehension about the unknown treatment. A significant impairment of cognitive functioning occurred after irradiation, which, the authors theorized, might be caused by nonspecific stress. The authors also found that the G-G's Hope Scale correlated with the course of disease. Hope scores obtained from the pretreatment verbal sample correlated with period of hospitalization and survival time. Higher initial hope scores were significantly associated with a shorter period of hospitalization and a longer survival time.

In another study examining the psychological correlates of radiotherapy treatment, Holland et al. [12] evaluated 20 women referred for radiotherapy following mastectomy. They were assessed using the G-G before their first radiotherapy treatment, during the 2nd week of treatment, and near the end of treatment, which was after approximately 4–6 weeks. There was a significant increase in hostility inward (depression) from pretreatment to the end of treatment, a significant increase in hostility outward (anger) at the 2nd week, and a significant decrease in mutilation anxiety during the treatment. Total anxiety, hope, and diffuse anxiety also decreased over time but not significantly. Important clinical applications of the results were to increase staff awareness of the patients' increased psychological distress when reaching the end of treatment. Staff who anticipate the response can plan for added emotional support around and following termination of therapy.

10.3.4.2 Use with Coronary Patients

Miller [31] utilized the G-G to compare 34 medical outpatients with a previous history of coronary artery disease with 34 medical outpatients free of coronary artery disease. Coronary patients were found to score significantly higher on overall anxiety and the Anxiety Subscales of Death, Separation, Shame, and Diffuse Anxiety. They were significantly more depressed (hostility inward) and exhibited significantly higher levels of ambivalent hostility than the noncoronary subjects. In addition, younger coronary patients scored consistently higher than older patients and controls on all of the G-G Scales. The impact of having a myocardial infarction, particularly in the younger patients, produced psychological disturbance in the form of anxiety and depression, as assessed by the G-G. The authors of this study commented favorably on the utility of the G-G and even developed a new scale, "achievement," scored from the verbal sample.

Leigh et al. [10] monitored the psychological impact of different environments in a coronary care unit. Patients in an "open," noisy, four-bedroom unit of a coronary care unit with individual private cubicles were assessed by means of the G-G, the Zuckerman Anxiety Scale, and a specifically devised questionnaire. Analysis of the verbal content analysis scales revealed that separation anxiety and covert hostility outward (which measures denied and displaced hostility) were significantly greater in the "closed" unit than in the "open" unit. Death anxiety and diffuse anxiety also tended to be higher in the "closed" unit. Shame anxiety, mutilation anxiety, and guilt anxiety, as well as overt hostility, tended to be higher in the "open" unit. Contrary to the authors' expectation, results indicated that patients in the "closed" unit did not have a reduction in anxiety levels as a result of this quiet environment. The authors also found that the risk of developing cardiac arrhythmias while on the coronary care unit (regardless of whether it was "open" or "closed") was significantly greater in patients who had higher levels of separation anxiety and hostility inward as well as lower levels of overt hostility. These "high-risk" scales significantly differentiated those patients who later developed cardiac arrhythmias while on the unit from those who did not, suggesting that certain affective states may be associated with a higher incidence of cardiac arrhythmias following myocardial infarction. The authors noted that the G-G provided more sensitive quantitative data on affective states than the self-report inventories, neither of which yielded any significant results.

Gottschalk et al. [32] employed the G-G to evaluate ten male patients with angina who had a history of coronary artery disease. They were studied in a randomized, double-blind crossover study of marijuana. Patients were given the G-G immediately before and after smoking a marijuana cigarette and a placebo marijuana cigarette (on a successive morning). They were also assessed at four half-hour intervals afterward. Though no significant changes in emotional state occurred after marijuana smoking, a significant increase in cognitive and intellectual impairment occured 0.5 h after patients smoked the marijuana cigarette. Significant psychophysiological correlations occurred between hostility-inward and -outward scores, anxiety scores, and blood pressure during placebo marijuana smoking. These significant correlations did not occur, however, during marijuana smoking. Apparently, the effects of marijuana on the central nervous system and peripheral cardiovascular system account for the negation of psychophysiological correlations.

10.3.4.3 Use with Other Medically Ill Patients

The effects of perphenazine on psychological variables were monitored in subjects hospitalized with various dermatological diseases [33]. In a double-blind, placebo crossover study, it was found that the psychoactive drug did indeed effect a significant decrease in outward hostility. The authors concluded that the G-G appears to be of significant sensitivity to accurately assess the effect of psychoactive drugs on mental processes.

In a study of hypertensive outpatients, a group of subjects with the diagnosis of essential hypertension scored significantly higher on both hostility outward and hostility inward than did a group of ambulatory medical outpatients with diagnoses such as bronchial asthma or ulcer [34]. The hypertensive and nonhypertensive female patients were differentiated more in terms of hostility inward, whereas the two male groups were distinguished by differing levels of hostility outward. However, the authors noted that while the hypertensive subjects talked into the tape recorder, the mean systolic blood pressure rose 6.7 mmHg. This level was significantly higher than that of the nonhypertensive subjects, which actually decreased by 4.9 mmHg. The mean diastolic blood pressure of the hypertensive subjects rose 2.1 mmHg; this level was also significantly higher than that of the nonhypertensive subjects, which decreased by 2.5 mmHg. Evidently, emotional tension (as measured by blood pressure response) rose in the hypertensive subjects during the assessment procedure, whereas the nonhypertensive subjects became more relaxed. This finding again points to the extreme sensitivity of the G-G to immediate emotional state.

A later study, again with hypertensive subjects [35], examined the effect of hydrochlorothiazide on affect in relation to blood pressure. When the subject was taking a placebo, significant positive correlations occurred between hostility-inward levels and average systolic and diastolic blood pressures, and significant negative correlations occurred between hostility-outward levels and blood pressure. These significant psycho-physiological correlations did not occur when the subjects were taking hydrochlorothiazide (a finding similar to that in the marijuana study cited previously). Results of the prior hypertension study [35] were corroborated when it was found that talking for 5 min into a tape recorder in the presence of another person increased the blood pressure of the hypertensive subjects.

Rad et al. [36] examined the theory of alexithymia by comparing 40 outpatients labeled "psychosomatic" (25 had either peptic ulcer or ulcerative colitis) with 40 "psychoneurotic" outpatients. The authors used the G–G in a novel manner: The first 1000 words spoken by the patient in a psychoanalytic interview were scored. Results confirmed the theory of restricted expression of feelings in psychosomatic patients. They expressed significantly lower levels of total anxiety, guilt anxiety, shame anxiety, separation anxiety, and diffuse anxiety than the neurotic group. The psychosomatic group also had significantly lower levels of hostility inward and ambivalent hostility than the neurotic group. The authors cited the following reasons for using the G–G: The instrument is based on psychoanalytic premises similar to the study's hypotheses, it is well validated, and it is adaptable to German. The authors did note, however, that schooling and occupational differences can influence scores.

10.4 Summary of Research

Table 3 presents an outline of the ten studies cited previously. Several observations can be made from Table 3:

1. Of the ten studies, three used evaluation measures in addition to the G–G; none of the other measures yielded significant results as compared to the G–G, which yielded significant results in all ten studies.
2. The G–G appears to be sensitive to pharmacological-physiological relationships [29, 32, 33, 35], treatment effects [12, 30], environmental effects [10], and psychological factors related to specific disease states [31, 34, 36].
3. The Anxiety and Hostility Scales appear to be the most frequently used and most valuable scales of the G–G for evaluation of medical patients.
4. The G–G is particularly suitable for longitudinal follow-up studies, as its test-retest reliability is excellent. Five of the studies [12, 30, 32, 33, 35] used the G–G in a repeated-measures design.
5. If one tentatively generalizes across studies, one can conclude that anxiety levels are highest when radiotherapy begins and subside as treatment continues [12, 30] and that disease states have their own specific associated emotional factors [31, 34, 36].

Figures 1 and 2 depict the overall levels of anxiety and hostility for the nonpharmacological studies reviewed in Table 3. The studies of Kaplan et al. [34] and Rad et al. [36] are not included because their scoring and methodological procedures differed greatly from those of the other studies.

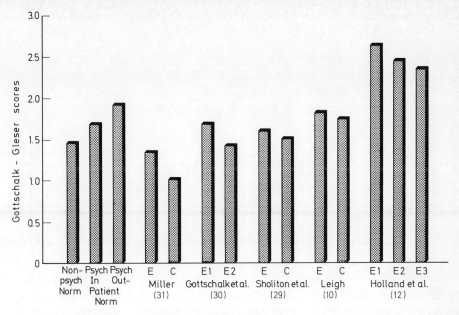

Fig. 1. Gottschalk-Gleser overall anxiety scores of five studies. *C*, comparison group; *E*, experimental group; *E1*, experimental group immediately before first treatment; *E2*, experimental group 2 weeks after treatment; *E3*, experimental group 6 weeks after treatment

It is evident from Fig. 1 that the anxiety levels of the medically ill in these studies exceed, in most cases, the nonpsychiatric norm; in two studies they exceed the psychiatric inpatient norm. Reported levels of anxiety in the study by Holland et al. [12] exceed even the psychiatric outpatient norm levels.

Figure 2 depicts the levels of the three Hostility Scales for the same studies as compared to the nonpsychiatric norm (psychiatric norm levels for hostility are not available). The medically ill generally exhibit higher levels of hostility outward and ambivalent hostility and much higher levels of hostility inward (depression). The comparison of G–G scores from different studies to the norms is somewhat tenuous because of variability in procedure and instructions. Nevertheless, use of the G–G with the medically ill appears to confirm clinical observations of pathological degrees of mood state in the medically ill.

10.5 Conclusions

The G–G has demonstrated sensitivity to the immediate mood states of patients with several different medical diseases. Environmental stresses such as treatment of disease and physical structure of room can, as evaluated by the G–G, have significant psychological effects on patients. In addition, the G–G appears to avoid many of the pitfalls of self-report and observer-rated measures.

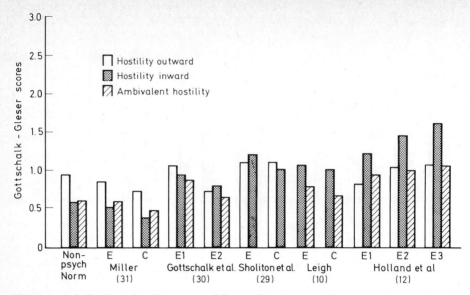

Fig. 2 Gottschalk–Gleser hostility scores of five studies. *C*, comparison group; *E*, experimental group; *E1*, experimental group immediately before first treatment; *E2*, experimental group 2 weeks after treatment; *E3*, experimental group 6 weeks after treatment

A problem of the G–G method is the effect of the evaluation instrument itself, the tape recorder. Talking into a tape recorder, in addition to the unstructured nature of the task, can be anxiety provoking and has been shown to elevate blood pressure levels [34, 35]. Certain population groups, such as the elderly or some minorities, who have little experience talking into a tape recorder or who have speech difficulties, may be especially prone to anxiety effects. Thus, the very evaluation of mood state itself may alter mood state, in particular, anxiety. In addition, some patients may be reluctant to comply with the G–G procedure because of its anxiety-provoking nature, though none of the studies cited in this review have noted such a problem.

The versatility of assessing many different mood states is an important advantage of the G–G technique. One is not limited by a priori hypotheses regarding specific mood states. The G–G reflects a full range of affect in addition to cognitive functioning and an elevation of schizophrenia. Furthermore, the specificity of type of anxiety is a unique feature of this instrument that is particularly relevant to the medically ill. Death, separation, mutilation, guilt, and shame are all types of anxieties seen in medically ill patients.

The advent of newer, more modern medical-technological advances will bring new machinery, treatment modalities, and treatment settings that may evoke adverse psychological reactions in patients. An instrument, such as the G–G, which can appropriately evaluate psychological reactions to modern medicine, can prove very useful in clinical research settings.

References

1. Cohen J, Cullen JW, Martin L (eds) (1981) Psychosocial aspects of cancer. Raven, New York
2. Holland JC (1973) Psychological aspects of cancer medicine. In: Holland JF, Frei E (eds) Cancer Medicine. Lea and Febiger, Philadelphia
3. Krug SE (ed) (1977) Psychological assessment in medicine. Institute for Personality and Ability Testing, Champaign
4. Prokop CK, Bradley LA (eds) (1982) Medical psychology: contributions to behavioral medicine. Academic, New York
5. Stone GC, Cohen F, Adler NE (eds) (1979) Health psychology. Jossey-Bass, San Francisco
6. Strain JJ (1978) Psychological interventions in medical practice. Appleton-Century-Crofts, New York
7. Strain JJ, Grossman S (1975) Psychological care of the medically ill: a primer in liaison psychiatry. Appleton-Century-Crofts, New York
8. Weiss SM, Herd JA, Fox BH (eds) (1981) Perspectives on behavioral medicine. Academic, New York
9. Holland JC, Plumb M, Yates J, Harris S, Tuttolomondo A, Holmes J, Holland JF (1977) Psychological response of patients with acute leukemia to germ-free environments. Cancer 40: 871–879
10. Leigh H, Hofer MA, Cooper J, Reiser MF (1972) A psychological comparison of patients in "open" and "closed" coronary care units. J Psychosom Res 16: 449–457
11. Forester BM, Kornfield DS, Fleiss J (1978) Psychiatric aspects of radiotherapy. Am J Psychiatry 135: 960–963
12. Holland JC, Rowland J, Lebovits A, Rusalem F (1979) Reactions to cancer treatment: assessment of emotional response to adjuvant radiotherapy as a guide to planned intervention. Psychiatr Clin North Am 2: 347–358
13. Mitchell GW, Glicksman AS (1977) Cancer patients: knowledge and attitudes. Cancer 40: 61–66
14. Peck A, Boland J (1977) Emotional reactions to radiotherapy treatment. Cancer 40: 180–184
15. Peterson LG, Popkin MK (1980) Neuropsychiatric effects of chemotherapeutic agents for cancer. Psychosomatics 21: 141–153
16. Gershon ES, Cromer M, Klerman GL (1968) Hostility and depression. Psychiatry 31: 224–235
17. Gottschalk LA, Gleser GC (1969) The measurement of psychological states through the content analysis of verbal behavior. University of California Press, Los Angeles
18. Gottschalk LA, Kaplan SM, Gleser GC, Winget CM (1962) Variations in magnitude of emotion: a method applied to anxiety and hostility during phases of the menstrual cycle. Psychosom Med 24: 300–311
19. Ivey ME, Bardwick JM (1968) Patterns of affective fluctuation in the menstrual cycle. Psychosom Med 30: 336–345
20. Gottschalk LA, Biener R, Noble EP, Birch H, Wilbert DE, Heiser JF (1975) Thioridazine plasma levels and clinical response. Compr Psychiatry 16: 323–337
21. Gottschalk LA, Stone WN, Gleser GC (1974) Peripheral versus central mechanisms accounting for anti-anxiety effect of propanol. Psychosom Med 36: 47–56
22. Stone WN, Gleser GC, Gottschalk LA (1973) Anxiety and beta adrenergic blockade. Arch Gen Psychiatry 29: 620–622
23. Gottschalk LA, Springer KJ, Gleser GC (1961) Experiments with a method of assessing the variation in intensity of certain psychological states occurring during two psychotherapeutic interviews. In: Gottschalk LA (ed) Comparative psycholinguistic analysis of two psychotherapeutic interviews. International Universities Press, New York

24. Gottschalk LA (1977) Recent advances in the content analysis of speech and the application of this measurement approach to psychosomatic research. Psychother Psychosom 28: 73–82
25. Gottschalk LA (1978) Content analysis of speech in psychiatric research. Compr Psychiatry 19: 387–392
26. Gottschalk LA (1979) The content analysis of verbal behavior: further studies. Halstead, New York
27. Gottschalk LA (1982) Manual of uses and applications of the Gottschalk-Gleser verbal behavior scales. Res Commun Psychol Psychiatry Behav 7: 273–327
28. Gottschalk LA, Winget CN, Gleser GC (1969) Manual of instructions for using the Gottschalk-Gleser content analysis: anxiety, hostility, and social alienation-personal disorganization. University of California Press, Los Angeles
29. Sholiton L, Wohl T, Werk E (1963) The correlation of two psychological variables, anxiety and hostility with adrenal cortical function in patients with lung cancer. Cancer 16: 223–230
30. Gottschalk LA, Kunkel R, Wohl TH, Saenger EL, Winget CN (1969) Total and half body irradiation: Effect on cognitive and emotional processes. Arch Gen Psychiatry 21: 574–580
31. Miller CK (1965) Psychological correlates of coronary artery disease. Psychosom Med 27: 257–265
32. Gottschalk LA, Aronow WS, Prakash R (1977) Effect of marijuana and placebo-marijuana smoking on psychological state and on psychophysiological cardiovascular functioning in anginal patients. Biol Psychiatry 12: 255–266
33. Gottschalk LA, Gleser GC, Springer KJ, Kaplan SM, Shanon J, Ross WD (1960) Effects of perphenazine on verbal behavior patterns. Arch Gen Psychiatry 2: 632–639
34. Kaplan SM, Gottschalk LA, Magliocco EB, Rohovit D, Ross WD (1961) Hostility in verbal productions and hypnotic dreams of hypertensive patients. Psychosom Med 23: 311–322
35. Gottschalk LA, Gleser GC, D'Zmura T, Hanenson IB (1964) Some psychophysiologic relations in hypertensive women. Psychosom Med 26: 610–617
36. Rad MV, Drucke M, Knauss W, Lolas F (1979) Alexithymia: anxiety and hostility in psychosomatic patients. Psychother Psychosom 31: 223–234
37. McNair DM, Lorr D (1964) An analysis of mood in neurotics. J Abnorm Soc Psychol 69: 620–627
38. Weissman AD, Worden JW (1976–77) The existential plight in cancer: significance of the first 100 days. Int J Psychiatry Med 7: 1–15
39. Worden JW, Sobel HJ (1978) Ego strength and psychosocial adaptation to cancer. Psychosom Med 40: 585–592
40. Derogatis LR, Lipman RS, Covi L (1973) The SCL-90: an outpatient psychiatric rating scale-preliminary report. Psychopharmacol Bull 9: 13–27
41. Craig TJ, Abeloff MD (1974) Psychiatric symptomatology among hospitalized cancer patients. Am J Psychiatry 131: 1323–1327
42. Derogatis LR, Abeloff MD, McBeth CD (1976) Cancer patients and their physicians in the perception of psychological symptoms. Psychosomatics 17: 197–201
43. Derogatis LR, Abeloff MD, Melisaratos N (1979) Psychological coping mechanisms and survival time in metastatic breast cancer. JAMA 242: 1504–1508
44. Wider A (1948) The cornell medical index. Psychological Corporation, New York
45. Beder OE, Weinstein P (1980) Explorations of the coping of adolescents with orofacial anomalies using the Cornell Medical Index. Prosthet Dentistry 43: 565–567
46. McKegney F, Gordon R, Levine S (1980) A psychosomatic comparison of patients with ulcerative colitis and Crohn's disease. Psychosom Med 32: 153–160
47. Goldberg DP (1972) The detection of psychiatric illness by questionnaire. Maudsley monograph no. 21. Oxford University Press, London
48. Jones RA, Murphy E (1979) Severity of psychiatric disorder and the 30-item general health questionnaire. Br J Psychiatry 134: 609–616

49. Tennant O (1977) The general health questionnaire: a valid index of psychological impairment in Australian populations. Med J Aust 2: 392–394

50. Beck AT, Ward CH, Mendelson M, Mock J, Erbaugh J (1961) An inventory for measuring depression. Arch Gen Psychiatry 4: 561–571

51. Plumb M, Holland JC (1977) Comparative studies of psychological function in patients with advanced cancer – I. Self reported depressive symptoms. Psychosom Med 39: 264–276

52. Lyon JS (1977) Management of psychological problems in breast cancer. In: Stoll BA (ed) Breast cancer management early and late. Yearbook Medical, Chicago

53. Spielberger CD, Gorsuch RL, Lushene RE (1970) Manual for the state-trait anxiety inventory. Consultant Psychologists, Palo Alto

54. Gentry WD, Foster S, Haney T (1972) Denial as a determinant of anxiety and perceived health status in the coronary care unit. Psychosom Med 34: 39–44

55. Spielberger CD, Wadsworth AP, Averbach SM, Dunn TM, Taulbee ES (1973) Emotional reactions to surgery. J Consult Clin Psychol 40: 33–38

56. Auerbach SM (1973) Trait-state anxiety and adjustment to surgery. J Consult Clin Psychol 40: 264–271

57. Zung WK (1965) A self-rating depression scale. Arch Gen Psychiatry 12: 63–70

58. Steuer J, Bank L, Olsen EJ, Jarvik LF (1980) Depression, physical health, and somatic complaints in the elderly: a study of the Zung self-rating depression scale. J Gerontol 35: 683–688

59. Cattell RB, Scheir IH (1963) Handbook for the IPAT anxiety scale questionnaire (self-analysis form). Institute Personality Ability Testing, Campaign

60. Schonfield J (1972) Psychological factors related to delayed return to an earlier life style in successfully treated cancer patients. J Psychosom Res 16: 41

61. Endicott J, Spitzer RL (1972) Current and past psychopathology scales (CAPPS): rationale, reliability and validity. Arch Gen Psychiatry 27: 678–687

62. Plumb M, Holland JC (1981) Comparative studies of psychological function in patients with advanced cancer II. Interviewer-rated current and past psychological symptoms. Psychosom Med 43: 243–254

63. Gorzynski JG, Lebovits AH, Holland JC, Vugrin D (1981) Psychosexual risk factors in testicular cancer. Psychosom Med 43: 89–90

64. Derogatis LR (1977) SCL-90 manual-I. Johns Hopkins University School of Medicine, Baltimore

65. Hamilton M (1967) Development of a rating scale for primary depressive illness. Br J Soc Clin Psychol 6: 278–296

66. Schwab JJ (1967) Hamilton rating scale for depression and medical inpatients. Br J Psychiatry 113: 83–88

67. Morris T, Greer HS, White P (1977) Psychological and social adjustment to mastectomy: a two-year follow-up study. Cancer 40: 2381–2387

68. Greer S, Morris T, Pettingale KW (1979) Psychological response to breast cancer: Effect on outcome. Lancet 785–787

Table 1. Examples of self-report inventories used with medically ill patients

Instrument	Mood states	Total no. of items	Response format	Developers	Examples of use in medically ill	Problems of use in medically ill
Multidimensional						
Profile of mood states	Tension, depression, anger, vigor, fatigue, confusion, total mood disturbance	65	Five-point adjective rating scale	McNair, Lorr [37]	Weissman, Worden [38]; Worden, Sobel [39]	Normative data limited to psychiatric outpatients and students
Symptom Checklist	Depression, anxiety, hostility	Original, 90; short, 45	Five-point scale of distress	Derogatis et al. [40]	Craig, Abeloff [41]; Derogatis et al. [42]; Derogatis et al. [43]	Several symptom dimensions such as "paranoid ideation" not present in most medically ill samples
Cornell Medical Index	Inadequacy, depression, anxiety, sensitivity, anger, tension	195	Yes/no format	Wider [44]	Beder, Weinstein [45]; McKegney et al. [46]	Many items evaluate dimensions other than mood state
General Health Questionnaire	Depression, anxiety	Several forms: 12, 20, 30, 36, 60, and 140 items	Four-point scale	Goldberg [47]	Jones, Murphy [48]; Tennant [49]	Based on psychiatric diagnostic criteria
Single affect						
Beck Depression Inventory	Depression	Original, 21; short, 13	Four-point scale	Beck et al. [50]	Plumb, Holland [51]; Lyon [52]	Limited to one affect
Spielberger State – Trait Anxiety Inventory	Anxiety	20	Four-point scale	Spielberger et al. [53]	Gentry et al. [54]; Spielberger et al. [55]; Auerbach [56]	Limited to one affect
Zung Self-Rating Depression Scale	Depression	20	Four-point scale	Zung [57]	Gentry et al. [54]; Steuer et al. [58]	Limited to one affect
Institute Personality Ability Testing Anxiety Scale	Anxiety	40	True/false format	Cattell, Scheir [59]	Sholiton et al. [29]; Schonfield [60]	Limited to one affect

Table 3. Studies using the Gottschalk-Gleser Verbal Content Analysis Scales (G-G) with medically ill samples

Authors	Subject sample	Objectives	Other psychological measures	Measures yielding significant results	G-G Scales used	Significant G-G findings
Cancer studies						
Sholiton et al. [29]	Lung cancer compared to chronic nonneoplastic diseases (e.g., heart disease/ulcer)	Emotional factors and adrenocortical hyperfunction	Clinical Rating Scale; IPAT Anxiety Scale	G-G	A, HI, HO	HI and HO correlated with overall plasma steroid levels in both groups
Gottschalk et al. [30]	Metastatic cancer, solid tumors	Cognitive and emotional factors and total- vs half-body irradiation assessed over time	Halstead Battery; Reitan tests; WAIS	G-G	A, HI, HO, AH, H, CII	CII after irradiation; pretreatment A > posttreatment A; higher pretreatment H associated with shorter period of hospitalization and longer survival time
Holland et al. [12]	Breast cancer with positive axillary nodes	Emotional factors and radiotherapy assessed over time	None	G-G	A, HI, HO, AH, H, As	HI and HO increased over time; mutilation A decreased over time
Coronary studies						
Miller [31]	Coronary artery disease compared with nondisease group by age and sex	Psychological factors and coronary artery disease	None	G-G	A, HI, HO, AH, As	Coronary patients had higher A, HI, AH; younger coronary patients scored consistently higher than older patients on all scales
Leigh et al. [10]	Patients in closed CCU compared to open CCU	Psychological comparison of CCU environments	Zuckerman Anxiety Scale; questionnaire by authors	G-G	A, HI, HO, AH, As	Closed CCU patients had higher separation A and covert HO

Table 3. (continued)

Study	Population	Focus			Measures	Results
Gottschalk et al. [32]	Coronary artery disease	Marijuana smoking, psychological and physiological states	None	G-G	A, HI, HO, AH, CII, SAPD	CII after marijuana smoking; in absence of marijuana psycho-physiological correlations occur
Other studies						
Gottschalk et al. [33]	Dermatological diseases (hospitalized)	Effects of perphenazine	None	G-G	A, HI, HO	Perphenazine reduced HO
Kaplan et al. [34]	Essential hypertension outpatients compared with medical outpatients (e.g., asthma)	Hostility of hypertensive patients	None	G-G	HI, HO	Hypertension group had higher HI, HO
Gottschalk et al. [35]	Essential hypertension outpatients	Psychophysiological relations among blood pressure, affect, and hydrochlorothiazide	None	G-G	A, HI, HO, AH	Positive correlation between HI and blood pressure; negative correlation between HO and blood pressure; all correlations disappear with hydrochlorothiazide
Rad et al. [36]	Psychosomatic outpatients (e.g., peptic ulcer, asthma) compared with "neurotic" outpatients	Alexithymia in psychosomatic patients	None	G-G	A, HI, HO, AH, As	Psychosomatic patients had lower A, HI, AH, separation A, guilt A, shame A, and diffuse A

IPAT = Institute Personality Ability Testing; A = total anxiety; HI = hostility inward (depression); HO = hostility outward; WAIS = Wechsler Adult Intelligence Scales; AH = ambivalent hostility; H = hope; CII = cognitive intellectual impairment; As = anxiety subscales; CCU = coronary care unit; SAPD = social alienation – personal disorganization.

11 Affective Content of Speech and Treatment Outcome in Bruxism*

Susana Aronsohn, Fernando Lolas, Arturo Manns, and Rodolfo Miralles

11.1 Introduction

Bruxism, the nonfunctional clenching and grinding of the teeth, and its associated my-ofascial pain dysfunction (MPD) syndrome have been explained either on the basis of mechanical (i. e., occlusal disharmonies) or psychological factors [5]. No definite conclusions regarding psychological characteristics have been reached by means of conventional psychometric testing. An alternative approach is furnished by content analysis of verbal behavior, which attempts to measure psychological states on the basis of the content of communication. Thus, inferences may be drawn from on-line information provided by the subject's speech behavior. The Gottschalk-Gleser method was designed to specify and quantify different kinds of emotions, taking into consideration the surface meaning as well as the "deeper layers of meaning embedded in the content" [7]. Clear-cut instructions are available for the coding and scoring of verbal samples according to content analysis scales of affect.

As stated by Lebovits and Holland [11], this method provides a systematic approach for the study of the psychological aspects of medical illness, without the drawbacks of interference of the subject's own state or the need of clinical skill posed by self- or observer-report scales. Characteristic speech patterns might be used to indicate intrapsychic modes of functioning.

The aim of this work was to gather information on the psychological profile of a group of patients affected by bruxism and MPD syndrome and its relation to dental treatment outcome (occlusal splint). Aside from conventional psychometric testing, verbal analyses of spontaneous speech and nonverbal behavior were evaluated to delineate the psychological characteristics. It was hypothesized that certain combinations of physical signs plus psychological makeup might predispose patients to chronicity and thus make them refractory to dental treatment alone [9].

* This research was partially supported by a project from the Departamento de Desarrollo de la Investigacion, University of Chile.

11.2 Method

11.2.1 Subjects

The study involved 15 patients (13 females and 2 males), aged 16–45 years, who met the following criteria [2, 10, 14]: spontaneous facial pain in the preauricular area, painful tenderness to palpation in the masticatory muscles, alteration of mandibular dynamics (mandibular deviation and/or restricted opening), clicking or popping sounds of the temporomandibular joints, and bruxism (grinding or clenching of the teeth).

11.2.2 Psychological Assessment

Inmediately after selection and before any dental treatment, subjects were administered a set of psychological tests and went through a semistandardized video-recorded interview. Questions were aimed at finding out mainly about physical complaints and subjective and expressive aspects of emotional behavior.

Psychological assessment included administration of the Eysenck Personality Inventory Form A [4], Beck [1] and Zung [17] Depression Inventories, and the Alexithymia Questionnaire, both in the original Beth Israel Hospital version (1973) as well as in a quantitated form [12].

11.2.3 Verbal Behavior

Content analysis was performed on the verbal transcripts of the interview. The Gottschalk-Gleser method was used to quantify the following:
1. *Anxiety:* measures "free" anxiety classified into six subtypes: death, mutilation, separation, guilt, shame, and diffuse or nonspecific anxiety.
2. *Hostility:* measures three types of a transient rather than enduring affect. According to the direction of this affect, the subtypes of Hostility-Directed-Outward, Hostility-Directed-Inward, and Ambivalent-Hostility Scales are defined. All three scales assign higher weights to scorable verbal statements communicating hostility that is more likely to be experienced by the speaker himself.

Scores on each of the Hostility and Anxiety Scales as well as on the total Anxiety Scale were obtained.

11.2.4 Nonverbal Behavior

Self-manipulative and illustrative behaviors as defined by Ekman [3] were scored. Self-manipulative behavior is defined as any movement in which one part of the body comes into contact with another part of the body of the same person. These acts are independent from speech, and it has usually been assumed that they reveal feelings of anxiety. Illustrative behavior is directly linked to speech and is used to stress what the person is trying to communicate; it has been related to excitement and has been found to diminish in depressed subjects [3].

Frequency and duration of self-manipulative as well as frequency of illustrative behaviors were independently evaluated by two observers woh attained an interrater correlation of 0.80.

Verbal as well as nonverbal behavior was analyzed on the basis of three 3-min samples from the initial, middle, and last part of the interview.

11.2.5 Dental Procedure

All patients were treated with a maxillary occlusal splint. Its use was restricted to 3 h/day discontinuously and all night for 3 weeks to avoid extrusion of the posterior teeth.

The patients were evaluated before and after treatment as follows:
1. A clinical questionnaire was conducted in which the signs and symptoms of each patient were transcribed (see Table 1) on a scale of 0 to 3 (0, absence; 3, presence). Intermediate values indicated degrees of improvement (1, overt; 2, slight). Based on this scale, a mean value of 20 signs and symptoms was obtained for each patient before and after treatment.

Table 1. Clinical questionnaire. Signs and symptoms scores before and after treatment in patients with MPD syndrome[a]

Patients	Initial	Final
	$\overline{x}$	$\overline{x}$
1	2.85	0.62
2	2.55	0.50
3	2.10	0.12
4	1.80	0.40
5	2.70	0.15
6	2.55	0.45
7	1.50	0.07
8	2.85	0.87
9	2.55	1.80
10	1.65	0.07
11	1.65	0.50
12	3.00	0.20
13	2.40	0.37
14	1.65	0.60
15	2.50	0.60

[a] 0, absence; 1, overt improvement; 2, slight improvement; 3, presence

Table 2. Myoarticular palpation scores before and after treatment in patients with MPD syndrome[a]

Patients	Initial	Final
	$\overline{x}$	$\overline{x}$
1	4.12	1.81
2	3.50	0.48
3	2.71	0.51
4	3.83	0.68
5	4.48	0.43
6	2.79	0.95
7	3.78	0.55
8	4.55	2.45
9	4.86	4.86
10	4.17	0.12
11	2.94	0.48
12	5.00	0.43
13	2.86	0.66
14	3.37	1.59
15	4.18	0.98

[a] 0, absence; 1, slight; 2, intermediate; 3, moderate; 4, overt; 5, intense

2. Myoarticular palpation was performed to quantify the bilateral painful tenderness to palpation of the mandibular and neck muscles as well as of the temporomandibular

joints (see Table 2) on a scale of 0 to 5 (0, absence; 1, slight; 2, intermediate; 3, moderate; 4, overt; 5, intense). A mean value for the total myoarticular symptomatology (seven muscles and temporomandibular joints) was obtained for each patient before and after treatment.

The symptomatology tests were performed by two examiners, one in charge of the clinical questionnaire and the other of the myoarticular palpation. A double-blind procedure was used.

11.3 Results

Scores obtained in the psychological assessment of patients afflicted with bruxism are shown in Table 3. Nonverbal behavior as expressed in self-manipulative and illustrative movements reached total mean frequency values of 2.97 and 7.08/min, respectively. These preliminary data may serve for future characterization of such sample since no normative data are available at present.

Table 3. Average scores and SD for psychometric indicators in a sample of patients suffering from bruxism ($n = 15$)

Eysenck Personality Inventory		Beck	Zung	Alexithymia	Questionnaire
Extraversion	Neuroticism			Classical	Quantified
12.60 ± 1.90	14.86 ± 4.99	10.2 ± 9.0	47.73 ± 15.35	1.75 ± 1.86	24.66 ± 5.87

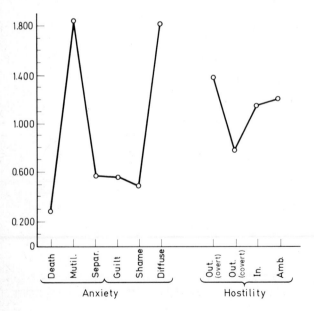

Fig. 1. Verbal content analysis scores for the Anxiety and Hostility Scales in the whole sample.

Verbal content analysis scores are presented as a profile in Fig. 1. Similar data presentation can be found in Lolas and von Rad [13]. It should be noted that patients suffering from bruxism show on average a significantly higher score regarding mutilation ($t = 11.4$; $df = 15$; $p < 0.01$) and diffuse anxiety ($t = 3.59$; $df = 15$; $p < 0.01$) than separation anxiety. This may indicate that complaints are focused on somatic aspects.

The mean scores on the Overt-Hostility, Covert-Hostility, Hostility-Directed-Inward, and Ambivalent-Hostility Scales were 1.371, 0.783, 1.135, and 1.191, respectively.

11.3.1 Initial Examination

Scores on the clinical questionnaire showed a correlation coefficient of 0.54 with the initial myoarticular palpation (Spearman rho).

No further significant correlations were found between either one of these evaluations and psychological variables.

11.3.2 Further Findings

Indices of the percentage of symptoms derived from the clinical questionnaire and the myoarticular disturbances that persisted after treatment were calculated by dividing the initial score (before treatment) into the final score (after) and multiplying by 100. These data are presented in Table 4.

Persistent subjective symptomatology correlated with Beck's depression score ($r = 0.446$) and negatively with the verbal and nonverbal expression of emotions: total hostility ($r = -0.667$) and self-manipulative behavior ($r = -0.429$). The score of per-

Table 4. Percentage of persisting subjective symptomatology and myoarticular disturbance after dental treatment.

Subjective symptomatology	Patients	Myoarticular disturbance	Patients
4.2	10	0.0	10
4.6	7	46.2	9
5.5	5	52.9	14
5.7	3	56.1	1
6.6	12	56.0	6
15.4	13	76.3	15
17.6	6	77.0	13
19.6	2	81.2	3
21.7	1	83.9	4
22.2	4	84.4	11
24.0	15	85.5	8
30.3	11	86.9	2
30.5	8	90.3	5
36.3	14	91.4	12
70.5	9	97.2	7

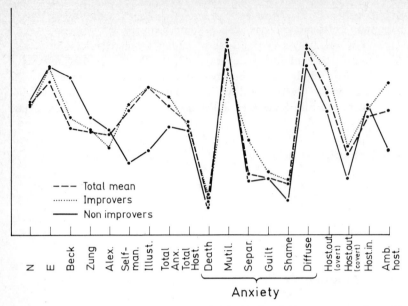

Fig. 2. Psychological assessment, mean nonverbal and verbal content scores in profile form for a sample of patients suffering from bruxism. Non-normalized data do not permit comparison between scales. *N*, neuroticism scores; *E*, extraversion scores (Eysenck Personality Inventory); *Self-man*, self-manipulatory movements; *Illus*, illustrative movements.

sisting myoarticular disturbances also correlated negatively with the total verbal expression of hostility ($r = -0.889$).

Finally, a total mean score of persisting symptomatology was calculated for each subject from the above-mentioned percentage scores based on the clinical questionnaire and the extent of myoarticular disturbances upon palpation. After ranking the subjects, the most improved (9.2% or below) and the least improved (32.6% or above) were selected to compare their psychological profiles with the mean of the entire group, as may be seen in Fig. 2. Differences between improvers and nonimprovers were compared by means of the Mann Whitney U test: improvers exhibited significantly more self-manipulatory behaviors ($U = 1$; $df = 4/4$; $p < 0.04$) during the interview and also expressed more ambivalent hostility ($U = 2$; $df = 4/4$; $p < 0.10$).

11.4 Discussion

The inquiry into personality characteristics of patients with MPD syndrome has been addressed at two main issues: (1) the identification of emotional components common in such patients and (2) the detection of clues about why certain patients fail to respond to conventional dental therapy.

The first question has been extensively pursued, psychological factors being widely acknowledged. On the Minnesota Multiphasic Personality Inventory, personality profiles have been found similar to those of patients with other somatic diseases, such as ulcer, colitis, low back pain, and hypertension [15, 16].

Our study has focused mainly on the fact, pointed out by Laskin [10], that "there are some emotional components of MPD syndrome which the dentist must take into consideration if effective treatment of the MPD syndrome is to be achieved." In this connection, Greene [8] observed that nonresponding MPD syndrome patients are quite similar psychologically to patients with chronic low back pain and headache. However, previous studies have made no attempt to investigate psychological makeup other than by questionnaires or conventional paper-and-pencil tests.

Normative data on verbal affect scores in an interview setting are not available. However, a preliminary comparison may be attempted between our data and normative scores for adults in 5-min speech samples elaborated by Gottschalk [6]. Patients afflicted by bruxism present increased hostility scores in overt, covert, and ambivalent expressions as they score above the 80th percentile on all three scales. Further, the group as a whole also presents increased mutilation and diffuse anxiety in the content of speech as compared with the other subtypes of anxiety.

From our results, a subgroup of nonimprovers can be classified on behavioral bases. Their self-manipulatory behavior, which has been associated with the expression of anxiety or discomfort in a social situation [3], was significantly decreased.

Verbal content analysis of these patients revealed a strong relation between reduction of pain and symptomatology due to dental treatment and the expression of verbal hostility: subjects with higher expression of hostility in the interview were precisely those with greater change after treatment.

In summary, verbal content analysis of patients suffering from bruxism revealed increased expression of hostility as well as mutilation and diffuse anxiety. The latter fits well with what would be intuitively expected in the sense of excessive worry about somatic functioning in this type of patient.

However, the subgroup of patients resistant to treatment presented decreased self-manipulatory and hostile speech behaviors. Hence, the possibility of success in treatment seems directly related to the capability of emotional expression through verbal and nonverbal channels.

A more specific relation seems to exist between speech utterances and symptomatology than conventional psychopathological labels (such as hysteria, psychopathy, etc.) would be able to account for. Thus, the Gottschalk-Gleser method appears to be a valuable alternative procedure since it seems to have prognostic value for an issue which is not yet definitely settled. Providing a more "molecular" and operational definition of psychological aspects relevant to assessment, it avoids umbrella terms, such as psychopathy or stress, and suggests more directly measurable empirical referents for prognosis and evaluation of treatment outcome.

References

1. Beck AT, Ward GH, Mendelson M, Mock JE, Erbaugh JE (1967) An inventory for measuring depression. Arch Gen Psychiatry 4: 561–571
2. Brooke RI, Stenn PG, Mothersill KJ (1977) The diagnosis and conservative treatment of myofascial pain-dysfunction syndrome. Oral Surg 44: 844–852
3. Ekman P, Friesen WV (1972) Hand movements. J Commun 22: 353–374
4. Eysenck NJ, Eysenck SE (1964) Manual of the Eysenck personality inventory. University of London Press, London
5. Glaros AG, Rao SM (1977) Bruxism: a critical review. Psychol Bull 84: 767–781
6. Gottschalk LA (1982) Manual of uses and applications of the Gottschalk-Gleser verbal behavior scales. Res Commun Psychiatry 7: 1–20
7. Gottschalk LA, Winget CN, Gleser GC (1969) Manual of instructions for using the Gottschalk-Gleser analysis scales: anxiety, hostility and social alienation-personal disorganization. University of California Press, Berkeley
8. Greene CS, Olson RE, Laskin DM (1982) Psychological factors in the etiology, progression and treatment of MPD syndrome. JADA 105: 443–448
9. Heiberg AM, Helöe B, Krogstad BS (1978) The myofascial pain dysfunction: dental symptoms and psychological and muscular function. An overview. A preliminary study by team approach. Psychother Psychosom 30: 81–97
10. Laskin DM (1969) Etiology of the pain-dysfunction syndrome. J Am Dent Assoc 70: 147–155
11. Lebovits AH, Holland JC (1983) Use of the Gottschalk-Gleser verbal content analysis scales with medically ill patients. Psychosom Med 45 (4): 305–320
12. Lolas F (1981) The quantitation of alexithymia: observations and perspectives. Proceedings of the 13th European conference on psychosomatic research, Istanbul. pp 431–438
13. Lolas F, von Rad M (1977) The Gottschalk-Gleser affective profile. Res Commun Psychol Psychiatry Behav 2: 321–324
14. Manns A, Miralles R, Adrian H (1981) The application of audiostimulation and electromyographic biofeedback to bruxism and myofascial pain-dysfunction syndrome. Oral Surg 52: 247–252
15. Millstein-Prentky S, Olson RE (1979) Predictability of treatment outcome in patients with myofascial pain-dysfunction (MPD) syndrome. J Dent Res 58 (4): 1341–1346
16. Schwartz RA, Greene CS, Laskin DM (1979) Personality characteristics of patients with myofascial pain-dysfunction (MPD) syndrome unresponsive to conventional therapy. J Dent Res 58: 1435–1439
17. Zung WWK (1965) A self-rating depression scale. Arch Gen Psychiatry 12: 63–70

12 Psychological States in Patients with Diabetes Mellitus*

Linda L. Viney and Mary T. Westbrook

12.1 Introduction

Diabetes mellitus differs from many other chronic diseases in that it is accepted medical practice to involve patients suffering from it in monitoring and treating their own condition [1, 2]. This is especially so if the diabetes is of the insulin-dependent type [3], for which patients are required, when possible, to learn to administer injections of insulin to themselves. Even patients with non-insulin-dependent diabetes are encouraged by medical and nursing practitioners to test their own blood sugar levels, take care of parts of their bodies which are made especially vulnerable by the disease, such as their feet, and to have an understanding of the disease process and how it affects them. Often these skills are developed and supported through self-help groups, such as the Diabetic Associations throughout Australia, and publications about diabetes for nonprofessionals, such as their magazine *Diabetes Conquest*. Encouragement of active participation in their treatment by patients through information-seeking and through mastery of illness-related skills is relatively rare among current chronic illness management practices in our society [4–7].

The aim of this paper is to explore the psychological states of patients with diabetes mellitus. Little information about them is available. More work concerned with patients' psychological states associated with other chronic diseases has been reported. *Uncertainty*, for example, has proved to be common, especially initially [8–10], so, too, have *anxiety* [11–16] and *depression* [17–20]. Chronic illness and consequent disability can also lead to frustration and thus to *anger* [21–24]. This anger can be expressed either directly or indirectly. Both forms have been identified in patients with chronic illness [25], and both have been found to increase with increased disability [20]. These negative emotions represent a range of reactions to the stresses of chronic illness, as well as other factors.

Some psychological states of patients might be expected to be related to whether they are involved as active participants in their own treatment. *Helplessness* is a reaction which is very common among chronically ill patients [25–28]. It has, however, not been associated with successful rehabilitation, although feelings of *competence* have [29–31]. Chronically ill people, given the stresses they face [32–35], would express relatively few *good feelings*, but they have been shown to express more than people who are not ill [25, 36, 37].

---

* The work reported here was funded by the Australian Research Grants Committee, Grant No. 77/5046 R.

From this information, a series of propositions was generated about the characteristics of the pattern of psychological states associated with diabetes mellitus. It was predicted that diabetics would, in accordance with previous observations [38], express much anxiety and depression, together with anger resulting from the frustrations of their restricted life style [1, 2]. In contrast, and because of their active participation in their own treatment, they were expected to show little uncertainty and helplessness and many feelings of mastery. Because of their somewhat isolating life style [2], they were expected to experience little sociability. Finally, because their disease, while leading to attacks of hyperglycemia, does not as often lead to sudden death as do some other chronic diseases, good feelings were not expected to be as common for them as for ill people who were appreciating life while under threat of death [36].

These propositions were examined by testing a series of hypotheses. The first of these concerned differences in the psychological states of diabetics and patients diagnosed as having other chronic diseases. No significant differences between disease groups have yet been demonstrated [39]. The second concerned differences in the psychological states of diabetics and people who have had no diagnosed chronic diseases. These procedures were designed to enable identification of a pattern of psychological states associated with diabetes mellitus. Once this was done, the variability of this pattern was to be examined by testing for differences according to sex, recency of onset, mulitplicity of health problems, and hospitalization vs at-home status of the diabetic patients. Differences according to sex have been found in one study [40], but not another [25]. Recency of onset has been observed to be a relevant factor [38]. The effect of multiple health problems has not been investigated, but they were considered likely to increase the stress-related reactions of diabetics. Hospitalization has been shown to affect patients' psychological states considerably [16, 31, 41, 42].

12.2 Method

12.2.1 Research Participants

Three groups of people participated in this research project: a group of 73 diabetic patients, another of 114 patients with other chronic diseases, and a third of 54 people for whom no chronic diseases had been diagnosed. The percentile distributions of their sex, age, marital status, and educational attainments are given in Table 1. Three-quarters of the *diabetic* group were insulin dependent. This group had equal proportions of men and women and more older than younger people. Two-thirds of them were married. Few had completed high school. The *group with other chronic diseases* matched them in its distribution for these four variables. The match of the *group without chronic diseases* was good for marital status and educational attainments, but not for sex and age. It contained more men and more older people. This lack of matching will be considered later with regard to the appropriateness of different forms of statistical analysis.

More than one-third of the diabetic group had been diagnosed within the past year; almost two-thirds had multiple problems, and equal proportions were hospitalized or at home when they were interviewed. Patients in the second group were also interviewed

Table 1. Percentile distributions of sex, age, marital status, and educational attainment for the groups of diabetics, those suffering from other chronic diseases, and those with no chronic disease

Group	Diabetics	Other chronic diseases	No chronic disease
Sex			
Male	51	48	68
Female	49	52	32
Age (yrs)			
<30	15	13	32
30–40	11	9	16
40–50	21	20	20
50–60	19	21	14
60>	34	37	18
Marital status			
Married	66	67	63
Not married	34	33	37
Educational attainment			
Primary school	32	29	25
Mid-high school	48	44	40
High school	8	12	15
Tertiary	12	15	20

while in the hospital or at home. They were defined as suffering from chronic diseases if the disease had lasted at least 6 months or had caused a permanent disability [43]. In terms of the International Classification of Diseases [44], their primary diagnoses included disorders of the circulatory system, neoplasms, and diseases of the genitourinary, respiratory, digestive, musculoskeletal, and nervous systems. There were also a number of paraplegics and quadraplegics who had been victims of accidents. People in the third group without chronic disease were selected for the best possible matching from a sample participating in a study of life transitions other than illness. Any people with diagnosed chronic disease were screened out of this gruop.

12.2.2 Assessment of Their Psychological States

The psychological states of the research participants were assessed in the following way. A young woman psychologist, introduced as from the nearby university and studying people's reactions to life experiences, conducted each interview. As part of the interview schedule, each research participant was asked to talk about "your life at the moment – the good things and the bad." No more structure was added to these instructions. With the permission of the research participants, their responses were tape-recorded, and the records were then transcribed. Content analysis was applied to the transcripts, in the form of content analysis scales representing the nine different psychological reactions. These content anaylsis scales have demonstrated interjudge reliability and construct validity for a range of populations, some of which are similar to those considered in this study [45, 46]. They have been succesfully used to assess reactions to many types of stress [47, 48]. They have proved especially appropriate in assessing reactions to disease and disability [16, 18, 20, 31, 49, 50]. Each scale score includes a correction factor which reduces bias otherwise introduced by the different lengths of the responses of research participants.

To assess *uncertainty,* the Cognitive Anxiety Scale [51] was used. This scale has been designed to measure a type of anxiety which appears when people have difficulty in making sense of what is happening to them. There is evidence that it does so. For example, its scores differentiate effectively between reactions to situations which are not new. The comments from the research participants which were scored on this scale included references to new experiences (e.g., "Diabetes is hard to get used to at first") and events which are not considered meaningful because of lack of information (e.g., "It's the kind of disease where you never know what is going to hit you next").

Other types of *anxiety* can also be assessed by content analysis scales. The Total Anxiety Scale [45, 52, 53] has been shown to be responsive to experimental manipulations of stress as well as to correlate with self-ratings and psychiatrists' ratings of anxiety and physiological arousal. It taps anxiety from a number of sources: Death Anxiety (e.g., "I don't have long to last"). Mutilation Anxiety (e.g., I'm afraid that my kidneys are deteriorating"), Separation Anxiety (e.g., "You can become a social outcast"). Shame and Inadequacy (e.g., "I'm sorry I can't get about like I used to"), and Diffuse Anxiety (e.g., "I am pretty tense these days"). These six subscales – measuring anxiety about loss of life and bodily integrity, loneliness, guilt, embarrassment, as well as vague unease – were to be used, if differences were found for the Total Anxiety Scale, to identify the contributing sources of anxiety.

Depression was measured using a content analysis scale developed by the same team [45, 52, 53]. This Hostility-In Scale focuses on comments which are self-destructive and self-critical, that is, which direct anger at the self (e.g., "Everyone else has lost weight except me"), together with overt expressions of depression (e.g., "I feel sorry for myself sometimes") and feelings of deprivation (e.g., I'm pretty restricted in what I can eat"). The Hostility-Out Scale, which was used to measure *anger expressed directly,* focuses on comments indicating anger turned out onto the external world (e.g., "I hate those damn neddles," "I get very irritable at times"). The third scale of this group, the Ambivalent-Hostility Scale, was designed to assess *anger indirectly expressed,* that is, anger which has been disowned and projected onto others so that it bevomes anger directed at onself (e.g., "People are liable to be offended when you say I can't eat this and that"). Scores on all three scales have been found to be associated with ratings of relevant psychological states by self and others and with physiological arousal.

Feelings of *helplessness* and *competence* were assessed by two content analysis scales, which are related conceptually but, empirically speaking, are independent. They are Pawn and Origin Scales [54]. Research participants scored high on the Pawn Scale when they expressed lack of intention (e.g., "I was not really wanting to learn to give the injections"), lack of effort (e.g., "I wasn't really trying"), lack of ability (e.g., "There's nothing much I can do about it"), and pawn-like position as a victim of circumstances (e.g., "If you have a blackout, someone has to get the sugar into you quickly"). They scored high on the Origin Scale, in contrast, when they described themselves as having intention (e.g., "I like to get my first injection in very early in the day"), effort (e.g., "I try to stick to my diet"), ability (e.g., "You can live a normal life, if you want to"), and origin-like ability to create and rise above circumstances (e.g., "I have learned to cope with the diabetes"). Pawn Scale scores have been found to be associated with scores on the scales of negative and distressing emotions so far described but not to be associated with the more positive scales to come. This pattern of correlation is the reverse of that found for the Origin Scale.

Feelings of *sociability* involve experiencing oneself as participating in interpersonal interactions which are personally rewarding. Low scores on the Sociality Scale [55] indicate the experience of alienation from others. Its scores correlate with ratings of success in initiating and maintaining relationships. Comments about four kinds of interactions were scored on it: Solidarity, or helping interactions (e.g., "They come and asked me how to deal with the diabetes"). Intimacy, or attracting interactions (e.g., "The nurses were lovely"), Influence interactions (e.g., "My husband likes me to be home for the children after school"), and Shared Relationships, in which no particular type of interaction is specified (e.g., "When we go on holidays together..."). If differences were found for the Sociality Scale, these four subscales were used to identify the types of interaction involved.

Good feelings were also assessed. They were measured by the Positive-Affect Scale [56], which was scored when any positive feelings were expressed by the research participants. Its scores correlate positively with those from other positively toned scales and negatively with those which are more negative in tone. It is also interesting to note that women who are dealing with normal, developmental transitions, such as childbearing and relocating their family in a new community, have scored high on this scale [48]. The comments from these research participants which were scored on it included "I really am good at the moment" and "I'm glad the diabetes was diagnosed when it was."

Some comments on the effectiveness of this method of assessment for this research paper are now appropriate. Interjudge reliability was tested by having the authors independently score a random combination of three subsamples of 15 from each of the three groups of research participants before they received any other information about those participants. The resulting interjudge reliability coefficients were higher than 0.82 for all of the nine content analysis scales. Since these were established scales, and not newly created ad hoc content analysis categories, the validational networks of information available for each scale can be considered to provide appropriate support for their use in this study. The impression of both authors, based on their extensive use of the scales with the chronically ill, is that the responses of these groups, including those of the diabetics, were validly scored. Ceiling effects did not occur, as comparisons of their scale score distributions with those of other samples showed [48].

12.3 Results

The technique selected for the analyses of the data was multivariate analysis of variance (MANOVA), which made it possible to identify differences not occurring by chance among the large number of variables. The first series of hypotheses to be tested involved a comparison of the diabetic group with the group suffering from other chronic

Table 2. Means and standard deviations of content analysis scores for the groups of diabetics, those suffering from other chronic diseases, and those with no chronic disease

Group	Diabetics		Other chronic diseases		No chronic disease	
	M	SD	M	SD	M	SD
Cognitive Anxiety	1.25	0.82	1.12	0.61	0.94	0.63
Total Anxiety	2.38	0.97	2.42	0.73	1.28	0.67
Hostility In	1.27	0.84	1.44	0.75	0.70	0.48
Hostility Out	1.06	0.68	0.95	0.44	0.79	0.58
Ambivalent Hostility	0.92	0.52	0.88	0.45	0.60	0.35
Pawn	1.55	0.56	1.62	0.47	1.00	0.41
Origin	1.01	0.39	1.06	0.43	0.95	0.43
Sociality	0.43	0.19	0.41	0.18	0.41	0.21
Positive Affect	0.80	0.41	0.87	0.41	0.66	0.29
Anxiety Subscales						
Death Anxiety	0.58	0.37	0.55	0.31	0.46	0.35
Mutilation Anxiety	1.30	0.81	1.11	0.57	0.52	0.38
Separation Anxiety	0.83	0.63	0.93	0.61	0.50	0.34
Guilt	0.60	0.41	0.49	0.29	0.43	0.33
Shame	0.93	0.77	1.26	0.81	0.58	0.46
Diffuse Anxiety	1.07	0.67	0.99	0.56	0.69	0.50
Sociality Subscales						
Solidarity	0.25	0.17	0.23	0.15	0.13	0.10
Intimacy	0.13	0.14	0.15	0.11	0.09	0.09
Influence	0.08	0.06	0.08	0.06	0.07	0.06
Shared Relationships	0.26	0.16	0.22	0.16	0.32	0.22

diseases. The second compared the diabetics with the group with no chronic diseases. The third was concerned with differences within the diabetic group, comparing men with women, recent with not recent onset, mulitple with single health problems, and patients hospitalized with those who were caring for themselves at home. When any multivariate analysis yielded a significant finding, it was followed by univariate analysis of each scale score. Only the nine scales described were used initally, but if significant results ($p < 0.05$) were found for the Total Anxiety Scale or the Sociality Scale, their subscale scores were examined in subsequent analyses. The means and standard deviations for all of the content analysis scores are provided in Table 2.

The distributions of scores for the diabetic and other chronic disease groups shown in Table 2 do not indicate many marked differences between them. In fact, the MANOVA conducted on them did not yield a significant result ($F = 9.53$; $df = 9,185$; $p > 0.05$). None of the hypothesized differences were found in the pattern of scores for the diabetic and other chronic disease groups. No further analyses of these scores were carried out.

The second series of hypotheses required comparisons of the diabetic group with the group with no chronic diseases whose scores can also be found in Table 2. In this case the MANOVA result was significant (multivariate $F = 59.82$; $df = 1.125$; $p <$

0.001). The patterns of scores of these two groups were found to differ. The results of the subsequent univariate analyses of variance (ANOVAs) are presented in Table 3. They indicate that of the scores representing the psychological states, seven showed significant differences. They were those from the Cognitive Anxiety Scale, the Total Anxiety Scale, the Hostility-In Scale, the Hostility-Out Scale, the Ambivalent-Hostility Scale, the Pawn Scale, and the Positive-Affect Scale. Examination of the Total Anxiety Subscales also yielded a significant finding (multivariate $F = 52.10$; $df = 1,125$; $P < 0.001$). Their univariate analyses, also reported in Table 3, indicated that the difference for each one was significant. Analyses of the Sociality Subscales were also carried out because the mean subscale scores of Table 2 suggested that the nonsignificant result for the total scale might have occurred because of confounding effects among the subscales. Table 3 shows that for Solidarity and Intimacy, on both of which diabetics scored higher than the group with other chronic diseases, there were significant effects. There was also a significant effect for Shared Relationships, for which the difference was in the opposite direction.

The poor matching of these two groups for sex and age caused some questioning of these findings. Differences which appeared to be due to diabetes could have been due to other differences between the groups, such as sex and age. Analysis of covariance (ANCOVA) with a 2×2 design was therefore carried out with each set of scores for which

Table 3. Univariate analyses of variance comparing the content analysis scores of the groups of diabetics and those with no chronic disease

	Univariate F	$P <$
Set 1		
Cognitive Anxiety	5.05	0.05
Total Anxiety	50.27	0.001
Hostility In	20.35	0.001
Hostility Out	5.69	0.05
Ambivalent Hostility	14.99	0.001
Pawn	35.72	0.001
Origin	0.71	NS
Sociality	0.21	NS
Positive Affect	4.19	0.05
Set 2		
Death Anxiety	3.84	0.05
Mutilation Anxiety	42.66	0.001
Separation Anxiety	12.09	0.001
Guilt	6.10	0.05
Shame	8.64	0.01
Diffuse Anxiety	12.70	0.001
Set 3		
Solidarity	20.50	0.001
Intimacy	4.52	0.05
Influence	0.43	NS
Shared Relationships	3.84	0.05

significant group differences had been found. Sex was thereby introduced as a new factor, with age as a covariate. For none of the nine original scales, the six Anxiety Subscales, nor the four Sociality Subscales was there a significant group x sex interaction, and no sex differences were observed for any of them either. Sex differences were not, then, contributing to the group differences.

Age was found to be a significant covariate of five of the original seven scales (with $df = 1,122$ the Anxiety Scale, $F = 19.87$, $P < 0.001$; the Hostility-In Scale, $F = 38.36$, $P < 0.001$; the Ambivalent-Hostility Scale, $F = 20.31$, $P < 0.001$; and the Pawn Scale, $F = 19.87$, $P < 0.001$). The group effects for these variables, however, remained after these covariate effects were removed (with $df = 1.122$, the Anxiety Scale, $F = 45.61$, $P < 0.001$; the Hostility-Out Scale, $F = 4.31$, $P < 0.05$; the Ambivalent-Hostility Scale, $F = 54.20$, $P < 0.001$; and the Pawn Scale, $F = 88.53$, $P < 0.001$). No other significant group effects were found. Age was found to be a significant covariate among the Anxiety Subscale for Death Anxiety (with $df = 1,122$, $F = 10.42$, $P < 0.01$) and Mutilation Anxiety (with $df = 1,122$. $F = 36.97$, $P < 0.001$) only. The group effects were retained for these scores after the covariate effects were removed (with $df = 1,122$, $F = 3.95$, $P < 0.05$ and $F = 104.73$, $P < 0.001$, respectively), as they were for guilt and shame (with $df = 1,122$, $F = 51.76$, $P < 0.001$ and $F = 49.02$, $P < 0.001$, respectively). The significant group effect was not retained for that score, but those for Intimacy (with $df = 1,122$, $F = 7.20$, $P < 0.01$) and Shared Relationships (with $df = 1, 122$, $F = 17.75$, $P < 0.001$) were.

These findings suggest that, of the original results, those relating to scores on the Anxiety, Hostility-In, Hostility-Out, Ambivalent-Hostility, and Pawn Scales do not represent age differences. The same can be said for the Anxiety Subscales in relation to Death Anxiety, Mutilation Anxiety, Guilt and Shame, and for the Sociality Subscale of Initmacy. The hypotheses concerning these scores were supported.

The third series of hypotheses involved comparisons within the diabetic group. The comparison of diabetic women with diabetic men yielded no significant pattern of differences (multivariate $F = 7.26$; $df = 9.63$; $P > 0.05$); nor did that of diabetic patients whose onset had been within 1 year of the interview with those whose onset had been earlier (multivariate $F = 7.36$; $df = 9,63$; $P > 0.05$). The comparison of patients having multiple health problems with those with single health problems did not produce significant findings ($F = 3.94$; $df = 9,63$; $P > 0.05$); nor did that of patients interviewed in the hospital with those interviewed at home ($F = 10.51$; $df = 9,63$; $P > 0.05$). The pattern of psychological states experienced by diabetics appeared to be consistent across patients experiencing different disease-related events.

The results were, in summary, that the hypotheses about differences between the diabetic group and the group with other chronic diseases found no support. Those hypotheses tested by comparisons of the diabetic group with the group having no chronic diseases found some support. Scores on the Total Anxiety Scale, Hostility-In Scale, Hostility-Out Scale, and Ambivalent-Hostility Scale differed as predicted, as did those of four of the Anxiety Subscales and one of the Sociability Subscales. Scores on the Cognitive Anxiety Scale, Pawn Scale, and Origin Scale did not, nor did those on the total Sociability Scale or Positive-Affect Scales, although for Sociality, this was due to the confounding of differences in different directions of scores on its subscales. No support was found, either, for the hypotheses about differences among diabetic patients.

12.4 Discussion

The application of the content analysis scales to open-ended responses from the research participants enabled us to assess their psychological states without being unduly obtrusive or suggesting particular states to them, as questionnaires or some interview schedules do. All of the participants proved sufficiently verbally fluent in terms of both quantity and quality of their responses to make use of this method appropriate. No difficulties were encountered in achieving agreement in the scale scores between independent judges. In the case of the diabetics, some readers may consider that to be dependent on regular doses of insulin would necessarily induce a particular psychological state, for example, helplessness. This was not so. While some diabetics who spoke of their self-administered injections did emphasize their helplessness (e.g., "I can't avoid that neddle each day"), others maintained a more positive state while considering a similar personal experience (e.g., "I'm glad I only have on shot a day"). Their psychological states were apparent, regardless of the content of their responses.

The pattern of psychological states associated with diabetes which emerged from these analyses included considerable anxiety, depression, and anger expressed both directly and indirectly. These were probably responses to stress, as at least one of the diabetic research participants stated. She had been diagnosed as an insulin-dependent diabetic within the past year and had, as yet, no other health problems. She said: "Oh, I go up the wall with it. It's just like crawling up the wall and not being able to get down. But it's not getting me anywhere, feeling sorry for myself; because nobody wants you if you are going to complain about your illness all the time." Distress and frustration were key elements, not only of her reactions but those of her fellow diabetics.

The other key element, which has already been noted, was anxiety. Four different sources of this anxiety proved to be important for diabetics. Fear of loss of life was one. As another research participant said, almost cheerfully. „Seventy years ago. I'd have been dead by now"; and he moved on from this expression of death anxiety to praise the development of insulin. Fear of loss of bodily integrity was another source of anxiety. This mutilation anxiety was identifed in these concerns: "The long-term prospects for diabetics are not good. We can lose our sight. We have trouble with our feet. And we are more likely than our friends to have heart attacks." These threats to their physical well-being were balanced for diabetics by threats to their psychological well-being. Their self-esteem was threatened, giving rise to feelings of guilt. As one woman said: "I hate having to be the center of attention in my family. I ought to be looking after them. I usen't to be like this. I feel bad about it." The second threat was to the respect they had received from others and led to feelings of shame. As one elderly man suffering from a diabetes-related eye condition sighed: "I just stay around here. There's nothing I can do ... I can't read ... I'm nearly blind. I have to ask for help for people to read my letters and things. I feel embarrassed ..."

Other psychological states experienced by the diabetics were more positive. Although they did, as predicted, describe fewer shared interactions which they enjoyed (such as "We want to ..." and "... and that is what happened to us"), they showed a heightened sense of intimacy. The kind of interaction which they often described as rewarding to them was one involving admiring, respecting, and loving others and being admired, respected, and loved by them. As one newly diagnosed woman reported:

"Having this happen has really made me value my family. They are so good to me. My husband is marvelous! And the children – they just couldn't be better. They all seem to care about me so much. And I care so much about them…" This statement illustrates, too, how the increased importance of a few significant relationships can be linked with considerable expression of good feelings and enjoyment. The findings concerning good feelings from this research project have been somewhat equivocal, but they have provided some support for the proposition that diabetics may not differ from people with other chronic diseases in this psychological state. Diabetics may also experience more enjoyment of life than people who are not threatened by disease and disability, although this is accompanied by many negative emotions.

The propositions about the effects on diabetics of the encouragement given by health care professionals to participate actively in their own treatment were not supported in this study. Diabetic patients were as uncertain as patients with other chronic diseases and expressed no more feelings of competence. In fact, one of the other important states consisted of feelings of helplessness. It seemed that although most of the patients with diabetes were involved in monitoring their own glucose levels and many in injecting themselves with insulin and thus exerting some control over the effects of their condition, they still felt overwhelmed by it. As another diabetic said: "I had no idea it was coming on. It hit me, just like that! You have to watch yourself all the time. Your whole life starts to revolve around it. You always have to carry an apple or a biscuit. My whole life revolves around the clock and what I can do in the time." Life as a diabetic has an irony about it, which was captured in one diabetic's comment: "You can forget you are a diabetic, as long as you never forget you are a diabetic."

This pattern of psychological states associated with diabetes mellitus in which there was considerable distress in the form of anxiety, depression, and frustration-related anger and feelings of helplessness and hopelessness, and yet some enjoyment of close relationships, has been found to be consistent. It did not vary according to the sex of the patients, nor whether they were interviewed when hospitalized or when caring for themselves at home, nor did it vary with recency of onset nor with multiplicity of health problems [31]. The pattern could not be said, however, to be characteristic of diabetics only. Koch and Molnar [57] found no consistent pattern of reaction to diabetes, while Lohman et al. [58] found diabetics not to differ psychologically from patients with hemophilia and chronic renal failure. It may be that this pattern of psychological states is associated with all chronic diseases. The pattern identified here has been found to be associated with poor rehabilitation for patients with other chronic diseases. This finding suggests that an approach to patients which is concerned with their psychology as well as their physiology would be helpful. This approach would develop their recognition and expression of stress-related feelings [59]. It would encourage the enjoyment they already have of close relationships but add to it involvement in social and community acitivites [49]. Last, but not least, it would strengthen their ability to assess accurately their physiological condition, their sense of active participation in their own treatment, and their control of their own metabolism, thereby developing their ability to cope with both the physiological and psychological effects of diabetes mellitus.

12.5 Summary

The psychological states of patients with diabetes mellitus were compared with those of patients suffering from other chronic diseases and people with no diagnosed chronic diseases. These states were assessed by applying content analysis scales to transcripts of their descriptions of their current experiences. Analyses of the diabetics' scale scores revealed a pattern characterized by much anxiety, depression, anger expressed both directly and indirectly, together with feelings of helplessness. The sources of anxiety which proved to be of most importance to them were fears of death and bodily mutilation, as well as guilt and shame. They experienced little sense of sharing with most people around them, although they showed considerable enjoyment of close relationships with family and friends. This pattern of psychological states did not vary with the sex of the patients or whether they were interviewed in a hospital or at home nor with recency of onset or multiplicity of health problems. It was similar to the pattern of patients with other chronic diseases but differed significantly from that of the healthy group.

Acknowledgment
The authors wish to acknowledge the contribution of Carol Preston to the collection and analysis of these data which were made available, inpart, by patients of the Wollongong Hospital and members of the Illawarra Branch of the Diabetic Association of New South Wales.

References

1. Strong JA, Baird JD (1971) Diseases of the endocrine system. In: Davidson S, McLeod J (eds) The principles and practice of medicine. Churchill Livingstone, London
2. Tattersall R (1981) Diabetes in adolescence. Inter Med 8: 624
3. Keen H (1981) The nature of the diabetes syndrome. Int Med 8: 587–589
4. Anderson ND (1981) Exclusion: a study of depersonalization in health care. J Human Psychol 21: 67–78
5. Janis IL, Rodin J (1979) Attribution, control and decision-making: social psychology and health. In: Stone GC et al (eds) Health psychology – a handbook. Jossey-Bass, San Francisco
6. Mechanic D (1977) Illness behavior, social adaptation and the management of illness. J Nerv Ment Dis 165: 79–85
7. Taylor SE (1979) Hospital patient behavior: reactance, helplessness or control. J Soc Iss 35: 156–184
8. Bard M, Sutherland AM (1977) The psychological impact of cancer. American Cancer Society, New York
9. Farber IJ (1978) Hospitalized cardiac patients: some psychological aspects. NY State J Med 43: 2045–2049
10. Rosenbaum EH (1975) Living with cancer. Prager, New York
11. Byrne DG, Whyte HM Dimensions of illness behavior in survivors of myocardial infarction. J Psychosom Res 22: 485–491
12. Holland JC, Rowland J, Lebovits A, Rusalen R (1979) Reactions to cancer treatment, Psychiatr Clin North Am 2: 347–350
13. Lewis FM, Bloom JR (1978–79) Psychosocial adjustment to breast cancer: a review of selected literature. Int J Psychiatry Med 9: 1–17

14. Moos RH, Tsu VD (1977) The crisis of physical illness: an overview. In: Moos RH (ed) Coping with physical illness. Plenum, New York
15. Viney LL (1984) Loss of life and loss of bodily integrity: two different sources of threat for people who are ill. Omega 15: 207–222
16. Viney LL, Westbrook MT (1982a) Patterns of anxiety in the chronically ill. Br J Med Psychol 55: 87–95
17. Holland JC, Rowland J, Lebovits A, Rusalen R (1979) Reactions to cancer treatment. Psychiatr Clin North Am 2: 347–350
18. Maguire GP, Lee EG, Bevington DJ, Kucherman CS, Crabtree R (1978) Psychiatric problems in the first year after mastectomy. Br Med J 1: 963–965
19. Stocksmeier V (1976) Medical and psychological aspects of coronary heart disease. In: Stocksmeier V (ed) Psychological approaches to the rehabilitation of coronary patients. Springer, Berlin Heidelberg New York
20. Viney LL, Westbrook MT (1981b) Psychological reactions to chronic illness-related disability as a function of its severity and type. J Psychosom Res 25: 513–523
21. Hackett TP, Cassem NH, Wishnie HA (1968) The coronary care unit: an appraisal of its psychologic hazards. N Engl J Med 279: 1365–1370
22. Pritchard MJ (1981) Temporal reliability of a questionnaire measuring psychological response. J Psychosom Res 25: 63–66
23. Skelton M, Dominian J (1973) Psychological stress in wives of patients with myocardial infarction. Br Med J 2: 101–103
24. Viney LL (1972) Reactions to frustration in chronically disabled patients. J Clin Psychol 28: 164–165
25. Westbrook MT, Viney LL (1982) Psychological reaction to the onset of chronic illness. Soc Sci Med 16: 899–905
26. Abrams RD, Finesinger JE (1953) Guilt reactions in patients with cancer. Cancer 6: 317–322
27. Cassell EJ (1976) The healer's art. Penguin, Middlesex
28. Le Shan L (1977) You can fight for your life. Evans, New York
29. Albrecht GL, Higgins PC (1977) Rehabilitation success: the interrelationships of multiple criteria. J Health Soc Behav 18: 36–45
30. Shontz FC (1975) The psychological aspects of physical illness and disability. Macmillan, New York
31. Viney LL, Westbrook MT (1982b) Psychological reactions to chronic illness: do they predict rehabilitation? J Rehabil Coun 13: 38–44
32. Blumberg B, Flaherty M, Lewis J (eds) (1980) Coping with cancer. US Department of Health and Human Services, Washington DC
33. Cohen F, Lazarus RS (1979) Coping with stresses of illness. In: Stone C, et al (ed) Health psychology – a handbook. Jossey Bass, San Francisco
34. Hamburg DA (1974) Coping behavior in life threatening circumstances. Psychother Psychosom 23: 13–25
35. Wortman CB, Dunkel-Schetter C (1979) Interpersonal relationship and cancer: a theoretical analysis. J Soc Iss 35: 120–155
36. Hamera EK, Shontz FC (1978) Perceived positive and negative effects of life threatening illness. J Psychosom Res 22: 419–424
37. Kinsman RA et al (1976) A scale for measuring attitudes towards respiratory illness and hospitalization. J Nerv Ment Dis 163: 160–165
38. Engelmann MW (1976) The diabetic client. In: Turner FJ (ed) Differential diagnosis and treatment in social work. Free Press, New York
39. Viney LL, Westbrook MT (1980) Psychosocial reactions to heart disease: an application of content analysis methodology. Proceedings of the Geigy symposium on behavioral medicine, Melbourne. Geigy, Melbourne

40. Nathanson CA (1975) Illness and the feminine role: a theoretical review. Soc Sci Med 9: 57–62
41. Lucente FE, Fleck S (1972) A study of hospitalization anxiety in 408 medical and surgical patients. Psychosom Med 34: 304–312
42. Volicer BJ (1978) Hospital stress and patient reports of pain and physical status. J Hum Stress 4: 28–37
43. Australian Bureau of Statistics (1979) Australian health survey, 1977–1978. Canberra
44. World Health Organization (1975) International classification of diseases. 9th edn. Geneva
45. Gottschalk LA, Gleser GC (1969) The measurement of psychological states from the content analysis of verbal behavior. University of California Press, Berkeley
46. Viney LL (1981) Content analysis: a research tool for community psychologists. Am J Common Psychol 9: 269–281
47. Westbrook MT, Viney LL (1977) The application of content analysis scales to life stress research. Aust Psychol 12: 157–166
48. Viney LL (1980) Transitions. Cassell, Syndney
49. Viney LL (1983) Images of illness. Krieger, Malabar
50. Viney LL, Westbrook MT (1981a) Measuring patients' experienced quality of life: the application of content analysis scales in health care. Community Health Stud 5: 45–52
51. Viney LL, Westbrook MT (1976) Cognitive anxiety: a method of content analysis for verbal samples. J Pers Assess 40: 140–150
52. Gottschalk LA (1979) The content analysis of verbal behavior: further studies. Medical and Scientific, New York
53. Gottschalk LA, Winget CN, Gleser GC (1969) Manual of instructions for using the Gottschalk-Gleser content analysis scales. University of California Press, Berkeley
54. Westbrook MT, Viney LL (1980) Measuring people's perceptions of themselves as origins and pawns. J Pers Ass 44: 157–166
55. Viney LL, Westbrook MT (1979) Sociality: a content analysis for verbalizations. Soc Behav Pers 7: 129–137
56. Westbrook MT (1976) Positive affect: A method of content analysis for verbal samples. J Con Clin Psychol 44: 715–719
57. Koch MF, Monar GD (1974) Psychiatric aspects of patients with unstable diabetes mellitus. Psychosom Med 36: 57–67
58. Lohmann R, Voges B, Meuter F, Rath KU, Thomas W (1979) Psychopathology and psychotherapy in chronically ill patients. Psychother Psychosom 31: 267–276
59. Viney LL, Benjamin YM (1983) A hospital-based counseling program for medical and surgical patients. J Rehab Counsel 14: 30–34

13 Emotional Impact of Mastectomy*

Louis A. Gottschalk, and Julia Hoigaard

13.1 Introduction

The emotional impact of surgery on the human body has been widely examined. One study focused on the reactions of surgical patients to the prospect of surgical procedures in general and observed that patients who manifested mild to moderate fear before surgery had more favorable outcomes and fewer long-term postsurgical complications than patients who covered up or inhibited such fear [61]. Other studies have examined the effects of surgery on surface organs, such as the nose [19, 44], the face in general [7], and on body parts that are visible to others [13, 15, 20, 45]. Emotional reactions to surgical procedures involving organs inside the body have also been studied, but these have usually focused on one specific kind of disease or another, such as neoplastic, vascular, and other disturbances [40, 57, 58].

When one considers the affects aroused in response to surgical treatment, it becomes apparent that the nature of the disease process itself can call forth various responses, as for instance, the affects evoked by discovering one has cancer versus one has a hernia. The reactions aroused to surgical procedures involving body parts that distinguish an individual's sexual identity, such as the external genital organs or breast, are likely to precipitate unique emotional consequences [20].

There have been investigations of breast cancer and efforts to determine whether psychosocial causes or effects are involved in the course of this disease [11, 13, 49]. Some shortcomings of such studies have been the absence of control groups and impressionistic instead of objective assessments of emotions.

The present report concerns a psychososial study of the emotional impact of the surgical treatment of breast cancer using several different methods of measuring these emotions. The data were collected under the auspices of a cooperative study supported by the National Cancer Institute involving five institutions collaborating over several years in planning and collecting the data. Unfortunately, funds were not provided to these institutions by the National Cancer Institute for data analysis. The senior author of this present report was told the wealth of data obtained, including the use of the Gottschalk-Gleser Content Analysis Scales [24, 25, 27], that were not going to be analyzed. Relying on the Freedom of Information Act, a copy of the data was requested of the National Cancer Institute, and it was made available on electronic tape. This

---

* Previously published in modified form in *Psychiatry Research*, (1986) 17: 153–167 with permission of the authors and publisher.

paper will limit its report to an assessment of the measurements of emotional responses to surgery.

The National Cancer Institute was interested in assessing the psychological state, within the 1st year after surgery, of women who has undergone a unilateral radical mastectomy for stage I or stage II breast cancer and in determining whether patients who have experienced such a mastectomy for breast cancer have special emotional reactions that can be differentiated from the emotions of other groups of women exposed to the stress of surgery.

13.2 Methods

13.2.1 Sources of Subjects and Data Collection

Subjects for this study were obtained in approximately equal numbers by case finding activities at five participating institutions: Montefiore Hospital, Bronx, NY; Peter Bent Brigham Hospital, Boston, MA; Midwest Research Institution, Kansas City, MO; West Coast Cancer Foundation, San Francisco, CA; and Stanford Research Institute International, Menlo Park, CA. Data collection was carried out by trained investigators at each institution following standardized and coordinated procedures. For the subjects reported on here, voluntary participants were screened from hospitals, clinics, and doctors, and the likelihood of follow-up interviews was enhanced by selecting subjects who agreed to return for later evaluations and who were assured of travel expenses to enable them to do so.

13.2.2 Type of Subjects

Four groups of subjects were involved:

1. Women who had an undergone a unilateral mastectomy for stage I or stage II breast cancer 1–3 months prior to being interviewed. Women with stage III and stage IV breast cancer were excluded to eliminate the confounding effects of metastatic versus localized cancer as well as the effects of anticancer chemotherapy or radiotherapy.

2. Women who had undergone a biopsy for benign breast disease 1–3 months before being interviewed. This group was included to determine the psychological effect, if any, of a negative surgical biopsy for breast cancer.

3. Women who had undergone a cholecystectomy 1–3 months before being interviewed. Inclusion of this group of women provided an opportunity to examine what psychological effect surgery on an internal organ for a noncancerous condition might have.

4. Healthy women who had not had a major surgical intervention within 2 years before being interviewed. In this group, women were excluded who had ever undergone a mastectomy, had undergone a biopsy within the past 2 years, had undergone cholecystectomy within the past 5 years, had suffered a serious illness or disability, or had received psychiatric therapy. These women were obtained by a screening technician from each test site, by using a standardized interview, and by telling women in the mastectomy group the following: "As I mentioned earlier, the purpose of this study is to

compare women who have had breast surgery with women who have had other kinds of surgery and with those who have had no surgery recently. Since we would like all the women in the study to be of similar backgrounds, I was wondering if you have friends who would be willing to be in this study too?"

13.2.3 Other Exclusion Criteria for Subjects

Subjects were also excluded from this study – on a self-report basis – if they were younger than 30 or older than 69 years of age, were not English speaking, had undergone other surgery in addition to a mastectomy, biopsy, or cholecystectomy, had had a bilateral mastectomy performed, had a stage III or IV breast cancer, had undergone a bilateral biopsy, needle biopsy, or more than one biopsy, had undergone a biopsy or cholecystectomy positive for cancer, had had a previous mastectomy or previous breast biopsy, had cancer of any kind, had evidence of metastasis diagnosed since the mastectomy, had received hormonal therapy, had obtained psychiatric treatment for more than 2 months, or had a recent history of drug or alcohol abuse or a depression.

13.2.4 Tests Administered

13.2.4.1 Symptom Checklist 90 Analogue.

The Symptom Checklist 90 Analogue (SCL) [12] is an interviewer rating scale on which the subject is rated along nine dimensions of psychopathology and one overall measure of psychological disorder. The nine dimensions of psychopathology are: somatization, obsessive-compulsive, interpersonal sensitivity, depression, anxiety, hostility, phobic anxiety, paranoid ideation, and psychoticism.

13.2.4.2 Global Assessment Scale

The Global Assessment Scale (GAS) [17] is a psychiatric rating scale on which a clinically trained external evaluator selects the lowest range describing the subject's functioning over the past week on a hypothetical continuum of mental health illness.

13.2.4.3 Gottschalk-Gleser Content Analysis Scale

The Gottschalk-Gleser Content Analysis Scales [24, 25, 27, 30] are a combination of a self-report and rating scales. These are measures derived from the typescript of 5 min of tape-recorded speech elicited from each subject by purposely ambiguous instructions to talk for 5 min about any interesting or dramatic personal life experiences. These typescripts are scored by technicians trained to score the scales with a reliability of 0.85 or better. Thorough validation studies have been carried out on the Gottschalk-Gleser Scales used in this study, namely. Anxiety (including six Anxiety Subscales: Death, Mutilation, Separation, Guilt, Shame, and Diffuse Anxiety), Hostility (comprised of Hostility Outward, Hostility Inward, and Ambivalent Hostility), Hope, and Total Denial [23, 27, 31, 32, 33, 34, 35, 51, 59].

13.2.5 Procedure

The subjects ($n = 349$) were interviewed on two occasions:
1. Within a 1–3 month period after the initial contact was made by the data collection team
2. 10–12 months after the initial contact

Psychiatric interviews and ratings on the SCL-90 Analogue and GAS were carried out by qualified psychiatrists or psychologists.

Five-minute speech samples were elicited from the subjects according to standard instructions [25, 30], and scoring of these speech samples for anxiety, hostility, hope, and denial was done blindly by trained content analysis technicians.

13.2.6 Data Analysis

As explained above, a series of three psychosocial measures were administered to the four populations on two occasions. The measures consisted of three separate instruments: (1) the SCL-90 Analogue, (2) the GAS, and (3) the Gottschalk-Gleser Content Analysis Scales which contain four sets of subscales. The four sets of subscales measured four conceptual areas: Anxiety, Hostility, Hope, and Denial. Hence, there were six subsets in all (i.e., the SCL, the GAS, and four from the Gottschalk-Gleser instrument). Other information, such as the patient's age as well as the interval of time since surgery, was also collected.

The women had undergone surgery 2 months (mean 58.02 ± 22.38 days) before the initial testing and 11 months (mean 327.85 ± 30.03 days) before the second testing period. There was no significant difference among the surgical groups, by analyses of variance, in the time interval between surgery and testing.

The mean ages of the women across all four groups was as follows: mastectomy group ($n = 125$; age 51.60 ± 9.97), biopsy group ($n = 65$; age 45.54 ± 10.52), cholecystectomy group ($n = 75$; 51.59 ± 10.15), and healthy group ($n = 84$; 49.86 ± 9.89). These mean ages were significantly different between groups by analysis of variance (df 3, 345; $F = 6.93$; $P < 0.01$). No significant correlations between age and anxiety or hostility, as measured by the Gottschalk-Gleser Content Analysis Scales, were found in several other normative and psychiatric adult samples, except for one Subscale of Anxiety, namely, Death Anxiety, which tends to increase with age in samples with a wider age range [27]. The effect of age on death anxiety scores would be expected to show up only if there were a wider spread of mean ages across our groups. Nevertheless, the possible effects of age were controlled by using a multiple analysis of covariance.

Since the focus of the study was concerned with the effect of the various group conditions on the psychosocial measures and since these variables consisted of six separate conceptual areas, each of these areas was analyzed separately as recommended by Finn ([18] p. 7). In each case, the four populations were compared on one or more variables measured on two occasions controlling for the effects of age, that is, each of the analyses contained one between-subject factor (i.e., four populations), one within-subject factor (i.e., time 1 vs time 2), and one covariate (i.e., age). Since the GAS consists of a single variable, it was analyzed using a repeated measures analysis of covariance (ANCOVA). Since the other five analyses involved sets of variables, a multiple analysis of covariance with repeated measures (MANCOVA) was employed.

The underlying theoretical orientation assumed that various types of surgery were perceived by the patients to cause differing amounts of disfigurement. Furthermore, the four subpopulations were assumed to be effected differently on the psychosocial variables, that is, the mastectomy group was assumed to be most effected, followed by the cholecystectomy, the biopsy, and finally the healthy group.

For each of the six analyses, the omnibus group comparisons were followed by single degree-of-freedom tests to determine if the group differences followed the ordering described above. Since there were four groups, three single degree-of-freedom tests were employed to examine differences between adjacent pairs of means (i.e., mastectomy vs cholecystectomy, cholecystectomy vs biopsy, and biopsy vs healthy).

All the analyses were conducted using the SPSS-X procedure, MANOVA [54]. This procedure includes a special (UNIQUE) option, which permits every factor to be examined while controlling for all other factors. The UNIQUE option was employed in these analyses. The repeated measures portion of the analyses employed the conservative multivariate approach [9, 54]. The multivariate approach was used because Bartlett's test of sphericity was significant [4] in four of the six analyses.

13.3 Results

No significant effect of age was found on the psychological measures. The most consistent positive finding was that the mastectomy group reported higher levels of emotional distress than the other groups. Although this pattern was observed in all three measures and at both time periods, the reaction seemed to be stronger in the initial time period and seemed to have its greatest and most consistent effect on the Gottschalk-Gleser Content Analysis Scales.

13.3.1 Emotional Differences Between the Groups of Women After Surgery

The mastectomy group had significantly higher mean total anxiety scores on the Gottschalk-Gleser Content Analysis Scales than the biopsy group and healthy group 1–3 months (see Table 1) and 10–12 months after surgery (see Table 2). Death Anxiety and Mutilation Anxiety Subscale scores accounted for these differences; death anxiety scores from the mastectomy group significantly exceeded the same scores from the cholecystectomy and healthy groups, and mutilation anxiety scores from the mastectomy group significantly exceeded those scores from the biopsy, cholecystectomy, and healthy groups. Ambivalent hostility scores (references to others being hostile to the self) from the mastectomy group were significantly higher than these scores from the healthy group. In addition, anxiety denial scores and total denial (anxiety and hostility) scores obtained from the mastectomy group were significantly greater than these scores from all three other groups, and hopefulness scores (expression of positive hope) were significantly higher from the mastectomy group than from the healthy group.

Table 3. Differences between groups on GAS scores adjusted for age 1–3 months and 10–12 months after surgery (by ANCOVA)

Groups	n	1–3 months Means (S.D.)	10–12 months Mean (S.D.)
1. Mastectomy	125	70.76 ($\pm$12.63)	71.86 ($\pm$13.25)
2. Cholecystectomy	75	70.96 ($\pm$12.23)	72.32 ($\pm$11.51)
3. Biopsy	65	74.34 ($\pm$11.60)	72.12 ($\pm$12.46)
4. Healthy	84	78.08 ($\pm$ 8.99)	75.46 ($\pm$11.43)
Groups		$F=4.80$	
		$df=3,325$	
		$P<0.01$	
Time		$F=1.06$	
		$df=1,325$	
		$P=NS$	
Group x time		$F=3.48$	
		$df=3,325$	
		$p<0.05$	

Differences between group scores when combined over occasions

Group 1 > 2	$P=NS$
Group 2 > 3	$P=NS$
Group 1 and 2 < 4	$df=1,325$, $F=4.02$, $P<0.05$
Group 3 < 4	$df=1,325$, $F=4.20$, $P<0.05$

Table 4. Differences between groups on SCL-90 Analogue Anxiety and Depression Rating Scale scores 1–3 months and 10–12 months after surgery controlling for age (by MANCOVA)

Groups	n	Depression scores 1–3 months Mean (S.D.)	10–12 months Mean (S.D.)	Anxiety scores[a] 1–3 months Mean (S.D.)	10–12 months Mean (S.D.)
1. Mastectomy	123	21.70 ($\pm$19.54)	18.77 ($\pm$17.33)	21.70$\pm$19.54	24.03 ($\pm$15.08)
2. Cholecystectomy	74	15.96 ($\pm$15.77)	18.54 ($\pm$17.07)	15.96$\pm$15.77	20.45 ($\pm$14.67)
3. Biopsy	63	16.65 ($\pm$13.52)	18.77 ($\pm$17.33)	16.65$\pm$13.52	22.66 ($\pm$13.33)
4. Healthy	83	11.35 ($\pm$12.09)	15.48 ($\pm$15.97)	11.35$\pm$12.09	17.77 ($\pm$13.07)
Groups		$F=4.26$		$F=7.62$	
		$df=3,338$		$df=3,338$	
		$P<0.05$		$P<0.001$	
Time		$F=0.16$		$F=24.73$	
		$df=1,339$		$df=1,339$	
		$P=NS$		$P<0.001$	

[a] Only the SCL-90 anxiety rating changed significantly over the two time periods ($df=1,339$; $F=24.73$; $P<0.001$).

Differences between group scores when combined over occasions

	Depression scores	Anxiety scores
Group 1 > 2	$df=1,338$	$df=1,338$
	$F=5.86$	$F=6.46$
	$P<0.01$	$P<0.01$
Group 2 > 3	$P=NS$	$P=NS$
Group 3 > 4	$P=NS$	$P=NS$

The mastectomy, cholecystectomy, and biopsy groups had significantly lower scores on the GAS of emotional well-being than the healthy group over both testing periods, and the groups differed in their amount of change in the GAS over time (see Table 3).

The mastectomy group had a significantly higher mean anxiety and depression score than the healthy group and the other two surgery groups on the SCL-90 self-report scale 1–3 and 10–12 months after surgery (see Table 4).

The UNIQUE option of the MANCOVA showed that the Gottschalk-Gleser Scale scores were significantly most deviant for the mastectomy group, less deviant for the cholecystectomy group, and still less deviant for the biopsy group (see Tables 1 and 2). Over both occasions, the GAS and the SCL-90 scores showed a roughly similar step-wise distribution of psychopathological responses among the women receiving recent surgery as compared to the healthy group, with the mastectomy group having the most deviant scores (see Tables 3 and 4).

13.3.2 Changes in the Psychological Scores over Time in the Postoperative Period

To determine whether there were any significant changes in the various psychological measures from the initial testing occasion to the second occasion, MANCOVA was calculated for each individual on each measure. Table 3 indicates there was no change over time for the GAS, and Table 4 shows there was an increase in SCL-90 anxiety scores for all groups over time, for which no explanation can be offered. Table 5 reports the mean difference in Gottschalk-Gleser scores for each group, using a t-test for correlated means. The mean can be compared across groups, and the sign of the difference can be used to determine the direction of the change, a minus sign indicating a decrease in mean score.

Table 5. Differences between means of Gottschalk-Gleser psychological measures obtained on two occasions from four groups of women (by t-test for correlated means)[a]

Scales	Groups			
	Mastectomy	Biopsy	Cholecystectomy	Healthy
Content Analysis				
Death Anxiety	−0.102**	0.010	−0.160**	−0.030
Mutilation Anxiety	−0.203**	−0.069	−0.230**	−0.059
Separation Anxiety	0.021	0.103	−0.058	−0.007
Guilt Anxiety	0.053	0.054	−0.055	0.004
Shame Anxiety	−0.177**	−0.095	−0.132	−0.031
Diffuse Anxiety	−0.099	−0.078	−0.099	0.059
Total Anxiety	−0.267**	−0.010	−0.360**	−0.033
Hostility Out Overt	0.129**	0.136*	−0.016	0.043
Hostility Out Covert	0.082	0.073	−0.038	0.044
Hostility Out Total	0.181**	0.168	−0.009	0.059
Hostility In	0.070	0.146*	−0.046	0.069
Ambivalent Hostility	−0.050	0.005	−0.124*	0.091

Table 5. (continued)

Scales	Groups			
	Mastectomy	Biopsy	Cholecystectomy	Healthy
Hope (+)	−0.080*	−0.080	−0.030	−0.000
Hope (−)	−0.069	−0.108	−0.231	0.064
Total Hope	−0.110	−0.110	0.067	−0.104
Denial				
Anxiety	−0.050	−0.007	0.015	−0.006
Hostility Outward	−0.005	0.019	0.015	−0.034
Hostility Inward	−0.010	−0.012	−0.005	−0.002
Ambivalent Hostility	−0.005	−0.002	−0.009	−0.011
Denial Total	−0.050	−0.010	0.014	−0.026

* Significant at 0.05 level;   ** significant at 0.01 level.
[a] Minus sign indicates decrease in mean score.
   $df = 1,325$ for all values.

There were no significant changes in the average scores for the healthy group over time on the Gottschalk-Gleser Content Analysis Scales. Significant reductions in mean mutilation, shame, and total anxiety ($P < 0.01$) occurred in the mastectomy group and in death, mutilation, and total anxiety ($P < 0.01$) in the cholecystectomy group.

Mean overt hostility out and total hostility out increased significantly ($P0.01-05$) in the mastectomy and biopsy groups, but showed no significant changes in the other two groups. Mean positive hope scores decreased in the mastectomy group, and mean ambivalent hostility decreased in the cholecystectomy group. No significant changes occurred in denial scores.

Significant positive correlations between mean content analysis scores obtained from these two occasions indicate the stability of these scores. The more emotionally distressed individuals at the initial period tended to remain the more distressed at the second time of observation.

13.4 Discussion of Emotional Impact of Mastectomy

13.4.1 Measures of Psychological Responses

The available research data collected from these four groups of women indicate, using these different types of measures (two rating scales and a combination of a self-report and rating scale, namely, content analysis measures) that long-term adverse emotional effects result from a unilateral mastectomy for type I and type II breast cancer. These effects might best be categorized as a significant increase in emotional distress 1–12 months after surgery as compared with the emotional status of a group of women who have had a cholecystectomy for a noncancerous condition, a breast biopsy negative for cancer, or a group of healthy women who have had no cancer or other serious disease. The severity of the emotional impact, as adjudged by the measures derived from the content analysis of speech, appears to be roughly graded across the groups of women. The greatest emotional disturbance occurs among the women in whom both cancer and surgery is involved, somewhat less distress is experienced among those who had had surgery for a noncancerous condition or who had had a breast biopsy with a negative finding for cancer, and the least, if any, distress occurs among the healthy women.

Comparing the overall scores from the women in this study with average scores from a normative group ($n = 282$, 73 males and 109 females) of individuals [25, 27], the healthy group of women from this study were in the 43rd percentile for total anxiety and 59th percentile for ambivalent hostility, whereas the women from the mastectomy group were in the 65th percentile for total anxiety and 71st percentile for ambivalent hostility.

The significantly higher affect denial scores and positive hope scores, derived from the content analysis of speech, for the mastectomy group as compared with the healthy group, suggest that the mastectomy group copes with their emotional arousal by the psychodynamic mechanism of denial and by maintaining high levels of positive hopefulness. Since women were excluded from this study who had seen any psychotherapist, data are not availbale to determine whether such women do not use such coping mechanisms and, hence, have to seek professional help to deal with the emotions aroused by mastectomy.

The tendency in the mastectomy group for anxiety arousal and other emotional concomitants of surgery to decrease with the elapse of time suggests that some recovery from the arousal of distress takes place with the passage of time. On the other hand, the fact that the anxiety scores of the mastectomy group remained significantly elevated at the time of the second assessment over the scores of the healthy group indicates there is some durability and depth to the emotional scarring.

With respect to why the Gottschalk-Gleser Content Analysis Scales reveal more significant findings that the other psychological measures used in this study, the Gottschalk-Gleser Scales are presumably more sensitive and may have less measurement errors than the other measures.

13.4.2 Emotional Distress as a Cause Versus an Effect of Surgical Intervention for Medical Disease.

Although this was not a prospective study and, hence, did not measure the emotional status of these women before the need for surgery was diagnosed, we do not believe that the women who underwent some kind of surgery had significantly elevated emotional distress, as compared with the healthy group, before a medical disorder justifying surgical intervention was discovered. Our evidence for this conjecture is as follows:

1. The healthy women included in this study and in other American studies [25, 27] as well as studies of normative women in Australia [59] and in West Germany [51] had mean affect scores derived by the Gottschalk-Gleser content analysis method which are not significantly different from one another and are significantly lower than the postsurgical mean affect scores of these women; yet, many of these healthy women go on to develop breast cancer.

2. Some of the affect scores, e.g., anxiety, decreased significantly from the first postsur-

gical evaluation point to the second one; such a decrease would be unlikely if these measures had been elevated premorbidly.

3. Prospective studies of cancer or gallbladder disease are rare, but the few we know about have not demonstrated elevated measures of emotional distress as compared with control groups. Follow-up studies of the life course of Johns Hopkins medical students [56] noted no striking emotional characteristics among students who subsequently developed cancer; the only unusual characteristic noted was that the people who developed cancer were not close to parental figures when young. On the other hand, a 10-year prospective study of cancerogenesis in 1353 subjects in a Yugoslavian town of 14000 inhabitants found an increased number of traumatic life events evoking hopelessness or chronic excitement and a chronic blockage of expression of feelings [36, 37]. In any event, the rare prospective studies examining psychosocial factors in cancer neither support not refute the hypothesis that increased emotional distress of the kind measured in the present study are a causal agent in breast cancer. It is likely that the kinds of emotional distress observed in the present study constitute a response to the discovery of a disease process plus the effect of surgical intervention rather than a level of emotional turmoil that preceded the discovery of disease and the occurrence of surgery.

13.4.3 Physiological and Biochemical Concomitants of Mastectomy.

Direct measures of physiological and biochemical sequelae of the emotional impact of mastectomy were not part of this study supported by the National Cancer Institute. Yet, these biological concomitants of the emotional arousal involved with mastectomy are likely to be instrumental in, if not markers of, the success of the body's homeostatic defenses in coping with illness. Is there not some evidence from other studies using some of these psychosocial measures that provide clues concerning what is happening biochemically in the body when anxiety and hostility are aroused or denied?

There is information available that does have a bearing on the probable physiological and biochemical concomitants of the emotional distress evoked among these women. Gottschalk and his co-workers have reported, on the basis of two studies, that there is a significant positive correlation between anxiety scores, derived from the content analysis of verbal behavior, and reduction in skin temperature [21, 28]. Also, these investigators found a significant correlation between increases in anxiety scores and the elevation of systolic blood pressure and between elevated hostility-inward scores and increases in diastolic blood pressure [32, 42].

Investigations of the biochemical concomitants associated with the arousal of anxiety, as measured by the content analysis method, have revealed persisting biochemical effects. The elevation of plasma free fatty acids, after 9–12 h of fasting (an indirect and sensitive measure of adrenergic secretion), has been demonstrated to be significantly correlated with increased anxiety [31–34, 55]. Moreover, the elevation of plasma free fatty acids occurring 5–15 min after a venipuncture has been observed to be significantly higher in anxious subjects as compared to nonanxious individuals [31, 34]. In these studies, levels of plasma triglycerides and plasma cholesterol have also been found significantly correlated with elevated hostility scores [31]. In addition, serum dopamine-beta hydroxylase levels have been found to be significantly correlated with anxiety scores derived from verbal samples by Silbergeld et al. [52]. In summary, evidence from other studies supports the idea that the emotional arousal observed in the mastectomy group is accompanied by arousal of the central nervous system and its complex of connections to the involuntary nervous system such that the biological homeostasis of the woman's body is changed.

13.4.4 Stress, the Immune Response, and Cancer.

What needs to be investigated further is whether those women who have experienced the more extreme emotional distress in reaction to mastectomy are more vulnerable to the development of metastases or are protected from spread of the neoplastic disease. From the psychobiological point of view, there is evidence that the higher hope scores are, the longer the life span of terminal cancer patients receiving total- or half-body irradiation [22, 23, 35].

Some investigators [5, 8, 13] have reported that relatively high levels of anxiety and hostility are associated with increased survival time in patients with breast cancer. That women with breast cancer do, indeed, have considerable emotional distress, including anxiety, hostility, and depression, has been well substantiated by others [5, 8, 10, 38] as well as in the present study.

Ader has convincingly demonstrated in animal studies that holding genetic predisposition constant, early life experiences interact with subsequent social factors to increase susceptibility to gastric lesions [1, 2] and/or neoplastic disorders [3]. Other investigators [43, 47, 53] are confirming that various kinds of stress can suppress immunity in animals and, by this means, enhance tumor growth. These experimental studies have implicated impairment of the immune system as a major mechanism in the increased vulnerability to the spread of neoplastic disease with exposure to various stressors. Although human studies are just getting underway in this research area, recent studies have revealed that depression and other psychological reactions can decrease various assays of immune competence [6, 26, 29, 46]; and that life stresses are significantly associated with a higher incidence of neoplastic disorders in children [41] and adults [46]. Pettingale et al. [48] reported finding significantly higher levels of serum IgM 3 months postmastectomy in a group of women with breast cancer who coped with their condition by denial rather than by fighting spirit or stoic acceptance; how this relates to survival has yet to be established. Prospective human studies pinpointing pathogenic linkages between emotional distress − an impairment of immune competence − and the onset of cancer, while holding constant the type of cancer and genetic and environmental carcinogenic influences, are extremely difficult to design and more difficult to implement. More feasible would be following the course of various types of human cancer once they have developed and ascertaining the interaction of vulnerability stemming from early personal and social history, the emotionally disturbing effect of more recent life experiences, and the degree of competence of many facets of the body's immune system. Increasing evidence is accumulating which provides psychosocial and biomedical markers and/or predictors towards vulnerability to stress and disease [16, 26, 41, 50]. These markers are available to test hypotheses concerning the interaction of psychosocial and biomedical factors as these influence the course of neoplastic disease. So far, no one has systematically tested these.

That emotional distress may have survival value is a hypothesis that merits exploration. There is evidence that a lack of fear or minimal fear or anger in response to real threats to health, e.g., before surgery [58] or childbirth [60], is predictive of increased surgical complications and prolonged labor in birth of a first child. It would seem that low or excessive emotional distress in reaction to such stresses could be counterproductive and disabling, whereas an optimal and realistic arousal of emotions – accompanied by increased steroid secretion and other adaptive biological variables – could better prepare the body's defenses, including immune responses, to fight disease.

13.5 Summary

1. To learn about the effects of unilateral mastectomy, the emotional responses of four groups of women, aged 30–69, were compared with one another on two occasions, 1–3 and 10–12 months after surgery. The four groups were: (1) mastectomy group ($n = 125$): women who had undergone unilateral mastectomy for stage I or II breast cancer 1–3 months before being interviewed; (2) biopsy group ($n = 65$): women who had had a biopsy revealing benign breast disease 1–3 months before being interviewed; (3) cholecystectomy group ($n = 75$): women who had undergone a cholecystectomy 1–3 months prior to being interviewed; and (4) healthy group ($n = 84$): women who had not had a major surgical interventions within 2 years prior to being interviewed.

2. Three types of measures of emotions were used: (1) the SCL-90 Analogue, an interviewer rating scale; (2) the Global Assessment Scale (GAS), an interviewer rating scale; and (3) the Gottschalk-Gleser Content Analysis Scale, a combination of a self-report and psychiatric rating scale.

3. Significantly higher mean Gottschalk-Gleser content analysis scores were obtained from the mastectomy group on total anxiety, death and mutilation anxiety, ambivalent hostility (references to others being hostile to the self), total denial and anxiety denial, and hopefulness at both testing periods. These scores exceeded the same mean scores from the biopsy, cholecystectomy, and/or healthy groups.

Significant reductions occurred in mean total anxiety, mutilation, and shame anxiety in the mastectomy group and in total and death and mutilation anxiety in the cholecystectomy group over the 9-month interval between the first and second postsurgical testing.

4. The mastectomy group had a significantly higher mean anxiety and depression score than the healthy group on the SCL-90 self-report scale 1–3 and 10–12 months after surgery.

5. The mastectomy and cholecystectomy groups had significantly lower scores on the GAS of emotional well-being than the healthy group over both testing periods, and the groups differed in their amount of change in the GAS over time.

6. All measures, most prominently the Gottschalk-Gleser Scales, showed significantly more psychopathological emotional responses in the mastectomy group, somewhat less in the cholecystectomy group, and the least in the biopsy group.

7. These findings suggest greater sensitivity and less measurement error from the Gottschalk-Gleser Scales than from the SCL-90 Analogue or the GAS. Also, the con-

tent analysis scale scores indicate that denial of affect and the maintenance of positive hopefulness are major coping mechanisms associated with the emotional distress aroused among the women experiencing a mastectomy.

8. The implications of these findings are discussed, including suggestions for further studies.

Acknowledgment

The assistance of James T.Ashurst, Ph.D., Computing Facility, University of California, Irvine, CA in data analysis is hereby gratefully acknowledged.

We acknowledge the contributions of the following groups: Writing Committee for Psychological Aspects of Breast Cancer Study Group: Joan R.Bloom, Ph.D., University of California, Berkeley, Mary Cook, Ph.D., Midwest Research Institute, Jimmie Holland, M.D., Sloan-Kettering Cancer Center, Larry Muenz, Ph.D., National Cancer Institute, and Doris Penman, Ph.D., Sloan-Kettering Cancer Center; other members of the group and co-authors: Sophia Fotopoulis, Ph.D., Midwest Research Institute, Christopher Gates, M.D., Peter Bent Brigham Hospital, Benjamin Murawski, Ph.D., Peter Bent Brigham Hospital, and Daphne Panagis, Ph.D., Public Response Associates. Institutions involved in data collection under contract with the National Cancer Institute included Montfiore Hospital and Medical Center, Peter Bent Brigham Hospital, Midwest Research Institute, West Coast Cancer Foundation, and SRI International.

References

1. Ader R (1965) Effects of early experience and differential housing on behavior and suspectibility to gastric erosions in the rat. J Comp Physiol Psychol 60: 233
2. Ader R (1977) The role of developmental factors in suspectibility to disease. In: Lipowski J, Lipsitt DR, Whybrow PC (eds) Psychosomatic medicine: current trends and clinical applications. Oxford University Press, New York, p 58
3. Ader R (ed) (1981) Psychoneuroimmunology. Academic, New York, p 661
4. Anderson TW (1958) An introduction to multivariate statistical analysis. Wiley, New York
5. Bacon CL, Renneker R, Cutler M (1952) A psychosomatic survey of cancer of the breast. Psychosom Med 14: 453
6. Bartrop RW, Lazarus L, Luckhurst E, Kiloh LG, Penny R (1977) Depressed lymphocyte function after bereavement. Lancet 1: 834
7. Bercheid E, et al. (1982) The social and psychological implication of facial physical attractiveness. Clin Plast Surg 9: 289
8. Blumberg EM (1954) Results in psychological testing of cancer patients. In: Gingerelli JA, Kirkner FJ (eds) Psychological variables in human cancer. University of California Press, Berkeley
9. Brown MB, Engleman L, Frane JW, Hill MA, Jennrich RI, Toporek JD (1981) BMDP statistical software. University of California Press, Berkeley
10. Cope O (1971) Breast cancer: has the time come for a less mutilating treatment. Psychiatr Med 2: 263
11. Daltore PJ, Shontz FC, Coyne L (1980) Premorbid personality differentiation of cancer and non-cancer groups: a test of the hypothesis of cancer proneness. J Consult Clin Psychol 48: 388
12. Derogatis LR (1977) The SCL-90-R administration, scoring and procedures manual, vol I. Clinical Psychometrics Research, Baltimore .

13. Derogatis LR (1979) Breast and gynecologic cancers. Their unique impact on body image and sexual identity in women. Front Radiat Ther Oncol 14: 1
14. Derogatis LR, Abeloff MD, Mellisaratos N (1979) Psychological coping mechanisms and survival time in metastatic breast cancer. JAMA 242: 1504
15. Earle EM (1979) The psychological effects of mutilating surgery in children and adolescents. Psychoanal. Study Child. 34: 527
16. Elliott GR, Eisdorfer C (1982) Stress and illness. In: Elliott GR, Eisdorfer C (eds) Stress and human health analysis and implications of research. Springer Publishing, New York
17. Endicott J, Spitzer R, Fleiss J, Cohen J (1976) The global assessment scale. Arch Gen Psychiatry 33: 766
18. Finn JD (1984) A general model for multivariate analysis. Rinehart and Winston, New York
19. Furnas DW, et al. (1980) Reconstruction of the burned nose. J Trauma 20: 25
20. Goin MK, Goin JM (1981) Midlife reactions to mastectomy and subsequent breast construction. Arch Gen Psychiatry 38: 225
21. Gottlieb AA, Gleser GC, Gottschalk LA (1967) Verbal and physiological responses to hypnotic suggestion of attitudes. Psychosom Med 29: 172
22. Gottschalk LA (1966) Total and half body irradiation. Effect on cognitive and emotional processes. In: Saenger EL (ed) Metabolic changes in humans following total body irradiation. DASA 1844 progress report in research project DA-49-I46-XA-315, Defense Atomic Support Agency, Washington DC
23. Gottschalk LA (1974) A hope scale applicable to verbal samples. Arch Gen Psychiatry 30: 779
24. Gottschalk LA (ed) (1979) The content analysis of verbal behavior: further studies. Spectrum, New York
25. Gottschalk LA (1982) Manual of uses and applications of the Gottschalk-Gleser verbal behavior scales. Res Commun Psychol Psychiatry Behav 7: 273
26. Gottschalk LA (1983) Vulerability to stress. Am J Psychother 37: 5
27. Gottschalk LA, Gleser GC (1969) The measurement of psychological states through the content analysis of verbal behavior. University of California Press, Berkeley
28. Gottschalk LA, Springer KJ, Gleser GC (1961) Experiments with a method of assessing the variations in intensity of certain psychological states occurring during two psychotherapeutic interviews. In: Gottschalk LA (ed) Comparative psycholinguistic analysis of two psychotherapeutic interviews. International Universities Press, New York
29. Gottschalk LA, Welch WD, Weiss J (1983) Vulnerability and immune response. Psychother Psychosom 398: 23
30. Gottschalk LA, Winget CN, Gleser GC (1969) Manual of instructions for using the Gottschalk-Gleser content analysis scales. University of California Press, Berkeley
31. Gottschalk LA, Cleghorn JM, Gleser GC, Iacono JM (1965) Studies of relationships of emotions to plasma lipids. Psychosom Med 27: 102
32. Gottschalk LA, Gleser GC, D'Zmura T, Hanenson IB (1964) Some psychophysiological relationships in hypertensive women. The effect of hydrochlorothiazide on the relation of affect to blood pressure. Psychosom Med 26: 26–610
33. Gottschalk LA, Stone WN, Gleser GC, Iacono JM (1966) Anxiety levels in dreams: relation to changes in plasma free fatty acids. Science 153: 654
34. Gottschalk LA, Stone WN, Gleser GC, Iacono JM (1969a) Anxiety and plasma free fatty acids (FFA). Life Sci 8: 61
35. Gottschalk LA, Kunkel RL, Wohl T, Saenger E, Winget CN (1969b) Total and half body irradiation. Effect on cognitive and emotional processes. Arch Gen Psychiatry 21: 574
36. Grossarth-Maticek R (1980) Psychosocial predictors of cancer and internal diseases: an overview. Psychother Psychosom 33: 122
37. Grossarth-Maticek R, Kanazir DT, Schmidt P, Vetter H (1982) Psychosomatic factors in the process of cancerogenesis. Psychother Psychosom 38: 284

38. Gyllenskold K (1982) Breast cancer: the psychological effects of the disease and its treatment. Tavistock, New York
39. Holmes TH, Rahe RH (1967) The social readjustment rating scale. J Psychosom Res 11: 213
40. Howells JG (eds) (1974) Modern perspectives in the psychiatric aspects of surgery. Brunner/Mazel, New York
41. Jacobs TJ, Charles E (1980) Life events and the occurrence of cancer in children. Psychosom Med 42: 11
42. Kaplan SM, Gottschalk LA, Magliocco EB, Rohovit DD, Ross WD (1961) Hostility in verbal productions and hypnotic dreams of hypertensive patients: studies of groups and individuals. Psychsom Med 23: 311
43. Keller SE, Weiss JM, Schleifer SJ, Miller NE, Stein M (1981) Suppression of immunity by stress: effect of a graded series of stressors on lymphocytic stimulation in the rat. Science 213: 1397
44. MacGregor F (1979) After plastic surgery. Bergin, New York
45. Maguire P (1974) The psychological and social sequelae of mastectomy. In: Howell JG (ed) Modern perspectives in the psychiatric aspects of surgery. Brunner/Mazel, New York, p 390
46. Palmblad J (1981) Stress and immunologic competence in man. In: Ader R (ed) Psychoneuroimmunology. Academic, New York, p 229
47. Pavlides N, Chirigos M (1980) Stress-induced impairment of macrophage tumoricidal acitivity. Psychosom Med 42: 47
48. Pettingale KW, Philalithis A, Tee DE, Greer HS (1981) The biological correlates of psychological responses to breast cancer. J Psychosom Res 25: 453
49. Quint JC (1964) Mastectomy – symbol of cure or warning sign? Gen Pract 29: 119
50. Rahe RH (1977) Epidemiological studies of life changes and illness. In: Lipowski ZJ, Lipsitt DR, Whybrow PC (eds) Psychosomatic medicine: current trends and clinical applications. Oxford University Press, New York, p 421
51. Schofer G, Koch U, Balck F (1979) The Gottschalk-Gleser content analysis of speech, a normative study. In: Gottschalk LA (ed) The content analysis of verbal behavior: further studies. Spectrum, New York, p 97
52. Silbergeld S, Manderscheid RW, O'Neill PH, Lamprecht F, Ng L. K. Y. (1975) Changes in serum dopamine-beta-hydroxylase activity during group psychotherapy. Psychosom Med 37: 352
53. Sklar LS, Anisman H (1980) Social stress influences tumor growth. Psychosom Med 42: 347
54. SPSS Inc (1983) SPSS-X user's guide. McGraw-Hill, New York
55. Stone WN, Gleser GC, Gottschalk LA, Iacono JM (1969) Stimulus, affect and plasma free fatty acids. Psychosom Med 21: 331
56. Thomas CB, Duszynski KR (1974) Closeness to parents and family constellation in a prospective study of five diseases: suicide, mental illness, malignant tumor, hypertension, coronary heart disease. Johns Hopkins Med J 134: 251
57. Titchener JL, Zwerling I, Gottschalk LA, Levine M (1958) Psychological reactions of the aged in surgery. The reactions of renewal and depletion. AMA Arch Neurol Psychiatry 79: 63
58. Titchener JL, Zwerling I, Gottschalk LA, Levine M, Culbertson W, Cohen SF, Silver H (1957) Consequences of surgical illness and treatment. Interactions of emotions, personality, surgical illness, treatment, and convalescence. AMA Arch Neurol Psychiatry 77: 623
59. Viney LL, Manton M (1973) Sampling verbal behaviour in Australia. The Gottschalk-Gleser content analysis scales. Aust J Psychol 25: 45
60. Winget C, Kapp FT (1972) The relationship of the manifest content of dreams to duration of childbirth in primiparae. Psychosom Med 34: 313
61. Zwerling I, Titchener JL, Gottschalk LA, Levine M, Culbertson W, Cohen SF, Silver H (1955) Personality disorder and the relationship of emotions to surgical illness in 200 surgical patients. Am J Psychiatry 112: 270

Table 1. Differences between groups on Gottschalk-Gleser Content Analysis Scale mean scores controlling for age 1–3 months after surgery (by MANCOVA)

Groups	n	Death Anxiety	Mutilation Anxiety	Total Anxiety	Ambivalent Hostility	Anxiety Denial	Hostility Out Denial	Hostility In Denial	Total Denial	Positive Hopefulness
		Mean (SD)	Mean (SD)	Mean (SD)	Mean (SD)	Mean (SD)	Mean (SD)	Mean (SD)	Mean (SD)	Mean (SD)
1. Mastectomy	118	0.76 (±0.58)	1.07 (±0.74)	1.95 (±0.90)	0.74 (±0.47)	0.50 (±0.25)	0.35 (±0.12)	0.35 (±0.13)	0.55 (±0.29)	0.94 (±0.38)
2. Cholecystectomy	69	0.58 (±0.40)	0.79 (±0.63)	1.69 (±0.76)	0.65 (±0.40)	0.36 (±0.13)	0.32 (±0.10)	0.32 (±0.87)	0.40 (±0.17)	0.89 (±0.40)
3. Biopsy	64	0.61 (±0.40)	0.70 (±0.56)	1.62 (±0.81)	0.66 (±0.43)	0.35 (±0.13)	0.31 (±0.08)	0.31 (±0.11)	0.39 (±0.16)	0.82 (±0.44)
4. Healthy	78	0.58 (±0.43)	0.55 (±0.44)	1.41 (±0.70)	0.47 (±0.26)	0.35 (±0.13)	0.33 (±0.11)	0.30 (±0.64)	0.39 (±0.16)	0.78 (±0.33)
df 3.325, F		5.65	11.50	8.19	6.73	17.72	2.70	3.59	15.72	2.87
P		0.004	0.000	0.000	0.000	0.000	0.05	0.01	0.000	0.04

Table 2. Differences between groups on Gottschalk-Gleser Content Analysis Scale mean scores controlling for age 10–12 months after surgery (by MANCOVA)

Groups	n	Death Anxiety Mean (SD)	Mutilation Anxiety Mean (SD)	Total Anxiety Mean (SD)	Ambivalent Hostility Mean (SD)	Anxiety Denial Mean (SD)	Hostility Out Denial Mean (SD)	Hostility In Denial Mean (SD)	Total Denial Mean (SD)	Positive Hopefulness Mean (SD)
1. Mastectomy	118	0.66 (±0.54)	0.87 (±0.64)	1.69 (±0.77)	0.69 (±0.40)	0.45 (±0.21)	0.35 (±0.12)	0.34 (±0.12)	0.50 (±0.26)	0.86 (±0.35)
2. Cholecystectomy	69	0.52 (±0.26)	0.56 (±0.43)	1.33 (±0.59)	0.53 (±0.30)	0.37 (±0.17)	0.33 (±0.11)	0.31 (±0.76)	0.41 (±0.19)	0.81 (±0.35)
3. Biopsy	64	0.62 (±0.58)	0.63 (±0.48)	1.61 (±0.66)	0.67 (±0.42)	0.36 (±0.15)	0.33 (±0.11)	0.30 (±0.68)	0.40 (±0.17)	0.74 (±0.31)
4. Healthy	78	0.55 (±0.47)	0.51 (±0.35)	1.34 (±0.62)	0.58 (±0.37)	0.36 (±0.15)	0.31 (±0.07)	0.30 (±0.73)	0.37 (±0.15)	0.78 (±0.36)
df 3,325, F		5.65	11.15	6.95	3.50	6.92	2.89	4.70	7.66	3.79
P		0.004	0.000	0.0002	0.02	0.002	0.04	0.003	0.0001	0.05

Differences between group scores when combined over occasions (1–3 and 10–12 months after surgery)

Anxiety

Death	Group 1 > 2,	$df = 1,324$, $F = 13.96$, $P < 0.001$
Multilation	Group 1 > 2,	$df = 1,324$, $F = 21.34$, $P < 0.001$
Separation	Group 1 > 2,	$df = 1,324$, $F = 5.26$, $P < 0.05$
Diffuse	Group 1 > 2,	$df = 1,324$, $F = 3.82$, $P < 0.05$
Mutilation	Group 1 > 2, 3, 4,	$df = 1,324$, $F = 4.04$, $P < 0.05$
Separation	Group 1 > 2, 3, 4,	$df = 1,324$, $F = 5.38$, $P < 0.05$
Diffuse	Group 1 > 2, 3, 4,	$df = 1,324$, $F = 3.96$, $P < 0.05$

Denial

Anxiety	Group 1 > 2,	$df = 1,324$, $F = 28.52$, $P < 0.001$
Hostility Out	Group 1 > 2,	$df = 1,324$, $F = 9.72$, $P < 0.05$
Hostility In	Group 1 > 2,	$df = 1,324$, $F = 4.36$, $P < 0.05$
Total	Group 1 > 2,	$df = 1,324$, $F = 24.18$, $P < 0.001$

Hostility

Hostility Inward	Group 1 > 2,	$df = 1,324$, $F = 9.36$, $P < 0.01$
Ambivalent Hostility	Group 1 > 2,	$df = 1,324$, $F = 5.38$, $P < 0.05$
Ambivalent Hostility	Group 3 > 4,	$df = 1,324$, $F = 9.60$, $P < 0.01$
Hostility Inward	Group 1 > 2, 3, 4,	$df = 1,324$, $F = 4.96$, $P < 0.05$
Ambivalent Hostility	Group 1 > 2, 3, 4,	$df = 1,324$, $F = 8.34$, $P < 0.01$

Denial

Anxiety	Group 1 > 2, 3, 3,	$df = 1,324$, $F = 52.76$, $P < 0.001$
Hostility Out	Group 1 > 2, 3, 4,	$df = 1,324$, $F = 8.21$, $P < 0.01$
Hostility In	Group 1 > 2, 3, 4,	$df = 1,324$, $F = 4.95$, $P < 0.01$
Total	Group 1 > 2, 3, 4,	$df = 1,324$, $F = 49,41$, $P < 0.001$

14 Some Sources of Alienation for Drug Addicts*

Linda L. Viney, Mary T. Westbrook, and Carol Preston

14.1 Introduction

One major focus in research concerned with drug addiction has been the interpersonal relationships of the addicts, particularly within their family. Families of addicts have been variously depicted as showing extreme marital tension, family breakdown, ineffectuality of fathers, pathology of mothers, alcoholism, cruelty, and overdependent, overprotective relationships [1–5]. Some of these factors have been seen as causes of addiction, others as factors contributing to addiction. Some researchers emphasize the need for family reconciliation and family therapy, while others see separation and independence from families as necessary for the successful treatment of the addiction.

Another aspect of the addicts' relationships which has been a major focus of study has been peer groups. The research in this area suggests an inability of addicts to relate effectively to either peers or spouses [6–8]. Chambers [9] concluded that addicts fail to develop satisfactory friendships because they convert peer relations to dependency relationships. Interviews with addicts have revealed that they emphasize the need for support from relatives and drug-free friends and that they regard the giving up of former addicted friends and acquaintances as a necessary prerequisite to becoming drug free [10, 11].

Follow-up studies of addiction treatments suggest that a more favorable outcome occurs for addicts who have more contact with relatives and drug-free friends [12, 13]. However, this may not be the case for all addicts. Tokar and his colleagues [14] interviewed heroin addicts with long addiction histories who had tried giving up drug use. They found that the addicts commonly maintained that they did not get enjoyment from friends, love, or life in general. They felt unable to enter into prolonged, close friendships. Heroin had become their only source of satisfaction.

Whether addicts enter into individual therapy or family therapy, the relationships which they maintain or develop within or outside of treatment are an important consideration. An understanding of the way they perceive these relationships is necessary to help them to develop their ability to relate to others in mature and satisfying ways. Researchers have identified only three types of interpersonal interactions which are indicative of positive relationships. The first set consists of interactions involving solidarity, or interpersonal support, and the sharing of resources. The second has to do with intimacy, in which relationships are sources of affection and personal satisfaction. The third focuses on influence, or the sharing of dominant and submissive roles [15–17].

* This research was funded by Australian Research Grants Scheme, Grant No. 77/5046 R.

The aim of this research was to explore which types of interpersonal interactions are salient to addicts. It was expected from the literature review that the interactions reported by addicts would be limited to interactions in which the addicts felt others had influence over them (e.g., treatment staff, legal bodies, drug contacts) and that intimate or affectionate relationships would be absent from their experience, indicating alienation from others. A second aim of the study was to identify the relationship between evidence of such sources of alienation and the history of the addicts.

14.2 Method

Addicts' perceptions of their interpersonal interactions were assessed from an interview, which included an unstructured question about their current experience: "Will you talk about your life at the moment, the good things and the bad, what it's like for you now." The responses were tape-recorded and transcribed, and a content analysis scale designed to represent the three types of interaction was applied to the transcripts.

The scale used, the Sociality Scale, was developed to make explicit the interpersonal interactions people experience and to assess the extent to which they are currently experiencing satisfying relationships or alienation. The scale has been shown to have both interrater reliability and construct validity [18, 19] and has been used effectively in studies of many life events [20–22]. Four Subscales are included in the total score to identify references to supportive interactions (Solidarity, e.g., "My mother tries to help"), affectionate interactions (Intimacy, e.g., "My boyfriend's really good to me"), and influential interactions (Influence, e.g., "My parole officer persuaded me to come here"). In addition to these three recognized types of interactions, references to shared relationships in which the nature of the interaction is not clear (Other Shared Experiences, e.g., "We moved up north to get away from it all") are also scored. The Sociality Scale has been shown to correlate negatively with anxiety, anger, and depression and positively with happiness [23]. Low scores on the scale indicate alienation or a lack of positive interpersonal relationships [24].

The histories of the addicts were classified into four sets of variables. The first was a set of *demographic variables* including sex, age, marital status, and educational status. The second set *(addiction history)* was made up of age at first involvement with drugs, length of addiction, time since most recent drug intake, number of periods of abstinence, and length of abstinence periods. A third set was concerned with the use of two *other drugs,* marijuana and alcohol, and the addicts' perception of the effect of these drugs on their lives. The last set of variables *(social supports)* included the marital status of the addicts' parents, the kind of relationship each addict experienced with his or her parents, parents' knowledge of the addiction, the extent to which the addicts' peers were involved in drug taking, and the kind of relationship each addict had with his or her peers.

14.3 Samples

The addicts interviewed were 60 clients who attended a counseling and referral center for addiction in a small Australian city during a 6-month period. Only one addict refused to participate. At the request of the center staff, five others were not approached because of their physical or psychological condition. The addicts were interviewed individually at the center by a psychologist (C. P.) who was well-known to both addicts and staff. Information about their addiction history was provided by each client's counselor and the medical practitioner at the center.

The interview was conducted with 43 men and 17 women. Their ages ranged from 17 to 41 years, but most were relatively young ($\overline{X} = 24$ years). Their educational status was low: 51 had not completed high school (only nine had done so); 21 had no post-high school vocational training, and 22 had started such training but dropped out. Only six of the addicts were employed. The rest were receiving unemployment or sickness benefits. Twenty were living with their parents, 17 with a spouse or in a de facto relationship, 9 lived alone, and 14 with friends. Their drugs of addiction included some combination of heroin, barbiturates, LSD, Pethidine, amphetamines, and methadone. When interviewed, only 14 had been drug free for more than 2 or 3 days.

A group of 73 full-time and part-time university students from the same city, matched with the addict groups for sex and age, was also interviewed to provide an understanding of how addicts differ from other young people who are successfully involved in full-time employment and/or academic studies which precludes any major involvement with drugs of addiction.

Table 1. Means and standard deviations of content analysis scale scores of addicts and students

	Addicts		Students	
	$\overline{X}$	SD	$\overline{X}$	SD
Solidarity	0.13	0.11	0.18	0.12
Intimacy	0.08	0.06	0.09	0.08
Influence	0.06	0.05	0.06	0.04
Other Shared Experiences	0.16	0.12	0.27	0.21

14.4 Results

The addict sample was compared with the student sample using multivariate analysis of variance (MANOVA). The means and standard deviations of the sociality scores for both groups are shown in Table 1. The MANOVA yielded a significant multivariate F value ($F = 5.06$; $df = 4,133$; $P < 0.001$). Table 2 shows the pattern of differences identified by univariate analysis. Two of the Sociality Subscales yielded significant differences (Solidarity and Shared Experiences). In both cases the addicts scored lower.

Table 2. Univariate analysis of variance of content analysis scale scores for addict and student groups

	Addicts/Students	
	F	$P<$
Solidarity	5.00	0.03
Intimacy	0.42	
Influence	0.41	
Other Shared Experiences	12.11	0.001

The second aim of this study was to establish the extent to which these sociality scores, representing different sources of alienation, were related to the history of the addicts. Canonical correlation (CANONA) was used for the analysis of the relationship between four sets of history variables and the sociality scores. Significant canonical correlation coefficients were found for three of the four sets. The coefficients for each significant set are shown in Table 3.

Table 3. Correlation coefficients for sociality scores and addict's history

Addiction history $R^2 = 0.61$; $X^2 = 31.35$; $df = 20$; $P < 0.05$			
Age first involved	−0.34	Solidarity	0.51
Length of addiction	0.03	Intimacy	−0.43
Last used drug	0.32	Influence	0.17
Number of abstinence periods	−0.96	Other Shared Experiences	−0.6
Length of periods of abstinence			
Other drug problems $R^2 = 0.46$; $X^2 = 17.9$; $df = 8$; $P < 0.02$			
Alcoholism	−0.67	Intimacy	0.38
		Other Shared Experiences	0.53
Social supports $R^2 = 0.62$; $X^2 = 37.33$; $df = 20$; $P < 0.02$			
Parents' marriage	−0.57	Solidarity	1.04
Relationship with parents	−0.24	Intimacy	−0.34
Parents' knowledge of drugs	1.14	Influence	−0.25
Involvement of associates	0.11	Other Shared Experiences	0.34
Relationship with associates	0.38		

None of the Sociality Scales varied as a function of the addicts' age, sex, marital status, or educational status. For the second set (addiction history), there was a significant correlation. Fewer but longer periods of abstinence and earlier involvement were found to be related to reports of fewer intimate and other shared interactions but more solidarity statements. The third set (other drugs) was also significantly related to the sociality scores. A pattern of no perceived problems with alcohol but heavy involvement with marijuana smoking was associated with high scores for each of the four types of interaction. The last set of variables (social supports) yielded the following pattern. Addicts whose parents were least likely to know about their addiction and had a stable marriage, and whose relationships with associates were described as "superficial," expressed more solidarity and other shared relationships but few intimacy interactions.

14.5 Discussion

The differences found between the sources of alienation of addicts and of students of the same age will be discussed. Then, the relationship between the addicts' pattern of alienation and their history will be considered. Finally, some implications from this research for the treatment of addicts will be examined.

As predicted, the addicts in this study were reporting fewer positive interpersonal interactions than students of the same age and sex. The types of relationships which were particularly lacking for the addicts were those involving supportive interactions and other shared experiences. The greatest difference between the groups was in the area of shared interactions, which would have included a wide range of generally shared experiences from which the addicts seemed to be alienated. Even though each of the addicts was involved in a treatment program, which included the availability of a personal counselor, care from a medical practitioner, facilities for live-in detoxification, and group support, the addicts apparently did not perceive these potential interactions as sources of interpersonal support. This was one significant indicator of their alienation.

The importance of different sources of alienation varied according to other aspects of the histories of the addicts. Those who reported fewer, but longer periods of abstinence, especially those who had begun the addiction cycle earlier, were involved in fewer intimate, affectionate relationships and fewer shared experiences but more supportive relationships. It would appear that addicts who had been able to successfully abstain from drug use for considerable periods of time in their past did experience some of their relationships as helpful and supportive, but for them, intimate relationships and even other, generally shared experiences were minimal. For abstainers, these were important sources of alienation.

Another factor in the addicts' histories which related to their alienation was their use of alcohol and marijuana. Those who reported heavy, problematic use of alcohol experienced much alienation from each of the sources measured, while those reporting heavy use of marijuana reported more involvement in each type of interpersonal interaction. Marijuana use may be accepted as a more sociable and preferred activity than heavy alcohol use among drug addicts, many of whom view being "drunk" much more negatively than being "stoned."

Addicts who came from homes where the parents had a stable marriage and were unlikely to know about the addiction problem, and who said that their relationships with their peers were superficial, reported more supportive interactions and more unidentified but positive interactions, but fewer affectionate or intimate interactions. These addicts may have limited their interpersonal involvement to what was necessary to maintain their habit to keep their family and nonaddict friends unaware of their problems. While this choice seemed to result in more support from others and other shared interactions, it was at a cost to the addicts in terms of alienation from intimate, affectionate relationships.

For the addicts of this study, their perceptions of interpersonal interaction involved complex social processes, including relationships with the families and nonaddict friends and with treatment staff, as well as their associations with other addicts. For many of the addicts, it seemed important to keep these parts of their lives separate. Others, perhaps those from broken families and those more deeply involved in the drug subculture, experienced less support and less generally shared interactions. The addicts seemed only to feel supported if they had proven themselves able to abstain in the past or if they kept knowledge of their addiction relatively hidden. Intimacy or affectionate, close relationships were only associated with the drug subculture of marijuana smoking. Generally shared experiences were restricted in both the drug world and the "straight" world.

Several sources of alienation have, then, been identified by this research. However, the sense of alienation and loneliness felt by young addicts is probably best communicated by the addicts themselves:

> When I'm using I can talk to people. I've always been a bit shy, like ... but I've got to give it up because of the law ... and also my family. My family want me to get off it. I'd like to be able to make it, you know, and make different friends 'cause all the friends I had, they stay away from you when you're using. I wanted to go into the country and start again. My boyfriend and I were going to try and live out there, but now my boyfriend's probably going to jail, so I don't know what I'll do.
> I suppose I do it because it helps me forget about things all the time, 'cause everything's not too good now. The family's all deserted me – not that I blame them, like ... they tried. I was only out of here a day last time and I was locked up again. It couldn't be a much worse life, could it ... wakin' up ... ripping off doctors and chemists ... sleeping, waking up. I think I might as well be dead ... I think if I could just find a nice girl, you know ... but I guess I just fool myself with that.

The sense of alienation of addicts which has been tapped here throws some light on previous findings in which researchers, and addicts themselves, have concluded that addicts are unable to develop effective close relationships or to gain satisfaction from relating to others. The findings of this study suggest that for addicts relating to others is primarily aimed at maintaining the kind of help and support they need either to survive as a drug addict or to work toward a drug-free life. It follows that potentially rewarding relationships are experienced by addicts as conditionally supportive but essentially alienating.

Many of the clients in this study had made numerous attempts to give up drug taking, and some had done so a number of times. Helping addicts to move away from drug taking is, then, an insufficient long-term treatment goal. The life addicted clients are moving toward needs to include close friendships, which should result in an ability to care for others and to accept being cared about. Many young addicts may have achieved neither. An important focus of treatment must therefore be helping clients to interact with friends, family, and treatment personnel in ways which do not bring about an increased sense of alienation. Such alienation seems likely to contribute to their relapse to drug use.

Acknowledgment.
Thanks are gratefully expressed to the staff and clients of Kembla House.

References

1. Alexander B, Dibb G (1977) Interpersonal perception in addict families. Fam Process 16 (1): 17–33
2. Kaldegg A (1978) A study of young male heroin dependent patients. Part II: attitudes to father, mother and family as revealed in a sentence completion test. Br J Addic 68: 257–263
3. Kaufman E (1981) Familiy structures of narcotic addicts. Int J Addic 16 (2): 273–282
4. Noone RJ, Reddig RL (1976) Case studies in the family treatment of drug abuse. Fam Process 15 (3): 325–332
5. Stanton MD (1977) The addict as saviour: heroin, death and the family. Fam Process 16 (2): 191–197
6. Hart L, Kroch L (1975) Problems of adjustment reported among a group of heroin addicts. Int J Addic 10 (3): 433–441
7. Kaplan H, Meyerowitz J (1969) Psychosocial predictions of post institutional adjustment among male drug addicts. Arch Gen Psychiatry 20: 278–284
8. Rosenbaum M (1981) When drugs come into the picture, love flies out the window: women addicts' love relationships. Int J Addic 16 (7): 1197–1206
9. Chambers JL (1972) Need associations of narcotic addicts. J Clin Psychol 28 (4): 468–469
10. Frykholm B (1979) Termination of the drug career: an interview study of 58 ex-addicts. Acta Psychiatr Scand 59: 370–380
11. Sjoberg L, Olsson G (1981) Volitional problems in carrying through a difficult decision: the case of drug addiction. Drug Alcohol Depend 7: 177–191
12. Frykholm B, Grunne T, Huitfeldt B (1976) Prediction of outcome in drug dependence. Addict Behav 1: 103–110
13. Gossop M (1978) Drug dependence: a study of the relationship between motivational, cognitive, social and historical factors and treatment variables. J Nerv Ment Dis 166 (1): 44–49
14. Tokar J, Brunse A, Steffire V, Sodergren J, Napior D (1975) Determining what heroin means to heroin addicts. Dis Nerv System 36 (2): 77–81
15. Danzinger K (1976) Interpersonal communication. Pergamon, New York
16. Osgood CE (1970) Speculations on the structure of interpersonal intentions. Behav Sci 15: 237–254
17. Straus MA (1964) Power and support of the family in relation to socialization. J Marr Fam 26: 318–326
18. Viney LL (1983) The assessment of psychological states by content analysis of verbal communications. Psychol Bull 94: 542–563
19. Viney LL, Westbrook MT (1979) Sociality: a content analysis scale for verbalizations. Soc Behav Pers 7 (2): 129–137
20. Viney LL (1980) Transitions. Cassell, Sydney
21. Viney LL (1981 a) Content analysis: a research tool for community psychologists. Am J Commun Psych 9: 269–281

22. Viney LL, Westbrook MT (1981) Measuring patients' experienced quality of life: the application of content analysis scales in health care. Commun Health Stud 5: 45–52
23. Westbrook MT, Viney LL (1977) The application of content analysis scales to life stress research. Aust Psychol 12: 157–166
24. Viney LL (1981 b) An evaluation of an Australian youth work programme. Aust Psychol 16: 37–47

15 Content Analysis of Speech of Schizophrenic and Control Adoptees and Their Relatives: Preliminary Results*

Dennis K. Kinney, Bjørn Jacobsen, Birgitte Bechgaard, Lennart Jansson, Britta Faber, Eva Kasell, and Regina L. Uliana

15.1 Introduction

Gottschalk and Gleser [1] devised standard methods for verbal content analysis and for eliciting speech samples. Several scales with subscales have been developed that tap several different psychological dimensions. Of these, the Schizophrenic, or Social Alienation-Personal Disorganization *(SA-PD)*, Scale was developed to measure those themes and characteristics often found in speech samples from schizophrenic patients. Mean scores on this scale have been found to be significantly higher in samples of schizophrenic patients than in groups of patients with other psychiatric disorders or than in normal control groups [2]. Although other important and reliable systems for scoring the content and/or formal properties of speech samples have also been shown to distinguish schizophrenics from controls at a significant level (e.g., 3, 4), results from several previous studies suggested it would be valuable to investigate the SA-PD Scale in the present sample.

Thus, Gottschalk et al. [1, 5] have suggested that the SA-PD Scale may be measuring a relatively stable psychological "trait." Evidence suggesting that SA-PD Scale scores measure a heritable, as well as a stable, trait was reported by Arnold [6]. She obtained SA-PD Scale scores by analyzing speech samples collected from Gottesman and Shields' [7] previous study of an English sample of monozygotic and dizygotic twin pairs – at least one of whom in each pair had a diagnosis of schizophrenia. Arnold also found that SA-PD Scale scores were higher in her schizophrenic sample than in normal subjects or than in patients with other psychiatric disorders. Consistent with a high heritability for the SA-PD Scale scores, Arnold found that intraclass correlation coefficients for monozygotic twin pairs were significantly higher than for dizygotic pairs. Scores of the schizophrenics and their monozygotic co-twins were highly correlated, even if the co-twin was *not* schizophrenic. High SA-PD Scale scores tended to characterize schizophrenics (a) whose symptoms did not remit to the point that they were able to work and (b) whose monozygotic co-twin was either schizophrenic or, if not hospitalized, still psychiatrically abnormal.

---

* Printed in modified form in *Social Science and Medicine* (in press) with permission of the author and publisher. This research was supported in part by grants from the MacArthur Foundation (No. 81–171), from the NIMH (MH-36 088 and MH-31 154), and from the Foundations Fund for Research in Psychiatry.

These findings suggest that a "high" (i. e., deviant) SA-PD Scale score may be a behavioral marker of a genetic liability to schizophrenia, characterizing not only (a) schizophrenics whose monozygotic co-twin also tends to be ill but also (b) individuals who, though not meeting diagnostic criteria for schizophrenia, carry a genetic liability for the disorder. However, although highly suggestive, these twin data must be interpreted with caution since monozygotic twins (unless reared apart, which those studied by Arnold were not) are more likely to share similar environments than are singleton sibs or even dizygotic twins [8].

Samples of adopted schizophrenics and controls and their relatives offer a method for avoiding this confounding of genetic and environmental influences. By making use of such samples, the present study was designed to investigate whether (a) high SA-PD Scale scores would discriminate schizophrenic subjects from subjects with other psychiatric disorders or with no psychiatric disorder. Of still greater interest was the question of whether (b) high scores would particularly characterize schizophrenics especially likely to have a genetic liability for the disorder as well as (c) "schizotypal" subjects who – even though not meeting diagnostic criteria for schizophrenia – would display symptoms suggesting they may carry a high genetic liability for schizophrenia. A complementary question (d) was whether high scores would characterize the adoptive relatives of schizophrenics, as one might expect if the familial environment had been a significant factor in accounting for Arnold's twin data.

Several hypotheses were advanced for testing. First, it was hypothesized that the schizophrenic adoptees would have significantly higher SA-PD Scale scores than control adoptees (previously determined by Kety et al. [9] to have no institutional record of treatment for psychiatric problems).

A second hypothesis was that the schizophrenic adoptees would also have significantly higher scores than other subjects in the study sample who (a) had no psychiatric history or (b) who met the Research Diagnostic Criteria (RDC) of Spitzer et al. [10] for other psychiatric disorders, based on the Schedule for Affective Disorders and Schizophrenia-Lifetime Version (SADS-L) interview.

A third hypothesis was that among the schizophrenic adoptees, SA-PD Scale scores would be particularly high among those most likely to have a genetic liability for schizophrenia, as evidenced by their having a first-degree biological relative who either (a) had been previously diagnosed as having chronic or borderline schizophrenia by Kety et al., (b) met RDC criteria for schizophrenia on the basis of being interviewed in the present study, or (c) had "schizotypal" features discovered in the course of the SADS-L interview. The schizotypal features are those signs and symptoms previously identified by Spitzer and Endicott [10], from a review of cases previously diagnosed by Kety et al. [11] as lying within the "schizophrenia spectrum" of disorders that appear to be genetically related to schizophrenia. These schizotypal features (e. g., "bizarre ideation," "odd communication," ideas of reference) are those that characterize subjects who, though not meeting full criteria for schizophrenia, were diagnosed by Kety et al. as having borderline or latent schizophrenia – diagnoses that Kety et al. found to be highly concentrated among the biological relatives of the schizophrenic adoptees. In DSM-III [12], the term "schizotypal personality disorder" is used to label subjects characterized by these schizotypal features.

Because these schizotypal features had previously been identified by Kety et al. as characterizing subjects with schizophrenia-like syndromes and were highly concentrated among the biological relatives of the schizophrenic adoptees, we hypothesized that individuals with at least one schizotypal feature would be particularly likely to be carrying a genetic liability for schizophrenia, even though they did not meet full diagnostic criteria for schizophrenia. A corollary hypothesis was that nonschizophrenics with schizotypal features would have significantly higher scores than subjects with no psychiatric history or those with diagnoses other than schizophrenia. We further hypothesized that nonschizophrenic subjects with schizotypal features who also were biological relatives of schizophrenic probands would have particularly high scores compared with biological control relatives without schizotypal features or schizophrenia.

In the studies described earlier by Gottschalk et al. [2], and Arnold [6], it was the highly deviant or "schizophrenic" scores on the SA-PD Scale – those outside the range typically shown by normal control subjects – that seemed to be particularly significant, that is, their samples of schizophrenics showed a very wide range of scores, with the majority of schizophrenics having SA-PD Scale scores that overlapped the range of scores displayed by normal control groups. Gottschalk, however, found that there was a large subgroup that had scores that were more extreme than those attained by virtually any of the subjects in nonschizophrenic comparison groups. A score of 5.0 or higher served as an approximate cut-off score demarcating this subgroup of high-scoring schizophrenics. Similarly, in Arnold's data, a threshold of approximately 5.0 points seemed to distinguish two subgroups of schizophrenics, with those schizophrenics scoring 5.0 or above particularly likely to show unremitting symptoms and to have a co-twin who was also schizophrenic. We therefore further hypothesized that in our sample variation in SA-PD Scale scores below 5.0 would be less important than whether or not a subject had a truly "extreme" or deviant score of 5.0 or above.

Finally, we hypothesized that high SA-PD Scale scores would reflect primarily the operation of genetic rather than environmental factors in the transmission of schizophrenia so that the SA-PD Scale scores for the adoptive relatives of schizophrenic adoptees would *not* be higher than in the adoptive relatives of controls.

15.2 Method

The present study sample was drawn from a larger, national sample of adopted schizophrenics and adopted control subjects and their relatives previously ascertained by Kety et al. [9, 13, 14]. This national sample of schizophrenics identified by Kety et al. consisted of all schizophrenics born in Denmark between 1924 and 1947 and adopted by families to whom they were not biologically related. For each schizophrenic or "index" adoptee (proband), a control adoptee with no record of psychiatric disorder was selected, matched for age, sex, and socioeconomic status of the adoptive home. Most of the adoptees were separated from their biological families shortly after birth, and they and their adoptive relatives had little or no contact with the adoptees' biological relatives. The relatives of schizophrenic and control probands placed for adoption in the city and county of Copenhagen were the subject of an earlier interview study [14]. Subjects in the present study comprise the "provincial" subsample, consisting of adoptees placed for adoption in the rest of Denmark and their respective biological and adoptive parents, siblings, and half-siblings. All adoptees and their relatives 18 years old or over and residing in Scandinavia were invited to participate; over 90% of this total sample agreed to be interviewed.

Subjects were interviewed by one of two Danish psychiatrists using a research diagnostic interview instrument of demonstrated reliability and validity, the SADS-L, which is designed for making diagnoses according to the RDC of Spitzer et al. [10]. After completing the interview, subjects were asked to provide a speech sample following the standard procedure of Gottschalk and Gleser [1], in which the subject is instructed to talk for 5 min about any interesting or dramatic personal life experience she or he has had, while being tape-recorded. Interview and speech samples were obtained by interviewers who were blind as to the subject's familial relationship to a schizophrenic or control proband.

The taped speech samples were transcribed verbatim and scored for SA-PD by a bilingual Danish psychologist trained in using the SA-PD Scale. To demonstrate the reliability of study ratings on the SA-PD Scale, a second rater, who was also a native Dane fluent in English, learned to score protocols on the SA-PD Scale. These two raters each independently scored transcripts of speech samples from a dozen subjects. Good interrater reliability was achieved ($r = 0.92$; $P < 0.001$). Those transcribing and rating the protocols were kept blind as to the diagnostic status of subjects and their familial relationships to control or schizophrenic probands. Following the guidelines suggested by Gottschalk and Gleser [1], all protocols with stories of at least 70 words were scored.

Two different types of statistical analyses were carried out to test each of our hypotheses. First, t-tests were conducted to test for mean differences between groups. In addition, it was expected that a second, nonparametric test might be an even better test of the hypotheses. Fisher's exact test was therefore used to test for whether SA-PD Scales scores of 5.0 or greater were associated with being an index schizophrenic (particularly one with a schizophrenic or schizotypal biological parent or sib) or with having schizotypal features, particularly among schizophrenics' biological relatives.

15.3 Results

The data tended to confirm the hypotheses. First of all, the mean SA-PD Scale score for the index (schizophrenic) adoptees was indeed significantly higher than that for the control adoptees (means of $+1.96$ vs -2.76; $t = 3.94$; $df = 44$; $P < 0.0005$) (see Table 1). (All P values for t tests reported in this paper are two-tailed; all significant differences between means were also in the predicted direction).

The mean SA-PD Scale score was also significantly greater for the index adoptees than for (a) all subjects in the sample with no psychiatric history or for (b) the sample of subjects with other psychiatric disorders (who had means of -3.50 and -1.62 respectively; $t = 4.91$; $df = 215$; $P < 0.0005$ and $t = 3.09$; $df = 126$; $P < 0.003$ for respective comparisons with index adoptees). The mean for subjects with other psychiatric disorders was also significantly higher than for subjects with no psychiatric disorder ($t = 3.31$; $df = 303$; $P < 0.002$). Among the index adoptees, the mean score was indeed much higher among those with a first-degree biological relative who had either schiz-

Table 1. Social Alienation-Personal Disorganization Scale Scores in different groups

Subject group	Percent with score > 5.0		Mean	SD
Schizophrenic adoptees	30.0%	(6/20)	+1.96	4.70
Schiz. adoptees with schizophrenic or schizotypal[a] parent or sib	50.0%	(4/8)	+3.79	5.19
Schiz. adoptees' biological relatives with schizotypal features[a]	17.6%	(3/17)	−1.25	5.93
Subjects with other psychiatric disorders[a]	5.6%	(6/108)	−1.62	4.76
Subjects with no history of psychiatric disorder[a]	3.6%	(7/197)	−3.50	4.73
Control adoptees	0.0%	(0/26)	−2.79	3.48
Schizophrenic adoptees' adoptive relatives	0.0%	(0/29)	−3.65	4.50

[a] Based on the SADS-L interview

ophrenia or schizotypal features (mean of 3.79) than for index adoptees with *no* schizophrenic or schizotypal first-degree biological relative (mean of 0.74). Index adoptees with this positive family history had a significantly higher mean score than did (a) control adoptees ($t = 4.15$; $df = 32$; $P < 0.0005$), (b) subjects with other disorders, or (c) subjects with no disorder ($t = 3.08$; $df = 114$; $P < 0.004$ and $t = 4.25$; $df = 203$; $P < 0.0005$, respectively). By contrast, index adoptees with no such first-degree relative differed less markedly from control adoptees ($t = 2.74$; $df = 36$; $P < 0.01$), from the group with other psychiatric disorders ($t = 1.65$; $df = 118$; $P = $ NS), and from subjects with no psychiatric disorder ($t = 3.03$; $df = 207$; $P < 0.004$).

It should be noted that it was possible to obtain scoreable speech samples on only 20 of the 41 schizophrenic adoptees in the provincial sample. Those adoptees for whom speech samples could not be obtained tended to be those with more severe symptoms so that if it had been possible to obtain SA-PD Scale scores for all index adoptees, it is likely that the group differences we found would have been even greater than they were.

Nonschizophrenic subjects with schizotypal features had a SA-PD Scale score mean of −1.64, which was much higher than for subjects with no psychiatric disorder ($t = 1.95$; $df = 225$; $P = 0.053$) and was very similar to the mean for subjects with other psychiatric disorders ($P = $ NS). Subjects who had schizotypal features and were also biological relatives of schizophrenic probands had a yet higher mean score of −1.25, which was greater than the mean of −2.66 for the comparison group of control adoptees' biological relatives without schizotypal features, although the difference was not statistically significant. The mean score for 29 adopted relatives of the schizophrenic adoptees was quite low (−3.65) – actually *lower* (less deviant) than the mean score of −1.49 for 34 adoptive relatives of the control adoptees ($t = −1.95$; $df = 61$; $P = 0.056$).

When SA-PD Scale scores were dichotomized as being greater than or equal to

+ 5.0 vs below + 5.0, our hypotheses were even more strongly confirmed. Table 1 displays the proportions of subjects in different groups with scores of 5.0 or above. It can be seen that among the 20 index adoptees for whom scoreable protocols could be obtained, 6 of 20 or 30% had scores of 5.0 or greater (hereafter referred to as "high" scores, for sake of brevity in exposition). This compared with (a) a high score rate of 0% among 26 control adoptees ($P = 0.004$, Fisher's exact test, one-tailed), with (b) 3.6% of the subjects in the entire sample with no psychiatric illness (based on the SADS-L interview) ($P = 0.0004$, exact test), and with (c) 5.6% of subjects having psychiatric disorders other than schizophrenia ($P = 0.004$, exact test).

Among those schizophrenic adoptees having a schizophrenic or schizotypal first-degree biological relative, 50% had high scores, which was significantly greater than for control adoptees, for all subjects with no psychiatric disorder, or for subjects with other psychiatric disorders (P values of 0.002, 0.0003, and 0.002, respectively; exact tests). By contrast, schizophrenic adoptees with no schizophrenic or schizotypal first-degree relative did *not* have a significantly higher proportion of high scores compared with these other groups ($P > 0.05$ in all cases). The proportion of high scores among subjects with other psychiatric disorders did not differ significantly from that in subjects with no apparent psychiatric disorder.

Among "schizotypal" subjects (i.e., nonschizophrenics with schizotypal features based on the SADS-L interview), 16.7% had high scores, which was a significantly greater proportion than for all subjects with no psychiatric disorder ($P = 0.012$, exact test) and also greater than for all subjects with other psychiatric disorders, although the P value did not quite reach the 0.05 level ($P = 0.061$, exact test). Among 17 schizotypal subjects who were also biological relatives of the schizophrenic adoptees, 3 (or 17.6%) had high scores compared with only 3 of 95 (or 3.2%) of the control adoptees' biological relatives with no schizotypal features ($P = 0.044$, exact test). Among the schizophrenic adoptees' adoptive relatives, 0 of 29 had SA-PD Scale scores > 5.0 compared with 2 of 34 control adoptees' adoptive relatives ($P = $ NS).

15.4 Discussion

On the whole, the results provide support for our hypotheses. Considering the difficulties of translating the Gottschalk-Gleser verbal content analysis system into another language and culture, the similarity of results to those reported earlier by Gottschalk et al. and Arnold is rather remarkable. The present study confirms in a Danish sample the results of these earlier studies done in the United States and Great Britain in finding that schizophrenics have higher mean SA-PD Scale scores than do either (a) control subjects with no apparent psychiatric disorder or (b) subjects with other psychiatric disorders.

Of even greater interest, the present results appear to confirm Arnold's finding that high SA-PD Scale scores are associated with those schizophrenics whose biological family history for schizophrenia suggests they are most likely to have a genetic liability for the disorder. Finally, we found evidence to support the hypothesis that the proportion of very high or deviant high SA-PD Scale scores is greater in individuals who, although not meeting full criteria for schizophrenia, nonetheless show "schizotypal" traits, suggesting they carry a genetic liability for schizophrenia that manifests itself in more subtle ways. The adoption study sample facilitated separation of genetic and environmental influences as most of the schizophrenic and control adoptees were separated from their biological parents shortly after birth and had little if any contact with their biological relatives. In summary then, our data did not suggest that environmental factors were major contributors to high SA-PD. Indeed, SA-PD Scale scores among the adoptive relatives of the schizophrenic adoptees were quite low and, in fact, lower than adoptive relatives of control adoptees. Our data thus suggest Arnold's twin findings were not attributable to the effects of postnatal environments which the twins shared in common. Rather, our results are consistent with other research suggesting that schizophrenia is an etiologically heterogeneous disorder and that a subgroup of schizophrenics may carry a particularly high genetic liability [15, 16].

It is notable that the SA-PD Scale scores, which emphasize speech content, appear in the present study (as in Arnold's twin study) to be tapping a heritable factor, whereas the data on our adoptive families do not appear at all suggestive of a significant influence of the familial environment. By contrast, twin and adoption study data involving measures that emphasize either formal or communicative aspects of speech have suggested stronger environmental and weaker genetic influences. For example, Berenbaum et al. [17] recently analyzed speech samples from essentially the same twin sample studied earlier by Arnold. The measure of Berenbaum et al., however, emphasized formal thought disorder, as opposed to the content emphasis of the SA-PD Scale, and empirical analyses indicated the two measures had little in common. Berenbaum et al. found evidence for significant familial influence, but *not* for genetic influence, on their thought disorder measures, and noted that their results are reminiscent of the finding by Wynne et al. [18] of elevated communication deviance in the adoptive parents of schizophrenics, which also points to a role for psychosocial processes.

The data from these different studies thus suggest that the SA-PD Scale, with its emphasis on themes of alienation from other people, may be tapping a relatively stable and heritable trait associated with schizophrenia. It is interesting in this regard that difficulties in interpersonal relations and competence have been found to be predictive of poor outcome in adult schizophrenics [19, 20]. Moreover, retrospective and high-risk studies (e.g., 21) suggest that interpersonal difficulties with young school peers are both (a) more common in children at increased risk for schizophrenia and (b) may tend to be associated with the kinds of attention deficits that other research has suggested may be genetic risk factors for schizophrenia.

A few notes of caution seem in order, however. It seems premature to use high SA-PD Scale scores clinically for identification of subjects with a genetic liability for schizophrenia. High SA-PD Scale scores do not appear to have an elevated prevalence among schizophrenics' nonschizophrenic relatives as a group [as seems to to be the case, for example, with dysfunctions of smooth pursuit eye movements (22)], but rather characterize only a relatively small group of biological relatives who themselves have schizotypal signs. Further work is needed to determine the sensitivity and specificity of high SA-PD Scale scores for etiological subtypes of schizophrenia or for schizotypal personality disorders.

Nonetheless, it is interesting that using blind ratings of relatively brief speech samples elicited by a single question, we obtained a pattern of significant results which complement previous studies and suggest that SA-PD Scale scores may be tapping a significant heritable factor in schizophrenia. Since schizophrenics' speech tends to become more disordered as an interview becomes longer or demands more decisions, it seems reasonable to expect that further refinement of the SA-PD Scale and its use with longer and more varied speech samples might yield even clearer differences among subgroups of schizophrenics and their relatives. The present study thus suggests that the Gottschalk-Gleser SA-PD Scale is a promising research tool for investigating genetic factors in the transmission of schizophrenia and their manifestation in deviant speech; this area clearly merits further careful investigation.

Acknowledgment

We thank Seymour S. Kety, David Rosenthal, Fini Schulsinger, and Paul Wender for making the adoption study sample available for this study, and the adoptees and their families for their participation. We thank Seymour S. Kety and Louis A. Gottschalk for their helpful advice; Maria E. Benet, Sandra M. Cole, Ann P. C. Merzel, and Karen L. Spritzer for research assistance; and Anette Ganz and Maureen Medeiros for typing the speech transcripts and manuscript, respectively.

References

1. Gottschalk LA, Gleser GC (1969) The measurement of psychological states through the content analysis of verbal behavior. Universities of California Press, Berkeley
2. Gottschalk LA, Gleser GC (1964) Distinguishing characteristics of the verbal communications of schizophrenic patients. Disorders of Communication. ARNMD 12: 100
3. Johnston MH, Holzman PS (1979) Assessing schizophrenic thinking. Jossey-Bass, San Francisco
4. Rochester S, Martin JR (1979) Crazy talk: a study of the discourse of schizophrenic speakers. Plenum, New York
5. Gottschalk LA, Uliana RL (1979) Profiles of children's psychological states derived from the Gottschalk-Gleser content analysis of speech. J Youth Adolesc 8: 269
6. Arnold KEO (1971) Language in schizophrenics and their twins. Dissertation, University of Minnesota
7. Gottesman II, Shields J (1972) Schizophrenia and genetics: a twin study vantage point. Academic, New York
8. Koch HL (1966) Twins and twin relations. University of Chicago Press, Chicago
9. Kety SS, Rosenthal D, Wender PH (1978) The biological and adoptive families of adopted individuals who became schizophrenic: prevalence of mental illness and other characteristics. In: Wynne L, (eds) The nature of schizophrenia. Wiley, New York, p 776
10. Spitzer RI, Endicott J, Robins F (1978) Research diagnostic criteria: rationale, and reliability. Arch Gen Psychiatry 35: 773
11. Kety SS, Wender PH, Rosenthal D (1978) Genetic relationships within the schizophrenia spectrum: evidence from adoption studies. In: Spitzer RL (eds) Critical issues in psychiatric diagnosis. Raven, New York, p 213
12. Diagnostic and Statistical Manual of Mental Disorders (DSM-III) (1980) 3rd edn. American Psychiatric Association, Washington DC
13. Kety SS, Rosenthal D, Wender PH, Schulsinger F (1968) The types and prevalence of mental illness in the biological and adoptive families of adopted schizophrenics. In: Rosenthal D (eds) The transmission of schizophrenia. Pergamon, Oxford, p 345

14. Kety SS, Rosenthal D, Wender PH, Schulsinger F, Jacobsen B (1975) Mental illness in the biological and adoptive families of adopted individuals who have become schizophrenic: a preliminary report based on psychiatric interviews. In: Fieve RR (eds) Genetic research in psychiatry. Johns Hopkins University Press, Baltimore, p 147
15. Matthysee S, Kidd KK (1978) Genetic principles in defining homogeneous subgroups of the schizophrenias. In: Akiskal H (eds) Toward a biological classification of psychiatric disorders. Spectrum, New York, p 155
16. Kinney DK (1983) Schizophrenia and major affective disorders (manic-depressive illness). In: Emery AH (eds) Principles and practice of medical genetics. Churchill Livingstone, Edinburgh, p 321
17. Berenbaum H, Oltmanns TF, Gottesman II (1985) Formal thought disorder in schizophrenia and their twins. J Abnor Psychol 94: 3
18. Wynne LC, Singer MT, Toohey ML (1976) In: Jorstad J et al. (eds) Schizophrenia 75: psychotherapy, family studies, research. Universitetsforlaget, Oslo, p 413
19. Garmezy N (1973) Competence and adaptation in adult schizophrenia and patients and children at risk. In: Dean SR (ed) Schizophrenia: the first ten dean award lectures MSS, New York, p 168
20. Goldstein MJ (1980) The course of schizophrenia psychosis. In: Brim OG Jr, (eds) Constancy and change in human development. Harvard University Press, Cambridge, p 325
21. Asarnow JR (1984) The Waterloo studies of interpersonal competence. In: Watt NF (eds) Children at risk for schizophrenia. Cambridge University Press, Cambridge, p 414
22. Holzman PS, Solomon CM, Levin S, Waternaux CS (1984) Pursuit eye movement dysfunctions in schizophrenia. Arch Gen Psychiatry 41: 136

16 Alexithymia and Affective Verbal Behavior of Psychosomatic Patients and Controls

Stephan Ahrens

16.1 Introduction

One of the main controversial topics currently being discussed within the field of psychosomatic medicine is the question of whether a personality structure of psychosomatic patients can be described which is distinct from that of somatic or psychoneurotic patients. Concepts of a specific personality structure have been developed on the basis of observational data. A central assumption of these concepts is that psychosomatic patients are unable to adequately perceive and comprehend affective behavior ("alexithymia," [1–3]; "pensee operatoire," [4, 5]; "psychosomatic phenomenon," [6–8]. As an example, Nemiah describes the course of an interview with a patient suffering from anorexia, who proved to be unable to localize feelings in her body or to describe them with adequate words. Therefore, she admitted to being nervous, when in reality she was hungry. Empirical investigations of this topic first began with the use of instruments in the tradition of personality trait assessment (for a review of this, see [9]), whereas von Rad et al. [10] concentrated on the study of psychosomatic patient's speech. The rationale of this second approach is based on the postulate of a decrease in affective verbal expression implied by the term "alexithymia." Von Rad et al. [10] were the first to use Gottschalk-Gleser content analysis of speech samples [11] for this purpose. In their study they used several kinds of experimental stimuli: Thematic Apperception Test (TAT) cards, unfinished stories, and an interview setting. Significant differences between psychosomatic patients vs psychoneurotic controls could only be found in respect to the interview setting.

This finding implies important consequences for the empirical study of alexithymia, which we followed up in the series of studies reported in this paper. To learn more about alexithymia, it seemed necessary to employ a methodology that would permit the recording of the patient's response to affective stimuli in an interpersonal context having high personal relevance. Also, it should permit in-depth analysis of verbal expression beyond the standardized format of questionnaires.

Given the methods capable of fulfilling these requirements, it is then possible to conduct experimental investigations in which stimuli are varied and patients from several clinical groups can be compared.

16.2 Method

The investigation was carried out as an experimental study in which the effects of systematic variation of affective stimuli were compared across several groups of patients. It was conducted in two stages, covering different clinical groups. The first stage (for details, see [12–15]) included three groups: psychosomatic, psychoneurotic, and somatic. In the second stage [16], two more psychosomatic groups were added.

16.2.1 Sample

A total of five clinical groups were studied. There were three groups of patients suffering from classic psychosomatic disease: duodenal ulcer ($n = 42$), Crohn's disease ($n = 22$), and ulcerative colitis ($n = 22$). These clinical diagnoses were confirmed by endoscopy. To provide ample experimental control, two nonpsychosomatic groups were also studied: psychoneurotic patients ($n = 22$) who were selected on the basis of clinical diagnoses which ruled out psychosomatic complaints and somatic patients ($n = 31$) who suffered from accidental somatic afflictions such as fractures. All patients received outpatient treatment at the time of the study.

No attempt was made to parallelize groups on the basis of socioeconomic statistics for we wanted to work with an undistorted sample of patients as they occur in the various clinical groups. We did nevertheless collect such data (age, sex, educational level, professional training, income) and compared the groups. No significant differences were found, but the group of ulcer patients tended to have a lower educational level and a higher income. This fits in with the well-known idea of an "ambitious ulcer personality." Nevertheless, it is not plausible to assume any systematic influence of this characteristic on what was quantified in our measurements; with respect to the first stage of our investigation, this was further checked in a control study [17, 18].

The control study involved the measurement of cognitive processing of affective stimuli which were not bound to any specific situation. The stimuli consisted of several photos showing different kinds of facial expressions. These had been defined and tested by Schüle [19] who found them to be distinct examples of general, everyday types of expression. There were no differences between the three experimental groups in the present study with respect to the patients' response to these stimuli [17]. Furthermore, intellectual performance level and verbal creativity were compared for the three groups using the Performance Testing System developed by Horn [20] and the Verbal Creativity Test developed by Schoppe [21]. Again, there were no differences between the groups. On the basis of these results, any influence of general, nonspecific personality/performance-related variables on our experimental data can be ruled out, and thus the effects found may be interpreted as situationspecific.

16.2.2 Material

Our stimuli were short silent films. These were designed to show human interaction of a kind which was highly relevant to the subjects on a personal level. The independent variable for systematic variation was the quality of affective behavior of that interaction. High personal relevance was achieved by selecting a scene that was well-known to the somatic and psychosomatic group: an examination of the upper part of the stomach by a physician. Systematic variation was made possible by producing two versions of the film: one in which the physician can be observed to be friendly and attentive and a second one in which the psysician acts in an unfriendly, matter-of-fact way. To guarantee a strong variation along the affective dimension without changing other aspects of the interaction in the film, the stimulus material was prepared under expert directions and supervision by actors from the "Kieler Schauspielhaus".

16.2.3 Procedure

Each of the five experimental groups was divided in half so that each individual patient was only shown one version of the film; this was done to avoid the possibility of contrast effects. The response to these stimuli was measured on two different levels: the first provided an opportunity for the patients to express their conscious cognitive processing of these stimuli, whereas the second was aimed at measuring unconscious, unintentional processes.

16.2.3.1 Level 1

On this level, cognitive attribution processes were measured. For this purpose, we used a modification of the semantic differential. It is a checklist of bipolar adjective pairs developed by Hofstätter [22], which had been tested and standardized by that author in a great number of studies.

The subjects were prompted to check this list with the question: "Wie haben Sie den Arzt erlebt?" (What was your impression of the physician?) These adjective pairs were combined into two scales (PP1 = Emotionality, PP2 = Activity) so that group comparisons could be performed for the two scores. These scores provide overall information on cognitive attribution of adjectives to the physician's behavior.

16.2.3.2 Level 2

On this level, we used the content analysis of speech samples developed by Gottschalk and Gleser [11]. In contrast to the first level of measurement, this level was meant to record and quantify the unconscious dimension of affective expression of the patient's verbal response. For this purpose, we used the Gottschalk-Gleser Hostility Scales, which had been adapted to the German language by Schöfer [23] and which had been validated in this version by Koch [24]. Speech samples were elicited by the instruction to describe one's feeling toward the physician in the interaction shown in the film.

16.3 Results

At the present time, it is only possible to report results from two separate analyses of data from the two stages of the investigation. Due to technical difficulties, the overall analysis of variance for all five groups will have to be reported at a later date. Still we feel that the two sets of results do converge sufficiently well to allow for a comprehensive overview. In the following, we shall report the two ANOVAs (3×2 and 2×2) for the two levels of measurement. For the purposes of illustration, we present multiple tables of univariate analyses, but these were confirmed by multivariate methods as well.

16.3.1 Level 1

In previous studies, data from the adjective checklist were factor-analyzed [25]. From these analyses, two dimensions were selected, and the items were grouped accordingly to form the basis of two scales giving stable measures for cognitive attribution. Thus, on this level there were two dependent variables (PP1 = Emotionality, PP2 = Activity) that were to be compared in respect to which version of the film was seen by the patients. One of the two ANOVAfactors was Version (friendly vs unfriendly), which was the same for both analyses. The other factor (Group) consisted of the three stages "psychosomatic vs psychoneurotic vs somatic" in the first and "ulcerative colitis vs Crohn's disease" in the second ANOVA.

Table 1. ANOVA table for two scales of the adjective checklist

Version		Groups				
		Ulcer	Somat.	Neurot.	Colitis	Crohn
PP1	Unfriendly	$\bar{x} = 3.1$	$\bar{x} = 3.4$	$\bar{x} = 3.4$	$\bar{x} = 4.75$	$\bar{x} = 4.20$
		$s = 0.94$	$s = 0.79$	$s = 0.76$	$s = 0.65$	$s = 0.67$
	Friendly	$\bar{x} = 2.6$	$\bar{x} = 1.7$	$\bar{x} = 2.1$	$\bar{x} = 3.40$	$\bar{x} = 3.31$
		$s = 0.49$	$s = 0.42$	$s = 0.49$	$s = 0.57$	$s = 1.00$
PP2	Unfriendly	$\bar{x} = 3.6$	$\bar{x} = 3.6$	$\bar{x} = 3.3$	$\bar{x} = 3.90$	$\bar{x} = 3.52$
		$s = 0.95$	$s = 0.85$	$s = 0.64$	$s = 0.66$	$s = 0.66$
	Friendly	$\bar{x} = 3.8$	$\bar{x} = 4.3$	$\bar{x} = 4.1$	$\bar{x} = 4.10$	$\bar{x} = 1.07$
		$s = 1.00$	$s = 0.67$	$s = 0.75$	$s = 0.63$	$s = 1.07$

Table 1 shows means and standard deviations for PP1 and PP2 scores for the five groups. Significance of differences was tested for the two factors Version and Groups. In the first ANOVA (for the three-group sample), there was a strong effect of Version (PP1: $F = 56.0$, $P < 0.001$; PP2: $F = 6.3$, $P < 0.05$), no effect of Groups (PP1: $F = 0.6$; PP2: $F = 0.7$), and some indication of an interaction of the two factors (PP1: $F = 5.5$, $P < 0.05$; PP2: $F = 1.1$). The interaction could be traced to different response patterns of the ulcer patients; unlike the two other groups, they did not clearly differentiate between the two versions of the film.

Results from the second study helped to further differentiate this. As in the case of the nonpsychosomatic groups from the first study, there was a strong effect of Version (PP1: $F = 24.06$, $P < 0.01$; PP2: $F = 8.64$, $P < 0.01$), and again there was no effect of Groups (PP1: $F = 2.08$; PP2: $F = 0.51$). There was one significant interaction (PP2: $F = 4.78$, $P < 0.05$) though; in their scores for PP2, patients from the ulcerative colitis group did not differ significantly in their response to the two versions of the film.

16.3.2 Level 2

On this level, ANOVA comparisons were performed for two Gottschalk-Gleser Scales, namely, Overt Hostility Directed Outward (OHDO) and Covert Hostility Directed Outward (CHDO). The selection of only these scales was necessary because of the way our speech samples differed from speech obtained by means of the Gottschalk-Gleser standard instructions (see [11]). Under our experimental conditions, the patient's affective response was channeled in a highly specific way in which outward aggression most certainly was the dominant theme. Table 2 shows means and standard deviations for these two scales.

Table 2. ANOVA table for Gottschalk-Gleser scores

Version		Groups				
		Ulcer	Somat.	Neurot.	Colitis	Crohn
OHDO	Unfriendly	$\bar{X} = 1.83$	$\bar{X} = 1.63$	$\bar{X} = 2.19$	$\bar{X} = 1.62$	$\bar{X} = 1.74$
		$s = 0.96$	$s = 0.98$	$s = 1.08$	$s = 0.61$	$s = 0.59$
	Friendly	$\bar{X} = 1.36$	$\bar{X} = 1.41$	$\bar{X} = 2.24$	$\bar{X} = 1.16$	$\bar{X} = 0.92$
		$s = 0.84$	$s = 0.63$	$s = 0.64$	$s = 0.80$	$s = 0.48$
CHDO	Unfriendly	$\bar{X} = 1.49$	$\bar{X} = 1.58$	$\bar{X} = 1.74$	$\bar{X} = 1.83$	$\bar{X} = 1.36$
		$s = 0.89$	$s = 0.98$	$s = 0.62$	$s = 0.79$	$s = 0.72$
	Friendly	$\bar{X} = 0.57$	$\bar{X} = 0.91$	$\bar{X} = 0.96$	$\bar{X} = 1.01$	$\bar{X} = 0.80$
		$s = 0.23$	$s = 0.78$	$s = 0.77$	$s = 1.22$	$s = 0.47$

OHDO, overt hostility directed outward; CHDO, covert hostility directed outward

The significance of differences was again tested in two analyses of variance for both studies. In the case of the first sample (three groups), there was an effect of Version for covert hostility (CHDO: $F = 17.1$; $P < 0.001$) and none for overt hostility (OHDO: $F = 1.0$). The factor Groups led to significant Fvalues in the case of overt hostility (OHDO: $F = 3.8$; $P < 0.05$) but not in the case of covert hostility (CHDO: $F = 1.0$). No interactions were found.

The other ANOVA previded even clearer results: There were significant effects of Version for both Gottschalk-Gleser Scales (OHDO: $F = 10.76$, $P < 0.01$; CHDO: $F = 7.52$, $P < 0.01$) and no effects of Groups (OHDO: $F = 0.08$; CHDO: $F = 7.52$, $P < 0.01$) and no effects of Groups (OHDO: $F = 0.08$; CHDO: $F = 1.70$), nor were there indications of interaction. The effects of Version could under all conditions be attributed to the unfriendly version of the film receiving higher scores, which is a confirmation of the intended experimental variation. The significant effect of Groups in the first study can be attributed to the fact that psychoneurotic patient's speech samples elicited by either version of the film received higher scores for overt hostility.

16.4 Discussion

Conscious cognitive attribution processes in response to experimental stimuli – friendly vs unfriendly films – were recorded on a checklist of bipolar adjective pairs. On this level, the psychosomatic patients' response to friendly vs unfriendly stimuli varied. Whereas the group of ulcerpatients did not show differential response toward the two versions of a film, colitispatients responded differentially on one scale only (PP1), and Crohnpatients were comparable to the two control groups. The failure to respond differentially can be interpreted as an indication of these patients' inability to adequately perceive or process the affective content of the films. As the results from this level show, this kind of inability is quite varied among the five groups.

The results of the second level of measurement nevertheless require this to be qualified. On that level, unconscious processing of the films' affective content was analyzed by means of the Gottschalk-Gleser technique of content analysis. This approach made it possible to gain a new perspective. None of the three groups of psychosomatic patients differed from somatic or psychoneurotic patients in their ability to register and respond to the differences of affective content. Patients from all groups showed significantly more covert hostility and separation anxiety toward the unfriendly physician in the film.

This demonstration of affective responsiveness of psychosomatic patients (duodenal ulcer) on an unconscious level is in sharp contrast to those concepts which claim psychosomatic patients to suffer from a deficit in their ability to adequately perceive and process affective stimuli.

However, even on the level of more conscious responses (adjective checklists), such concepts have to be questioned on the basis of the present results. Only the group of ulcer patients responded in a way which is in line with the traditional view of alexithymia. Colitis patients showed some responsiveness, and Crohn patients do not differ from controls. The fact that some psychosomatic patients did not differentiate well between friendly vs unfriendly films on the cognitive/functional level should therefore not be explained by postulating a deficit in perception and processing, but on the basis of the results from level 2 they should rather be seen as the outcome of specific defense mechanisms.

References

1. Sifneos PE (1973) The prevalence of alexithymic characteristics in psychosomatic patients. Psychother Psychosom 22: 255–262
2. Nemiah JC (1977) Alexithymia. Theoretical considerations. Psychother Psychosom 28: 199–206
3. Freyberger H (1977) Psychosomatik des erwachsenen Menschen. In: Freyberger H (ed) Psychosomatik des Kindesalters und des erwachsenen Menschen, Klinik der Gegenwart, vol 2. Urban and Schwarzenberg, München
4. Marty P (1976) Les mouvements individuels de vie et de mort. Payot, Paris
5. de M'uzan M (1977) Zur Psychologie des psychosomatisch Kranken. Psyche 31: 318–332
6. Stephanos S (1979) Das Konzept der "pensee operatoire" und das "psychosomatische Phänomen". In: v Uexküll Th (ed) Lehrbuch der Psychosomatischen Medizin. Urban and Schwarzenberg, München
7. Ahrens S (1983) Die psychosomatische Persönlichkeitsstruktur – Faktum oder Fiktion? Fortschr Neurol Psychiatry 51: 408–426
8. Nemiah JC (1972) Emotions and physiology: an introduction into physiology, emotion and psychosomatic illness. Ciba Found Symp 8: 15–29
9. Ahrens S, Deffner G (1985) "Alexithymia" – results and methods in a research field of psychosomatic medicine. Psychother Med Psychol 35: 147–159
10. von Rad M, Lalucat L, Lolas F (1977) Differences of verbal behaviour in psychosomatic and psychoneurotic patients. Psychother Psychosom 28: 83–97
11. Gottschalk LA, Gleser GC (1969) The measurement of psychological states through the content analysis of verbal behaviour. University of California Press, Berkeley
12. Ahrens S, Deffner G (1983) Empirische Befunde zur Affektverarbeitung bei Ulkuspatienten. Verh Dtsch Ges Inn Med 89: 558–560
13. Ahrens S (1983) Das psychosomatische Phänomen. Z Psychosom Med 29: 307–320
14. Ahrens S (1983) Die psychosomatische Persönlichkeitsstruktur – Faktum oder Fiktion? Fortschr Neurol Psychiatry 51: 409–426
15. Ahrens S, (1985) Alexithymia and affective verbal behaviour of three groups of patients. Soc Sci Med 20: 691–694
16. Ahrens S (1984) Affektverarbeitung. Z Psychosom Med 30: 201–213
17. Ahrens S (1981) Untersuchung kognitiver Funktionen bei Ulcuspatienten. In: Zander W (ed) Experimentelle Forschungsergebnisse in der psychosomatischen Medizin. Vandenhoeck and Ruprecht, Göttingen
18. Ahrens S (1981) Empirische Untersuchungen zum Krankheitskonzept neurotischer, psychosomatischer und somatisch kranker Patienten, T II. Med Psychol 7: 175–190
19. Schüle W (1976) Ausdruckswahrnehmung des Gesichtes. Fachbuchhandlung. Psychologie, Frankfurt
20. Horn W (1962) Das Leistungs-Prüfsystem (LPS). Hogrefe, Göttingen
21. Schoppe K-J (1975) Verbaler Kreativitätstest. Hogrefe, Göttingen
22. Hofstätter PR (1959) Zur Problematik der Profilmethode. Diagnostica 5: 19–24
23. Schöfer G (1980) Gottschalk-Gleser – Sprachinhaltsanalyse. Theorie und Technik. Studien zur Messung ängstlicher und aggressiver Affekte. Beltz, Weinheim
24. Koch U (1980) Möglichkeiten und Grenzen einer Messung von Affekten mit Hilfe der inhaltsanalytischen Methode nach Gottschalk und Gleser. Med Psychol 6: 81–94
25. Ahrens S (1983) Zur Affektverarbeitung von Ulcus-Patienten – ein Beitrag zur "Alexithymie" – Diskussion. In: Studt HH (ed) Psychosomatik in Forschung und Praxis. Urban and Schwarzenberg, München

17 Expression of Positive Emotion by People Who Are Physically Ill: Is It Evidence of Defending or Coping?*

Linda L. Viney

17.1 Introduction

Expression of positive emotion by patients hospitalized because of illness or injury is rarely expected by the medical and nursing staff who work with them, nor has such expression of good feelings and contentment been examined in any detail by researchers. Some evidence of this phenomenon is now emerging in the literature [1]. The more severe their illness, the more positive emotion patients express [2]. Yet, the less severe they perceive the handicaps induced by their illness to be, the more positive emotion they express [3]. It is possible to view positive emotion as a distortion of the distressed emotions which are more appropriate reactions to illness and injury [4]. It is also possible to see it as an indication of the high quality of life some patients can maintain in spite of coping with multiple stressors [5]. The expression of positive emotion has been found to be associated with both poor [6] and good [7] medical prognoses. Hence, it may be evidence of either defending or coping.

The use of defensive psychological processes by patients has been described as rigid and reality distorting [8]. It has been linked with passive surrender to illness or injury [9]. Denial is one form of defending by patients which has often been described. They may deny the illness or its effects, or the distress which is linked with it. Sigmund Freud defined denial as an unconscious mechanism used to deal with anxiety [10]. Anna Freud expanded the concept to include dealing with anger and negating reality [11]. This distorting mechanism has been further broadened to be seen as a way of escaping confrontation of events and their negative implications [12–15]. Most studies of the effects of denial by patients have focused on their anxiety. Some have shown it to be reduced [16–18]; others have not [19–21]. Others have pointed to its associations with unwanted effects, such as delay of treatment [22].

Coping, in contrast, is reality oriented and flexible [7]. It consists of activities which preserve psychological integrity and facilitate physical recovery [23]. It involves effective action which results in a sense of competence, as descriptions of coping by ill and injured people which focus on skills [24], problem-solving [25], and mastery [26] have

* Reprinted from the Journal of Psychosomatic Research (29 December 1985) with permission of the author and publisher. This research has drawn on funding from both the Australian Research Grants Scheme (Grant No. 77/15046R) and the Commonwealth of Australia Department of Health.

shown. Coping processes enable patients not only to keep distressing emotions within tolerable limits, but to maintain their self-esteem and to preserve the interpersonal relationships which are important to them [13].

If expression of positive emotion by hospitalized patients is assumed, on the one hand, to be evidence of defending, it is possible to generate a set of hypotheses about the psychological states of these patients. While their anxiety and directly expressed anger may be controlled by defending, other reactions to stress, such as uncertainty, depression, indirectly expressed anger, and helplessness, should be apparent. They should also rarely see themselves as competent or as participating in interpersonal relationships which are satisfying to them. If expression of positive emotion is assumed, on the other hand, to be evidence of coping, then a rival set of hypotheses is apparent. If this assumption holds, then patients who express much positive emotion should feel little uncertainty, depression, indirectly expressed anger, or helplessness, and they should see themselves as competent and participating in many satisfying relationships. These two opposing sets of hypotheses were tested by making comparisons within a large sample of patients between those who differed in their expression of positive emotion.

Several subsidiary hypotheses about the expression of positive emotion were also tested. It was hypothesized that, while patients' perceptions of handicaps in areas such as mobility, self-care, and leisure would not modify their expression of positive emotion, handicaps that affected relationships would. It was predicted, too, that the perceived availability of support from significant others, such as family and friends, and from hospital and community would moderate the expression of positive emotion. The possible moderating effects of patient demographic factors such as sex, age, marital status, occupation, and education on positive emotion were also explored. Finally, the data for two of the most common diagnostic groups, patients with gastrointestinal and cardiovascular problems, were reanalyzed to provide a test of the generalizability of the findings concerning positive emotion.

17.2 Method

17.2.1 Patient Sample

A sample of 507 hospitalized patients containing equivalent numbers of women and men was drawn for interview at three provincial hospitals. They ranged in age from 18 to 99 years, with the majority being over 50 years of age. Two-thirds of them had been living with a spouse up to the time of hospitalization. Their occupations were graded according to a scale of socioeconomic status [27] and proved to be predominantly low to middle class. Their educational histories were not, as might be expected, extensive. Almost half of these patients had finished six years of high school education but only a few had continued their education beyond that level. Most perceived themselves as having handicaps in mobility and in pursuing leisure activities while hospitalized, smaller numbers perceived themselves as having handicaps in self-care and relationships. They reported much support from their family and friends but less from their hospital and from community-based organizations (such as Meals-on-Wheels). More information about these characteristics of the sample is available in Table 1.

Table 1. Demographic, handicap, and support characteristics of the patient sample

Sex:	women = 49%;	men = 51%	
Age:	18–30 = 15%;	31–40 = 15%;	41–50 = 14%;
	51–60 = 20%;	61–99 = 36%	
Marital status:	married = 62%;	single or widowed = 38%	

Occupation: (1 = high occupational status)

1 = 2%;	2 = 4%;	3 = 8%;	4 = 12%
5 = 24%;	6 = 37%;	7 = 13%;	

Education:	primary = 42%;	mid-high school = 38%
	high school = 14%;	post-high school = 6%

Handicaps: (1 = severe)

Mobility	1 = 20%;	2 = 11%;	3 = 29%;	4 = 40%
Self-care	1 = 10%;	2 = 27%;	3 = 23%;	4 = 40%
Leisure	1 = 27%;	2 = 28%;	3 = 25%;	4 = 20%
Relationships	1 = 3%;	2 = 8%;	3 = 20%;	4 = 69%

Support: (1 = none)

Family/friends	1 = 7%;	2 = 15%;	3 = 78%	
Hospital/community	1 = 28%;	2 = 38%;	3 = 23%;	4 = 11%

Diagnostic categories:

Gastrointestinal	= 26%	Cardiovascular	= 24%
Genitourinary	= 15%	Endocrine	= 8%
Breast	= 9%	Respiratory	= 6%
Neoplasms	= 3%	Accidents	= 3%
Musculoskeletal	= 3%	Central nervous system	= 3%

All of the patients were hospitalized with severe and often painful illness or the mutilating effects of accidents. Many of those who were acutely ill were scheduled for exploratory or corrective surgery for problems such as gastrointestinal or back pain. Many women and men were hospitalized for surgery for genitourinary malfunctions. Another large group of patients were suffering from cardiovascular conditions, such as the results of myocardial infarctions or angina. Other chronically ill patients were suffering from diabetes and its complications, as well as progressive diseases of the nervous system, such as multiple sclerosis. A number of paraplegics and quadraplegics who were victims of accidents were also included, as were accident patients with fractures of limb bones as well as more minor spinal injuries. The percentages of the sample in each diagnostic category are given in Table 1.

17.2.2 Interview

All patients aged 18 years and over who were admitted to any of the three hospitals on randomly selected days during a 3-year period were approached by one of five female psychologists. A small number of patients who were assessed by senior nursing staff as too ill to communicate were excluded from the data collection. No patient who was approached refused to participate. The resulting response rate of 97% was considered satisfactory. The interviews took place at the bedside or in a day room adjacent to their ward. A standard interview schedule was employed. It included questions about the demographic, handicap, and social support information which have been reported elsewhere [28]. After the questions dealing with the first of these three sets of factors, a standard request was made of the patients: "I'd like you to talk to me for a few minutes about your life at the moment – the good things and the bad." Their responses were, with each patient's permission, recorded and later transcribed.

17.2.3 Appraisal of Positive Emotion and the Other Psychological States

Content analysis scales were applied to the resulting transcripts to gauge the extent of the emotions that have been described. This method has the rigor that the demonstrated interrater reliability and validity of the scales indicate [29–31], without any loss of the meaning intended by the patients. Such a loss is often incurred when structured questionnaires or rating scales are used [32]. These scales have been employed to assess emotional reactions to a wide range of crises, transitions, and other stressful events [2, 33, 34]. In this study the interrater reliability for each of the nine scales used proved to be 0.82 or higher.

Patients' expression of *positive emotion* was measured by the Positive-Affect Scale [35]. This required the scoring of references to or implications of good feelings and contentment (e.g., "My friends are very kind to me," and "When I am well, I enjoy playing the poker machines"). Like most of the scales described here, the Positive-Affect Scale is not ordinarily influenced by demographic factors. It has been shown to discriminate between the responses of people in enjoyable situations and those whose situations are not so enjoyable [33]. This content analysis scale was applied to assess the main variable in this research. The eight other content analysis scales which were used to measure the other psychological states included in the two sets of hypotheses will now be briefly described.

Uncertainty and anxiety were assessed as follows. The Cognitive Anxiety Scale was used to measure *uncertainty* [36]. It was designed to assess the emotion people experience when they have difficulty making sense of what is happening to them. References by patients to events that were new to them (e.g., "I've never been in hospital before") were scored on this scale. It has been shown to discriminate between responses to situations that are new and those that are not. The Total Anxiety Scale was used to measure *anxiety* [37–39]. This technique is based on subscales reflecting anxiety from a variety of sources (e.g., "I could have been killed" and "I get pretty tense these days"). The validity of this scale has been demonstrated by its relationships with ratings of anxiety by psychiatrists and self and with indices of physiological arousal.

Anger was appraised in all its forms. *Anger directly expressed* was measured by the Hostility-Out Scale, *anger indirectly expressed* by the Ambivalent-Hostility Scale, and *depression,* or anger turned in on oneself, by the Hostility-In Scale [37–39]. The first was scored when patients expressed destructive and critical thoughts toward others and the world (e.g., "I'm angry about not getting out of hospital"). The second was scored when they described others as blaming oneself (e.g., "That nurse is annoyed with me"). The third was scored when patients made statements blaming themselves or felt sad or deprived (e.g., "They never give me the medication I should have"). Validation of these scales has been based, again, on demonstrated relationships with ratings of anger and depression and with physiological arousal.

Feelings of *helplessness* and *competence* fluctuate with a sense of self-reliance. They were assessed by the Pawn and Origin Scales [40], which indicated whether patients were attributing events to forces beyond their control or to their own actions. For the Pawn Scale, statements expressing lack of intention (e.g., "I never meant to get ill") and lack of ability (e.g., "I'm not much good at tests") were scored. For the Origin Scale, comments showing intention (e.g., "I mean to get back to work soon") and ability (e.g., "I can do it if I want to") were scored. Scores on the Pawn and Origin Scales correlate positively and negatively, respectively, with the scores on the scales of distress already described.

High scores on the Sociality Scale indicate sociability [41]. This scale assessed whether the current experiences of patients included personal involvement in *positive interpersonal relationships*. There are three kinds of relationship which are scored: those in which the patient is the reactor (e.g., "The nurses help me a lot") and the initiator (e.g., "I made sure the bed was made properly by that aide") and those in which the role filled is not clear (e.g., "We talked for a while"). The total score has been shown to correlate negatively with the anxiety, anger, and depression scores, which have been described, and positively with positive emotion.

17.3 Results

The results of this research are best reported in two groups. The first group includes the rival sets of hypotheses about defending or coping. Multivariate analysis of variance (MANOVA) was used to test these hypotheses as well as to identify the types of sociability roles associated with different expressions of positive emotion. Where the multivariate F values proved significant, univariate F values are reported to identify which psychological states showed significant group differences. The second category of results includes those from tests of the association of degree of perceived handicap and support with patients' expression of positive emotion and of the extent to which this emotion varied as a function of demographic variables. Chi square tests were employed here. For all of these analyses, the sample was divided into quartiles to form four groups of those with high ($n = 130$; $\overline{X} = 1.61$; $S = 0.26$), moderately high ($n = 124$; $\overline{X} = 1.25$; $S = 0.28$), moderately low ($n = 126$; $\overline{X} = 0.97$; $S = 0.20$), and low ($n = 127$; $\overline{X} = 0.65$; $S = 0.17$) positive emotion.

The means and standard deviations of the other psychological state scores for these groups are shown in Table 2, together with the significant multivariate effects. There was a significant difference between the groups over all the psychological states, and the states for which this difference was most notable were competence and sociability. Helmert's contrasts revealed that the major finding for competence was that the group of patients with low positive emotion had lower competence scores than the other three groups. For sociability, however, it was the group with high positive emotion which showed significantly more sociability than the other three groups. Three other psychological states also showed findings approaching significance: depression, anger expressed indirectly, and helplessness. For depression and anger expressed indirectly, it was the group with high positive emotion which showed less than the other groups. These findings are in accord with the set of hypotheses which were based on the assumption that positive emotion is evidence of coping. For helplessness, however, the results were not so clear-cut. It was the two extreme groups (with high and low positive emotion) which expressed the least helplessness. There were no significant findings, as hypothesized, for anxiety and directly expressed anger. Only uncertainty did not show the predicted pattern of results.

Table 2. Means and standard deviations and *MANOVA* results for the psychological state scores of patients differing in their expression of positive emotion (high, moderately high, moderately low, and low)

Psychological states	Positive emotion							
	Moderately				Moderately			
	High		High		Low		Low	
	$\overline{X}$	S	$\overline{X}$	S	$\overline{X}$	S	$\overline{X}$	S
Uncertainty	1.06	0.78	1.20	0.64	1.24	0.72	1.21	0.72
Anxiety	2.21	1.05	2.29	0.77	2.42	0.89	2.22	0.70
Depression	1.03	0.65	1.21	0.68	1.28	0.85	1.16	0.62
Anger expressed directly	1.01	0.90	0.95	0.51	1.01	0.64	0.90	0.48
Anger expressed indirectly	0.72	0.43	0.85	0.43	0.87	0.53	0.84	0.49
Helplessness	1.47	0.64	1.60	0.53	1.55	0.54	1.43	0.50
Competence	1.18	0.76	1.07	0.41	1.02	0.39	0.96	0.41
Sociability	0.51	0.22	0.41	0.17	0.40	0.18	0.40	0.18

	F	df	P<
Multivariate group effect	2.59	24,1439	0.001
Univariate group effects			
Depression	2.38	3,503	0.07
Anger expressed indirectly	2.43	3,503	0.07
Helplessness	2.04	3,503	0.09
Competence	3.86	3,503	0.01
Sociability	10.03	3,503	0.001

Patients' perceptions of their handicaps and of the support available to them were considered next. Four areas of handicap were rated by patients on a four-point scale (see Table 1). No significant relationship with positive emotion was found for three of them (mobility, self-care, and leisure). Relationship handicaps, however, proved to be significantly associated with the expression of positive emotion, (chi square $= 18.23$; $df = 9$; $P < 0.03$). Less interference with relationships was associated with more expression of positive emotion. Patient's perceptions of the support available to them (see Table 1) were also considered in relation to their positive emotion. Both family- and community-based support proved to be significantly related to positive emotion (chi square $= 17.69$ and 18.00, respectively, and with $df = 9$; $P < 0.05$). In both cases, most positive emotion was expressed by patients who reported having most support. None of the associations between the demographic variables of sex and age, marital status, and the occupational status of the patients and their positive emotion proved to be significant. Finally, reanalysis of the data for the genitourinary and cardiovascular groups showed results similar to those for the main analysis (with multivariate $F = 2.01$, $df = 24,108$ and $F = 2.23$, df $= 24,98$, respectively, $P < 0.01$).

17.4 Discussion

The role of the positive emotion which is expressed by patients who are hospitalized because of illness and injury which is implicit in the results from this research will now be examined. This role will first be elaborated by reference to the rival assumptions that such emotion is evidence of defending or coping by patients. Then, the importance of satisfying interpersonal relationships to the patients' positive emotion will be considered. Finally, the implications of the role of positive emotion for patient management will be examined.

Some support has been found for the assumption that the expression of positive emotion by patients is evidence that they are effectively coping with their illness and hospitalization. It has proved to be associated with the sense of competence implicit in coping and with the maintenance of satisfying interpersonal relationships. Low levels of a distressing emotion such as depression and of indirectly expressed anger were found for those who express much positive emotion, indicating that their negative feelings were within tolerable limits. For helplessness, however, this may have been the case for some patients only. For others, however, positive emotion was found to be associated with many expressions of such helplessness. There was, then, some evidence for the passivity of defending in patients who expressed positive emotion. Also, the hypothesis concerning uncertainty was not supported. However, the balance of these findings, which generalized over the two largest diagnostic groups, favored the interpretation that patients who express much positive emotion are preserving their psychological integrity, as a basis for preserving their physical integrity. Their quality of life is, relative to other groups of patients, high.

It has been noted that reports of satisfying interpersonal relationships have been associated with much expression of positive emotion. The part played by such relationships in stimulating positive emotions in hospital patients has been highlighted by other findings as well. Of the four areas in which patients perceived illness-induced handicap, only interference with relationships led to less positive emotion, and little interference was associated with more positive emotion. Also: the support patients perceived as available from their family and friends, on the one hand, and their hospital and community, on the other, proved to be associated with considerable positive emotion.

Only some of the implications of these findings for the management of patients while they are hospitalized can be treated here. The sense of competence, the tolerable levels of distress, and the good interpersonal relationships which contribute to the psychological integrity of patients who are effectively coping with rather than merely defending against their physical problem should be among the goals which the hospital staff have in working with them. When these goals are achieved, this can be seen in the expression of positive emotion by patients. How else can this quality of life be encouraged in patients who lack it? Experiences of good interpersonal relationships help to generate positive emotions in patients, and these need not all be with family and friends. Hospital staff form an important source of relationships for patients. Improved relationships with staff could lead to their period of hospitalization being more often an opportunity for positive change and growth [42–45]. Humor can be an appropriate way of initiating positive emotion [1]. Humor can be triggered by the patients themselves. It can also be used by hospital staff, but this must be with sensitivity and gentleness, and an empathic understanding of each patient's psychological states. This is one important way in which staff may develop good relationships with patients.

Expression of positive emotion by patients may be associated with effective coping rather than with distorting negative emotions by defending against them. Its expression may suggest good quality of life. For both of these reasons, management of patients who are hospitalized because of illness or injury should and can include opportunities for them to identify and, if necessary, develop feelings such as happiness and harmony, laughter and love.

Acknowledgments

I would like to thank Ms. Sue Beattie, Ms. Yvonne Benjamin, Ms. Rosemary Caruana, and Ms. Carol Preston for their help with the data collection and analysis and the patients and staff of the Bulli, Port Kembla, and Wollongong Hospitals for their cooperation.

References

1. Viney LL (1983) Images of Illness. Krieger, Malabar
2. Westbrook MT, Viney LL (1982) Psychological reactions to the onset of chronic illness. Soc Sci Med 16: 899–965
3. Hamera EK, Shontz FC (1978) Perceived positive and negative effects of life threatening illness. J Psychosom Res 22: 419–424
4. Haan N (1977) Coping and defending. Academic, New York
5. Viney LL, Westbrook MT (1981 a) Psychological reactions to chronic illness-related disability as a function of its severity and type. J Psychosom Res 25: 513–523
6. Derogatis LR, Abeloff MD, Melisaratos N (1979) Psychological coping mechanisms and survival time in metastatic breast cancer. JAMA 242: 1504–1508
7. Brown J, Rawlinson M (1976) The morale of patients following open heart surgery. J Health Soc Behav 17: 134–144
8. Vaillant GE (1977) Adaptation to life. Little, Brown, Boston
9. Lipowski ZJ (1967) Review of consultation psychiatry and psychosomatic medicine. Psychosom Med 29: 201–225
10. Freud S (1935) A general introduction to psychoanalysis. Liverright, New York
11. Freud A (1948) The ego and the mechanisms of defence. Hogarth, London
12. Weisman AD (1972) On dying and denying. Behavioural Publication, New York

13. Hamburg DA (1974) Coping behavior in life threatening circumstances. Psychother Psychosom 23: 13–25
14. Janis IL (1974) Psychological stress. Academic, New York
15. Moos RH, Tsu VD (1977) The crisis of physical illness: an overview. In: Moos RH (ed) Coping with physical illness. Plenum, New York
16. Froese A, Hackett P, Cassem NH, Silverberg EL (1974) Trajectories of anxiety and depression in denying and nondenying acute myocardial infarction patients during hospitalisation. J Psychosom Res 8: 413–420
17. Sanders JB, Kardinal C (1977) Adaptive coping mechanisms in adult leukemia patients in remission. JAMA 238: 952–954
18. Meyerowitz BE (1983) Postmastectomy coping strategies and quality of life. Health Psychol 2: 117–132
19. Hackett TP, Cassem NH, Wishnie HA (1968) The coronary care unit: an appraisal of its psychologic hazards. N Engl J Med 279: 1365–1370
20. Miller WB, Rosenfeld R (1975) A psychophysiological study of denial following acute myocardial infarction. J Psychosom Res 19: 43–54
21. Billing E, Lindell B, Sedorholm M, Theorell T (1980) Denial, anxiety and depression following myocardial infarction. Psychosomatics 21: 639–645
22. Moses R, Cividali N (1966) Differential levels of awareness of illness: their relation to some salient features in cancer patients. N Y Acad Sci Ann 125: 984–994
23. Lipowski ZJ (1970) Physical illness and the individual and the coping process. Psychiatry Med 1: 91–101
24. Mechanic D (1974) Social structure and personal adaptation: some neglected dimensions. In: Coelho GV, Hamburg DA, Adams JE (eds) Coping and adaptation. Basic, New York
25. Cohen F, Lazarus RS (1979) Coping with the stresses of illness. In: Stone GC, Cohen F, Adler NE (eds) Health psychology – a handbook. Jossey Bass, San Francisco
26. Weisman AD, Worden JW (1976–77) The existensial plight in cancer: significance of the first 100 days. Int J Psychiatry Med 7: 1–15
27. Congalton AA (1969) Status and prestige in Australia. Cheshire, Melbourne
28. Viney LL, Westbrook MT (1984) Coping with chronic illness: strategy preferences, changes in preferences and associated emotional reactions. J Chronic Dis 37: 489–502
29. Viney LL (1984) Loss of life and loss of bodily integrity: two different sources of threat for people who are ill. Omega 15: 207–222
30. Viney LL (1981) Content analysis: a research tool for community psychologists. Am J Commun Psychol 9: 269–281
31. Viney LL, Westbrook MT (1981) Measuring patients' experienced quality of life: the application of content analysis scales in health care. Commun Health Stud 5: 45–52
32. Viney LL (1983) The assessment of psychological states through content analysis of verbal communications. Psychol Bull 94: 542–563
33. Viney LL (1980) Transitions. Cassell, Sydney
34. Viney LL (1983) Psychological reactions of young people to unemployment. Youth Soc 14: 457–474
35. Westbrook MT (1976) Positive affect: a method of content analysis for verbal samples. J Consult Clin Psychol 44: 715–719
36. Viney LL, Westbrook MT (1976) Cognitive anxiety: a method of analysis for verbal samples. J Pers Assess 40: 140–150
37. Gottschalk LA (1979) The content analysis of verbal behavior: further studies. Spectrum, New York
38. Gottschalk LA, Gleser GC (1969) The measurement of psychological states through the content analysis of verbal behavior. University of California Press, Berkeley
39. Gottschalk LA, Winget CN, Gleser GC (1969) Manual of instructions for using the Gottschalk-Gleser content analysis scales. University of Los Angeles Press, Berkeley

40. Westbrook MT, Viney LL (1980) Scales of origin and pawn perception using content analysis of speech. J Pers Assess 44: 157–166
41. Viney LL, Westbrook MT (1979) Sociality: a content analysis scale for verbalizations. Soc Behav Personal 7: 129–137
42. Viney LL, Clarke AM, Bunn TA, Benjamin YN (1985) Crisis intervention counseling: an evaluation of long-term and short-term effects. J Coun Psych 32: 29–39
43. Viney LL, Clarke AM, Bunn TA, Benjamin YN (1985) An evaluation of three crisis intervention counseling programmes for general hospital patients. Br J Med Psychol 58: 75–86
44. Viney LL, Clarke AM, Bunn TA, Benjamin YN (1985) The effects of a hospital-based counseling service on the physical recovery of surgical and medical patients. Gen Hosp Psychiatry 7: 294–301
45. Viney LL, Benjamin YN, Clarke AM, Bunn TA (1985) Sex differences in the psychological reactions of medical and surgical patients to crisis intervention counseling: source for the goose may not be sauce for the gander. Soc Sci Med 20: 1199–1205

18 Affective Content of Speech as a Predictor of Psychotherapy Outcome*

Fernando Lolas, Hans Kordy, and Michael von Rad

18.1 Introduction

Affective content of speech has been used as an aid in the psychological evaluation of patients undergoing psychopharmacological or psychotherapeutic treatment [4, 12]. One assessment procedure, the Gottschalk-Gleser method [5], has proved valuable in studying both transient changes in mood and enduring psychological characteristics. This eclectic method relies on the grammatical clause as a coding unit and can be applied by technicians working on written materials for scoring up to 16 psychological "dimensions." Most of the scales developed so far (particularly those measuring anxiety and hostility) have been externally validated and show some degree of stability over time and across situations [8].

The present report summarizes some of the results obtained within the framework of a follow-up project designed to evaluate the outcome of psychotherapeutic interventions. Among the instruments routinely employed for behavioral/psychodynamic evaluation both before and after treatment, a speech sample was elicited in a standardized manner (standard instructions of Gottschalk and Gleser) and the resulting text scored for different psychological dimensions. In the present study, protocols obtained before the beginning of treatment were scored for anxiety and hostility. The main aim of this work was to explore the prognostic relevance of Gottschalk-Gleser anxiety and hostility scores in terms of treatment outcome. To this end, outcome measures were studied in groups defined according to their initial Gottschalk-Gleser scores.

18.2 Method

Five-minute tape-recorded speech samples [5] were obtained from 98 patients during the first contact with the clinic before the beginning of psychotherapy. Verbatim protocols in response to the standard instructions were scored by a technician not familiar with the hypothesis under study and unaware of the patient's diagnoses or form of treatment. Anxiety and hostility scores, obtained by the usual procedure, were classified

---

* This study was performed while the senior author was on a leave of absence from the Faculty of Medicine, University of Chile, aided by the Alexander von Humboldt Foundation.

as "low", or "high" on the basis of published norms for the German language [13] and previous studies [8]. Within one-half standard deviation above and below the mean of this normative population was regarded as the middle area. The analysis of results in this study was limited to those subgroups scoring high and low in anxiety and hostility, that is, ≥ 0.5 standard deviation from the appropriate mean scores.

Patients were assigned to different forms of psychotherapeutic treatment: group therapy (46%), combined group and individual therapy (34%), individual therapy (9%), and psychoanalysis (7%) depending upon diagnosis (psychoneurosis and psychosomatic conditions, see Table 1) and other relevant variables [3, 9]. The first two treatment modalities comprise a period of inpatient care.

Table 1. Distribution of diagnoses ($n = 98$)

Psychoneurotic symptoms[a]	48% ($n = 46$)
Psychosomatic symptoms[a]	19% ($n = 18$)
Cardiac neurosis	9% ($n = 9$)
Ulcerative colitis	2% ($n = 2$)
Peptic ulcer	5% ($n = 5$)
Crohn's disease	2% ($n = 2$)
Anorexia nervosa	4% ($n = 4$)
Depressive neurosis	13% ($n = 12$)

[a] Complaints of either somatic or psychological nature, not meeting criteria for inclusion into one of the nosological entities listed below.

The outcome was evaluated at the end of treatment by six assessment procedures. Three of them were performed by therapists regarding symptoms (symptom rating) or goal attainment using a modification of the Goal Attainment Scaling method [7]: therapists provided an overall impression of goal attainment and an evaluation of that goal most related to what the therapist considered to be the main conflictual area of the patient.

Goals of the therapeutic undertaking and the "grain" of the scale were individually formulated for each case. The other three assessment procedures involved patient self-rating: changes in self-image as measured by the Giessen Personality Inventory [1], changes in complaints, as assessed by the Giessen Complaint Inventory [2], comprising 57 items, and a measure of the patient's own satisfaction with the results of the treatment.

Scores yielded by these instruments were transformed to five-point scales (worsening/no change/moderate success/good success/optimum success). Despite a certain degree of redundancy (Table 2), they were all scored separately, attempting to maintain "multidimensionality" in the assessment and refraining from computing a single "success score." For each of them, the probability of "worsening" or "no change" was interpreted as "risk of failure." "Chance of success" was defined as the probability of a patient falling into the two uppermost levels of the five-point scale. In this report we concentrate on the risk of failure in relation to high and low Gottschalk-Gleser anxiety and hostility scores. The latter were computed separately for each of the six forms of anxiety (shame, guilt, death, mutilation, separation, and diffuse) and four forms of hostility (hostility directed outward-overt and covert, hostility directed inward, and ambivalent hostility).

Table 2. Correlation coefficients (Spearman) between the six "dimensions" of change ($n=98$).

	Self-image	Complaints	Satisfaction	Symptoms	Individual goals
Self-image					
Complaints	0.40				
Satisfaction	0.15	0.11			
Symptoms	0.31	−0.01	−0.08		
Individual goals	0.41	0.32	0.36	0.42	
Main goal	0.11	0.33	0.27	0.31	0.69

For each of the outcome measures, risk of failure for the overall sample was compared with risk of failure within each of the subgroups defined according to the Gottschalk-Gleser content analysis method. No further specification of sample characteristics, such as treatment form, length of treatment, and socioeconomic variables, was made due to the number of patients studied.

Table 3. Increased ($+$) or decreased ($-$) risk ($P<0.1$ and $P<0.2$) of unsuccessful psychotherapy outcome in relation to Gottschalk-Gleser anxiety and hostility scores before treatment ($n=98$)

Gottschalk-Gleser Scale[a]	Range of scores	Dimensions of change					
		Symptoms	Individual goals	Main goal	Complaints	Self-image	Satisfaction
Separation Anxiety	High[b]						
	Low[c]	−	−	−			
Guilt Anxiety	High	+	+	+		+	
	Low						
Shame Anxiety	High					+	+
	Low						
Diffuse Anxiety	High	−	−				
	Low		+	+			+
Hostility Directed Outward Overt	High	+	+	+			
	Low	−	−	−	−		−
Ambivalent Hostility	High	+	+	+			
	Low	−	−				+

[a] Death Anxiety, Mutilation Anxiety, Hostility Directed Outward (Covert), and Hostility Directed Inward scores had no significant correlations with the measures of treatment outcome.
[b] High, >0.5 standard deviation above mean of normative population (13).
[c] Low, >0.5 standard deviation below mean of normative population (13).

18.3 Results

The main results of the study are that psychotherapy outcome can be predicted from Gottschalk-Gleser anxiety and hostility scores before treatment (see Table 3). Sub-groups scoring high and low on the Gottschalk-Gleser Anxiety and Hostility Scales are compared with risk of failure obtained for the whole subject sample in each assessment procedure. Results are shown only *in those cases where they reached reasonable significance* (10% and 20% chance probability was considered acceptable, given the different sources of data).

It can be observed that in almost all scales, with the exception of diffuse anxiety, high scorers tended to show an increased risk of treatment failure. Although this is more obvious in those assessment procedures depending upon therapists' evaluation (symptom rating and individual goal attainment), even in those outcome measures where statistical significance was not reached (hence, not depicted) the same trend was observed. On the other hand, low scorers consistently showed a pattern of reduced probability for treatment failure (reduced risk).

18.4 Discussion

A retrospective analysis of Gottschalk-Gleser anxiety and hostility scores from speech samples elicited before the beginning of psychotherapeutic treatment has shown a rather consistent pattern of relationships with six outcome measures. Since Gottschalk-Gleser Verbal Content Analysis Scales have been used in the context of diagnostic differentiations [10, 14] and in the assessment of mood change [4, 10], it is worth dealing with their possible application in studies of predictability of success or failure in psychotherapy.

It is not implied in this study that a single Gottschalk-Gleser assessment suffices for predicting psychotherapy outcome. It is well-known that affective content scores show moderate degrees of generalizability [5], are dependent upon situational and context-related factors [11], and show a moderate degree of stability over time and across situations [8]. Nevertheless, the rather consistent pattern of relations between extreme anxiety and hostility scores (low and high) and outcome measures may be considered as a useful suggestion for further research along this line. This is reinforced by the fact that the Gottschalk-Gleser method relies upon spontaneous communication and that it has been used in the assessment of short-term psychological change. On the other hand, there are at present not very many reliable predictors for success or failure of psychotherapeutic interventions.

A further limitation to the interpretation of these results comes from the fact that they are based on group assessments that do not take into account many sources of variance, such as diagnosis and treatment modality. In view of these uncontrolled influences, the consistency in the direction of the changes becomes all the more remarkable and suggests that at least part of the variance in the outcome measures might be related to the initial mood state of the patients involved.

As it has been shown, patients exhibiting higher affective scores tend to run a higher risk of treatment failure than those with low scores. This seems to contradict the assumptions and results of the Menninger Psychotherapy Research Project in which patients with a high initial level of anxiety benefited most from psychoanalytically oriented psychotherapy. Kernberg et al. [6] stated:

> ... that a high level of manifest anxiety (independently of whether the patient had high or low ego strength) is an indication of good prognosis for treatments conducted within the framework of psychoanalytic theory. More specifically, we found that the higher the Initial *Level of Anxiety*, the higher the *Global Improvement* and the higher the *Increase in Ego Strength*, both at Termination and at Follow-up. It needs to be stressed that the Initial *Level of Anxiety* refers only to the physical and/or psychic manifestations of anxiety and not to the character pathology or the various symptoms which were conceptualized originally as "averted anxiety". While the level of manifest anxiety thus has a significant value as a predictor of the outcome of treatment, the statistical analysis also suggested that the decrease in the level of manifest anxiety is a relatively weak indication of improvement in other areas of the patient's functioning.

The authors suggested that the painful experience of anxiety is an important aspect of motivation for treatment during its initial stages.

The reasons for the discrepancy between our results and those of Kernberg et al. [6] may stem in part from the different modes of operationalization of the construct "initial anxiety". We would like to emphasize that the assessment method employed here relies upon *monological* verbal expression and not on dyadic interaction. Moreover, the speech samples for the present study were collected after patients went through a psychometric test battery, thus making it possible that the contents of speech might have been influenced by material awakened by the previous testing. The influence of sequential testing upon Gottschalk-Gleser scores has not been ascertained, but it could be speculated that long-lasting personality variables are liable to imprint speech samples under the conditions of this study. The issue should be clarified on the basis of further examination of these data. It might also be speculated that therapists tend to rate success with patients scoring high in anxiety and hostility on a more stringent basis than the one adopted for low scorers. Another explanation might be that high scorers are the more disturbed patients, thus having less possibilities for a positive change under comparable circumstances.

It should be emphasized that all forms of therapy employed are psychodynamically oriented and hence either insightenhancing or anxietyprovoking. In the absence of processual indicators regarding the depth of regression or transference factors, it is not known at which point therapy was terminated in each case. Many of these factors might influence the relationship between speech content and outcome measures in an unknown way.

A sideresult of this study is worth mentioning for methodological reasons. It was not possible to always obtain a good response from patients at the end of treatment using the standard instructions for eliciting speech recommended by Gottschalk and Gleser [5]. Aside from preventing a before-after comparison of speech content scores, this suggests that the situation, purportedly neutral and projective-like, represents a burden to the patient when added to a standard test battery like the one employed in this study. Due to its unstructured character, it may well be that patients are uncertain about the evaluation or the features which will be considered. Since in other studies we have found that the diagnostic relevance of the method is more limited using the standard instructions than an interview protocol, more careful attention to the interplay of situational, subjective, and observer-dependent factors should be devoted in studies of its prognostic use.

References

1. Beckmann D, Richter HE (1972) Giessen-Test (GT). Huber, Bern
2. Brähler E, Scheer JW (1979) Skalierung psychosomatischer Beschwerdekomplexe mit dem Gießener Beschwerdebogen (GBB). Psychother Med Psychol 29: 14–27
3. Engel K, Haas E, v Rad M, Senf W, Becker H (1979) Heidelberg rating. Med Psychol 5: 253–268
4. Gottschalk LA (ed) (1979) The content analysis of verbal behavior. Further studies. Spectrum, New York
5. Gottschalk LA, Gleser GC (1969) The measurement of psychological states through the content analysis of verbal behavior. University of California Press, Los Angeles
6. Kernberg O, Burstein E, Coyne L, Appelbaum A, Horwitz L, Voth H (1972) Psychotherapy and psychoanalysis: final report of the Menninger foundation's psychotherapy research project. Bull Menninger Clin 36: 1
7. Kiresuk TJ, Sherman R (1968) Goal attainment scaling: a general method for evaluating comprehensive community mental health programs. Community Ment Health J 4: 443–453
8. Kordy H, Lolas F, Wagner G (1982) Zur Stabilität der inhaltsanalytischen Erfassung von Affekten nach Gottschalk und Gleser. Z Klin Psychol Psychother 30: 202–213
9. Kordy H, v Rad M, Senf W (1983) Success and failure in psychotherapy: hypotheses and results from the Heidelberg follow-up project. Psychother Psychosom 40: 211–227
10. Lebovitz AH, Holland JC (1983) Use of Gottschalk-Gleser verbal content analysis scales with medically ill patients. Psychosom Med 45: 305–320
11. Lolas F, v Rad M, Scheibler D (1981) Situational influences on verbal affective expression of psychosomatic and psychoneurotic patients. J New Ment Dis 169: 619–623
12. Marsden G (1971) Content analysis studies of psychotherapy: 1954 through 1968. In: Bergin A, Garfield SL (eds) Handbook of psychotherapy and behavior change. Wiley, New York
13. Schofer G, Koch U, Balck F (1979) The Gottschalk-Gleser content analysis of speech: a normative study (the relationship of hostile and anxious affects to sex, sex of the interviewer, socioeconomic class, and age). In: Gottschalk LA (ed) The content analysis of verbal behavior. Spectrum, New York
14. v Rad M, Drücke M, Knauss W Lolas F (1979) Alexithymia: a comparative study of verbal behavior in psychosomatic and psychoneurotic patients. In: Gottschalk LA (ed) The content analysis of verbal behavior. Spectrum, New York

19 Aggressiveness in Psychotherapy and Its Relationship with the Patient's Change: An Adaptation of the Gottschalk-Gleser Hostility Scales to the Portuguese Language

Paulo Belmonte de Abreu

19.1 Introduction

Today, more than ever, aggressiveness is an issue of concern due to its widespread manifestations within several levels of society. Its origins, its future, and the individual's relationship to and use of it have been extensively discussed elsewhere [1, 2]. It is known to be part of our daily life and when appropriately oriented to external reality, it can help an individual be more fulfilled and satisfied in this world.

As physicians, we have a double role to play: (1) to follow the studies on aggressiveness and, at the same time, (2) to help our patients deal with their own aggressiveness. For this purpose, without playing the external roles of social-controlling agents or individual-redeemer priests, we have to recognize and analyze aggressiveness in its biological, psychological, and social aspects. Physicians cannot simply limit their attention to aggressive acts, but they have an obligation to observe the corresponding mental representations of these behaviors and their verbal and preverbal manifestations to decide whether and how they should judiciously respond.

19.2 Bibliographic Review

Besides playing an important role in the life of animals [1], of normal people [2, p. 507], and of patients with psychiatric disturbances, aggressiveness is also present in the relationship of any physician with his patient, given the peculiar characteristics of this meeting which facilitates the transference of feelings, even hostile ones, to the therapist. Initially identified by Freud in 1897 [2] as a patient's resistance to treatment, it was later called negative transference since it involves the election of the physician as the object of the patient's aggressiveness.

Freud, in 1905 [2], in his article "Fragments of an Analysis of a Case of Hysteria," referred to the importance of the treatment of aggressiveness in psychotherapy, maintaning that it should be resolved through the analysis of the transference of the patient's hostile feelings to the therapist. Otherwise, the patient "breaks up very quickly with the physician who is not sympathetic to him, without giving the physician any time to influence him" [2, p. 999]. Later, authors such as Heigl [3] and Alexander and French [4] also emphasized the need for analysis of aggressiveness in the treatment, with varied recommendations concerning its approach. Wolberg [5] also contributed to the psychotherapy of aggression by indicating that when aggressiveness occurs, the therapist should accept the patient's hostile feelings and try to find their relevance to the present in terms of his past experiences, being careful not to make the patient feel guilty for these feelings. With this last remark, Wolberg pointed out the risk of iatrogenic factors blocking successful psychotherapy due to the therapist's improper understanding and mastering of the patient's hostility. Certainly, ignoring systematic interpretation of the patient's aggressive fantasies, especially the transference ones, may lead to the abandonment of treatment by the patient and may make the patient run the risk of fostering his fantasies of destructiveness.

19.3 Hypotheses

To investigate more objectively these viewpoints about the role and management of the patient's aggression in psychotherapy, the following features of psychotherapy were focused upon: the patient's expression of aggressiveness in the first psychotherapy session, the therapist's response to this expression, and the patient's symptomatic changes observed at the end of the 1st month of treatment. Three hypotheses were formulated, all referring to the expression of aggressiveness measured in the first session and the occurrence of symptomatic changes after 1 month of treatment.

Hypothesis 1 (H_1): The patient's expression of aggressiveness contributes to a positive change in the treatment.

Hypothesis 2 (H_2): The therapist's response varies according to the extent of aggressiveness expressed by the patient.

Hypothesis 3 (H_3): The therapist's response to the patient's aggressiveness causes significant changes in the patient.

19.4 Methods and Procedures

19.4.1 Patient and Therapist Selection

Because this was observational research, it was decided not to introduce modifications in the treatments. Hence, the approach was followed of determining the effect of variables considered to be important: sex similarity of the patient-therapist dyad, use of psychoactive drugs, role of the therapist in the selection and frequency of sessions, and duration of the patient's illness.

The patient-therapist dyads were obtained from the "Ambulatorio de Psiquiatria" of the "Hospital Universitario da PUC-RS (HUP)". This is a general hospital with 500 beds and an outpatient department encompassing 31 medical specialties with a monthly average flow of 7202 patients (data from 1980). The psychiatric outpatient department, which occupies 15 rooms of the outpatient service and has been operating since the hospital was first opened, has a monthly average flow of 1200 patients or

16.6% of the overall HUP outpatient flow. At the time of this research, consultation was provided by six 1st-year residents in psychiatry, eight 2nd-year residents, and seven psychiatrists who had completed the 2 years of residence. All the psychiatric consultations were private, with a 3-day waiting list. After selection of the patient, the treatment which best met the needs of both the patient and the psychiatry service was recommended [6].

The patients were selected on the basis of the following criteria: female patients aged 16–65 who were diagnosed by ICD-9 as having: neurotic disturbances (300.0-9), personality disorders (301 except 7 and 9), physiological disorders stemming from mental factors (306.0.9), syndromes and special symptoms not classified elsewhere (307.09 except 1), adjustment reaction (300.0 to 9), depressive disorders not classified elsewhere (311), and emotional disturbances specific to children and adolescents (313.0.9), excluding those who remained less than 1 month in outpatient treatment.

The therapists were chosen from among eight volunteers who offered to participate in this study. Two male and two female therapists were chosen, all residents in psychiatry. Assignment of the patients to therapists was routine and unbiased in that no one was given priority and the therapists did not select specific patients for this study.

19.4.2 Measures Used

The first psychotherapeutic interview of each patient was tape-recorded and typed. This typescript of the first psychotherapeutic session was subjected to content analysis as described below.

19.4.2.1 Assessment of the Patient's Aggressiveness

The content analysis method selected for measuring aggression was developed by Gottschalk and his co-workers [7, 8, 9]. The method consisted basically in the content analysis of the typescript of the first psychotherapeutic session according to the Gottschalk Hostility Scales (Appendix A).

These scales analyze the verbal content of the typed material according to three basic categories of Hostility: *Outward, Inward,* and *Ambivalent.* The content scored comprises verbal references to thoughts and destructive actions, taking the person who speaks as the referent. If the verbal reference involves hostility toward others, whether the agent of the hostility is the speaker or another person, the reference is scored on the Hostility-Outward Scale. With the Hostility-Inward Scale, verbal categories are counted in which the patient refers to the hostile contents by the self against the self. With the Ambivalent-Hostility Scale, verbal categories are counted in which hostility is expressed by others in relation to the self.

Each one of the three basic types of hostility includes thematic categories which are given different weights, ranging from the most intense and direct hostility (people killing or destroying others) to milder and more disguised forms (privation-threatened animals, inanimate beings and situations, suffering and anxiety, and also denial of hostility).

The final score is obtained by adding a factor (0.5) to correct for zero scores to the sum of weighted *(w)* frequency scores, dividing by the number of words spoken, multiplying by 100 (to give an index per 100 words), and then taking the square root of the corrected score, according to the formula proposed by Gottschalk and Gleser [7, 9].

$$\sqrt{\frac{100 \times (f_1 w_2 + f_2 w_2 + f_n w_n + 0.5)}{N \text{ (number of words)}}}$$

19.4.2.2 Therapist's Expression of Hostility (a Scale of Responses to the Patient's Aggressiveness) (Appendix B)

This therapist's scale of hostility was derived by the author from the Gottschalk-Gleser Hostility Scales with the aim of measuring the therapist's remarks that refer to the thematic categories of the patient's aggressiveness. This scale is divided into the same categories, thematic contents and people, employing the same methodology for the computing of results. The difference is that for coding purposes, the measurements should be seen as the therapist's responses to the patient's verbal behavior. This is the justification for the substitution of the statement in which "the therapist states that the person (or other) has or refers to a given affect or destructive action."

19.4.3 Scales of Change

19.4.3.1 Global Assessment Scale (GAS) [10] (Appendix C)

This scale ranges from 0 to 100, and comprises ten global functioning levels, including symptomatic aspect, defensive and integrated in the person, from the most severe grade of psychopathology and functioning disintegration to the highest level of integration. The rating of the subject's lowest level of functioning in the previous week is done by selecting the lowest range which describes his functioning on a hypothetical continuum of mental health illness, irrespective of the treatment the patient is receiving.

19.4.3.2 Scale of Symptoms: Physician Questionnaire (PQ) [11] (Appendix D)

This is a questionnaire with 25 items to be filled in by the physician responsible for the patient. In this research, only items 1–15 were used. Each one of these items has grades from 1 to 7 according to the intensity of occurrence (1, not present; 2, very mild; 3, mild; 4, moderate; 5, moderately severe; 6, severe; 7, extremely severe). The items from 1 to 6 describe symptoms in the emotional area, those from 7 to 14 in the somatic area, and 15 refers to the interpersonal relationship.

19.5 Observations

19.5.1 Data Collection

The selection of patients started on July 15, 1980, when the therapists received standard material and instructions for recording the first interview and also for filling out the Spitzer GAS (Appendix C) and the PQ (Appendix D). The latter two scales were completed after the first interview and again after 4 weeks of treatment.

Then the typescripts of the first psychotherapeutic session were prepared according to Gottschalk's instructions [7, 9], and segments equivalent to 25% of the number of lines of typescript (using a table of random numbers) were randomly selected from each interview. Each segment was numbered and given to each one of the coders, who did not know the therapist's and patient's identity. All coders were previously trained, by having them score 48 samples of the patient's expressions, according to Gottschalk's instructions and of the therapist's responses according to the author's instructions [7, 8, 9]. The coders' results were then compared, and only those yielding adequate agreement were accepted, according to the recommendations of Lolas and co-workers [12, 13].

The final scores on each of the three Hostility Scales for each patient and therapist were obtained using the formula proposed by Gottschalk and Gleser [7]. The total hostility (TH) value was obtained by combining the weights and frequencies for all types of hostility.

19.5.2 Examples

Patient. Case no. 3. On the second sample, the patient complained about her relationship with her husband, saying: "Then I blamed him, that he didn't want me and all these things. When we were fine, we thought it over and decided I was the one to be blamed, that he was too different and that this affected me a lot." In this part, two clauses were scored: (a) "Then I blamed him" (patient in relation to her husband – category Ic3: Overt Hostility Outward; the person criticizes adversely, depreciates, blames, or expresses anger and dislike toward other people) and (b) "we thought it over and decided I was the one to be blamed" The person in relation to herself – category Ib3: Hostility Inward; self-criticism, expressing anger or hatred to self, considering self worthless or of no value, causing oneself grief or trouble, or threatening to do so).

Therapist. Case no. 8. On the second sample, the patient talked about her fear that people thought she was mad, when the therapist said that "perhaps the fear is that I thought so" (that the patient was mad). This part was scored in category CI, theme a2 Ambivalent Hostility; the therapist states that the patient refers to other people, himself in this case, misunderstanding her (it suggests that the patient was afraid that the therapist thought she was mad).

19.6 Results

After 1 month 9 patients had improved with psychotherapy and seven were not changed or were worse, using GAS and PQ scores as criteria of symptomatic change. The scores for the therapist's aggressiveness were lower than those for the patient's aggressiveness. Significance tests were not made for this latter finding because it had not been included in the hypotheses.

19.6.1 Internal Controls

Fisher's test was used to test the relationship of the patient's varibables (income, age, and illness duration) and the therapeutic approach (use of medicines, similarity of sex of patient and therapist, role of therapist in the patient selection, and frequency of interviews) to the scores for global assessment change (GAS) and the patient's Gottschalk-Gleser total hostility scores. There were no significant findings at the 5% level of confidence for any of the 12 tests (6 with GAS and 6 with Gottschalk-Gleser total hostility scores).

The correlation between both scales of change was also calculated and the correlation was found to be: 0.88 ($n = 16$; $P < 0.01$).

19.6.2 Tests of Hypotheses (See Table 1)

The test of linear regression was applied with $P = .05$ and 14 df (critical correlation $= 0.50$).

H_1: Patient's total hostility scores (HTP) correlated with change in GAS scores ($r = 0.56$) and with change in PQ scores ($r = 0.51$).

With regard to the (PQ) partial scores on somatic cluster (cs), psychological cluster (cp), interpersonal relationship cluster (ri), a significant correlation occurred only between total hostility scores (HTP) and change in psychological cluster (cp) ($r = 0.65$). Amont the separate types of hostility, only the patient's hostility-outward scores correlated significantly ($r = 0.66$) with improvement in GAS scores.

H_2: Sixteen calculations of linear regression between the patient's and the therapist's hostility scales were made, and only one correlation was found to be significant: hostility-outward scores (HFP) correlated ($r = 0.57$) with the therapist's interpretations of hostility outward.

H_3: This hypothesis was that the therapist's response to the patient's aggressiveness causes significant symptomatic changes in the patient. The therapist's scores on references to the total hostility of the patients correlated significantly ($r = 0.50$) with improvement in PQ scores for the somatic cluster (cs). The patient's total hostility scores correlated ($r = 0.52$) with improvement in the PQ interpersonal relationship cluster (ri).

19.7 Conclusions

The analysis of the results, considering the limitations of the method used, makes the following conclusions possible:

H_1: 1. The expression of aggressiveness, as measured by Gottschalk-Gleser total hostility scores, in the first psychotherapy session can be considered as a factor predicting positive symptomatic changes observed in the patients after 1 month of treatment. 2. These changes occur both at a global assessment functioning and at a symptomatic level. In the latter, they occur mainly in symptoms involving the psychic area and in interpersonal relationships.

H_2: 1. The significant correlation found between the patient's hostility-outward scores and references of the therapist to this hostility outward shows that the therapist usually responds to the patient's expression of aggressiveness during the first therapy session by mirroring such references, that is, answering in the same way, when the hostility is outwardly directed. 2. This specificity does not occur with other forms of aggressiveness (hostility directed inward and ambivalent hostility), indicating that there is a greater variety of responses from the therapist when confronted with these other kinds of expression of aggressiveness. 3. No therapeutic approach variable (frequency of sessions, role of the therapist in patient selection, use of medication, therapist-patient sex similarity) nor patient characteristic (age, income, disease duration) was associated with a specific kind of aggressive response from the therapists or patients.

H_3: 1. The correlation found between the frequency of the references by the therapists to the total hostility of the patients and improvement in somatic concerns of the patient suggests that the response of the therapists may decrease the symptoms of the patient in the somatic area after 1 month of treatment. 2. No patient, therapist, or therapeutic approach factors were associated with the total or partial change in patients at the end of the 1st month of treatment.

19.8 Comments

The finding that the expression of aggressiveness by the patient provokes total and partial improvements, mainly in the psychic area, confirms the idea that there is a cathartic effect of psychotherapy. The finding that the expression of outward aggressiveness of a patient is associated with a response from the therapist dealing with the patient's outwardly directed hostility, which does not occur with aggressiveness verbalized by the patient as originating from other sources, shows that psychotherapists are more likely to work on aggressiveness when the patient acts as its agent or observer. There is a greater variation of therapist responses when the patient is self-aggressive or feels others have been aggressive toward him. Finally, the conclusion seems justified that the interpretation and neutral acceptance of the patient's hostility by the therapist provokes a decrease in the patient's symptoms involving both the somatic area and interpersonal relationships. The evidence appears to be that this kind of activity from the therapist makes possible the patient's expressing his conflicts less through his body and allows the patient to improve his relationship with other people.

These conclusions should be regarded with some reservations and should not be overgeneralized. A small sample of nonpsychotic patients was involved, in nonemergency situations, and in an institution with training and research objectives. In spite of the precautions taken in selection of the patient-therapist dyad, the possibility cannot be entirely rejected that the therapists might have been attracted by the opportunity of being involved in a research study, even without knowing its title or subject. It is also possible that the therapists who have collaborated on this research were somehow different from the average of the physicians of the psychiatric outpatient service in some special way, for example, they may have had a greater aptitude than others to carry out systematic psychotherapy on an outpatient basis. Furthermore, the number of significance tests used in this study make all conclusions in need of replication. At best, the conclusions can be considered valid only for female patients functioning at a neurotic level with an average within the 3rd decade, treated on an outpatient basis by physicians in psychiatric training having a psychodynamic orientation, and who are examined at the beginning and at the end of the 1st month of treatment.

The usefulness of the Gottschalk-Gleser Content Analysis Scales in studying some psychodynamics of psychotherapy has been illustrated.

References

1. Garattini S, Sigg EB (eds) (1968) Biology of aggressive behavior. Excerpta Medica, Amsterdam
2. Freud S (1973) Obras completas, 3rd edn. Biblioteca Nueva, Madrid
3. Heigl F (1967) Fatores de eficacia en la terapia psicoanalítica. Revista de psicoanalisis, psiquiatria y psicologia 7: 67–80
4. Alexander F, French T (1956) Terapeutica psicoanalítica. Paidos, Buenos Aires, p 284
5. Wolberg LR (1954) The technique of psychotherapy. Grune and Stratton, New York
6. Albuquerque MA, Pinto SL (1981) O curso de especializacão em Psiquiátria da PUC/RS. Rev da Associacão Psiquiatrica do Piauí 1: 78–84
7. Gottschalk LA, Gleser GC (1969) The measurement of psychological states through the content analysis of verbal behavior. University of California Press, Berkeley
8. Gottschalk LA (1979) The content analysis of Verbal behavior: further studies. Spectrum, New York
9. Gottschalk LA, Winget CN, Gleser GC (1969) Manual of instructions for using the Gottschalk-Gleser content analysis scales: anxiety, hostility, and social alienation-personal disorganization. University of California Press, Berkeley
10. Endicott J, Spitzer R, Fleiss J, Cohen J (1976) The global assessment scale. Arch Gen Psychiatry 33: 766
11. Rickels K, Howard K (1970) The physician questionnaire: a useful tool in psychiatric research. Psychopharmacologia 17: 338–344
12. Lolas F, Gottschalk LA (1978) El método de análisis de contenido de Gottschalk y Gleser en la investigación psiquiátrica. Acta Psiquiátr Psicol Am Lat 24: 247–256
13. Gottschalk LA, Winget CN, Gleser GC, Lolas FS (1984) Análisis de la conducta verbal. Editorial Universitaria, Santiago

Appendix A

Schedule 1

Hostility-Directed-Outward Scale: destructive, injurious, critical thoughts, and actions directed to others

I. Hostility Outward-Overt. Thematic categories

a 3* Self-killing, fighting, injuring other individuals, or threatening to do so

b 3 Self-robbing or abandoning other individuals, causing suffering or anguish to others, or threatening to do so

c 3 Self-adversely criticizing, depreciating, blaming, expressing anger, dislike of other human beings

a 2 Self-killing, injuring, or destroying domestic animals, pets, or threatening to do so

b 2 Self-abandoning, robbing domestic animals, pets, or threatening to do so

c 2 Self-criticizing or depreciating others in a vague or mild manner

d 2 Self-depriving or disappointing other human beings

a 1 Self-killing, injuring, destroying, robbing wild life, flora, inanimate objects, or threatening to do so

b 1 Self-adversely criticizing, depreciating, blaming, expressing anger or dislike of subhumans, inanimate objects, places, situations

c 1 Self-using hostile words, cursing, mention of anger or rage without referent

II. Hostility Outward-Covert. Thematic categories

a 3 Others (human) killing, fighting, injuring other individuals, or threatening to do so

b 3 Others (human) robbing, abandoning, causing suffering or anguish to other individuals, or threatening to do so

c 3 Others adversely criticizing, depreciating, blaming, expressing anger, dislike of other human beings

a 2 Others (human) killing, injuring, or destroying domestic animals, pets, or threatening to do so

b 2 Others (human) abandoning, robbing domestic animals, pets, or threatening to do so

c 2 Others (human) criticizing or depreciating other individuals in a vague or mild manner

---

* The numbers serves to give the weight as well as to identify the category. The letter also helps identify the category.

d 2 Others (human) depriving or disappointing other human beings

e 2 Others (human or domestic animals) dying or killed violently in death-dealing situation, or threatening with such

f 2 Bodies (human or domestic animals) mutilated, depreciated, defiled

a 1 Wild life, flora, inanimate objects injured, broken, robbed, destroyed, or threatening with such (with or without mention of agent)

b 1 Others (human) adversely criticizing, depreciating, expressing anger or dislike of subhumans, inanimate objects, places, situations

c 1 Others angry, cursing without reference to cause or direction of anger; also instruments of destruction not used threateningly

d 1 Others (human, domestic animals) injured, robbed, dead, abandoned, or threatened with such from any source including subhuman and inanimate objects, situations (storms, floods, etc.)

e 1 Subhumans killing, fighting, injuring, robbing, destroying each other, or threatening to do so

f 1 Denial of anger, dislike, hatred, cruelty, and intent to harm

Schedule 2

Hostility-Directed-Inward Scale: self-destructive, self-critical thoughts and actions

I. Hostility Inward. Thematic categories

a 4 References to self (speaker) attempting or threatening to kill self, with or without conscious intent

b 4 References to self wanting to die, needing or deserving to die

a 3 References to self-injuring, mutilating, disfiguring self, or threats to do so, with or without conscious intent

b 3 Self-blaming, expressing anger or hatred to self, considering self worthless or of no value, causing oneself grief or trouble, or threatening to do so

c 3 References to feelings of discouragement, giving up hope, despairing, feeling grieved or depressed, having no purpose in life

a 2 References to self needing or deserving punishment, paying for one's sins, needing to atone or do penance

b 2 Self-adversely criticizing, depreciating self; references to regretting, being sorry or ashamed for what one says or does; references to self mistaken or in error

c 2 References to feeling of deprivation, disappointment, lonesomeness

a 1 References to feeling disappointed in self; unable to meet expectations of self or others

b 1 Denial of anger, dislike, hatred, blame, destructive impulses from self to self

c 1 References to feeling painfully driven or obliged to meet one's own expectations and standards

Schedule 3

Ambivalent-Hostility Scale: destructive, injurious, critical thoughts and actions of others to self

II. Ambivalent Hostility. Thematic categories

a 3   Others (human) killing or threatening to kill self
b 3   Others (human) physically injuring, mutilating, disfiguring self, or threatening to do so
c 3   Others (human) adversely criticizing, blaming, expressing anger or dislike toward self, or threatening to do so
d 3   Others (human) abandoning, robbing self, causing suffering, anguish, or threatening to do so
a 2   Others (human) depriving, disappointing, misunderstanding self, or threatening to do so
b 2   Self-threatened with death from subhuman or inanimate objects, or death-dealing situation
a 1   Others (subhuman, inanimate, or situation) injuring, abandoning, robbing self, causing suffering, anguish
b 1   Denial of blame

Appendix B

Hostility Scale (Gottschalk and Gleser, modified by Abreu) Therapist's expression of hostility

I. Hostility outward: destructive and injurious thoughts and action directed to others

1. Hostility Outward-Overt (the patient toward others) – HFA

a 3   The therapist states that the patient kills, fights, injures other individuals, or threatens to do so

b 3   The therapist states that the patient robs or abandons other individuals, causes suffering or anguish to others, or threatens to do so

c 3   The therapist states that the patient adversely criticizes, depreciates, blames, expresses anger, dislike of other human beings

a 2   The therapist states that the patient kills, injures, or destroys domestic animals, pets, or threatent to do so

b 2   The therapist states that the patient abandons, robs domestic animals, pets, or threatens to do so

c 2   The therapist states that the patient criticizes or depreciates others in a vague or mild manner

d 2   The therapist states that the patient deprives or disappoints other human beings

a 1   The therapist states that the patient kills, injures, destroys, and robs wildlife, flora, inanimate objects, or threatens to do so

b 1   The therapist states that the patient adversely criticizes, depreciates, blames, expresses anger or dislike of subhumans, inanimate objects, places, situations

c 1   The therapist states that the patient uses hostile words, curses, mentions anger or rage without referent

2. Hostility Outward-Covert (others in relation to others than the patient) – HFC

a 3   The therapist states that the patient refers to others (human) killing, fighting, injuring other individuals, or threatening to do so

b 3   The therapist states that the patient refers to others (human) robbing, abandoning, causing suffering or anguish to other individuals, or threatening to do so

c 3   The therapist states that the patient refers to others adversely criticizing, depreciating, blaming, expressing anger, dislike of other human beings

a 2   The therapist states that the patient refers to others killing, injuring, or destroying domestic animals, pets, or threatening to do so

b 2   The therapist states that the patient refers to others abandoning, robbing domestic animals, pets, or threatening to do so c 2 The therapist states that the patient refers to others criticizing or depreciating other individuals in a vague or mild manner

d 2 The therapist states that the patient refers to others depriving or disappointing other human beings

e 2 The therapist states that the patient refers to others dying or killed violently in death-dealing situation, or threatened with such

III. Ambivalent-Hostility Scale: destructive, injurious, critical thoughts and actions of others to self

1. Ambivalent Hostility (others toward the patient)

a 3 The therapist states that the patient refers to others (human) killing or threatening to kill himself

b 3 The therapist states that the patient refers to others (human) physically injuring, mutilating, disfiguring himself, or threatening to do so

c 3 The therapist states that the patient refers to others (human) adversely criticizing, blaming, expressing anger or dislike toward himself, or threatening to do so

d 3 The therapist states that the patient refers to others (human) abandoning, robbing himself, causing suffering, anguish, or threatening to do so

a 2 The therapist states that the patient refers to others (human) depriving, disappointing, misunderstanding himself, or threatening to do so

b 2 The therapist states that the patient refers to being threatened with death from subhuman or inanimate object or death-dealing situation

a 1 The therapist states that the patient refers to others (subhuman, inanimate, or situation) injuring, abandoning, robbing

b 1 The therapist refers to the patient denying blame

Appendix C

Global Assessment Scale (GAS)*

Rate the subject's lowest level of functioning in the last week by selecting the lowest range which describes his functioning on a hypothetical continuum of mental health illness. For example, a subject whose "behavior is considerably influenced by delusions" (range 21–30) should be given a rating in that range even though he has "major impairment in several areas" (range 31–40). Use intermediary levels when appropriate (e.g., 35, 58, 63). Rate actual functioning independent of whether subject is receiving and may be helped by medication or some other form of treatment.

Name of patient (1st letters) .... HUP no ....
Outpatient dept. no .... Code no ....
Admission date .... Date of rating..............
Rater... Rating ....

100 No symptoms, superior functioning in a wide range of acitvities, life's problems
    never seem to get out of hand, is sought out by others because of his warmth and
 91 integrity.

90 Transient symptoms may occur, but good functioning in all areas, interested and
    involved in a wide range of activities, socially effective, generally satisfied with
 81 life, "everyday" worries that only occasionally get out of hand.

80 Minimal symptoms may be present but no more than slight impairment in func-
    tioning, varying degrees of "everyday" worries and problems that sometimes get
 71 out of hand.

70 Some mild symptoms (e.g., depressive mood and mild insomnia) or some diffi-
    culty in several areas of functioning, but generally functioning pretty well, has
    some meaningful interpersonal relationships, and most untrained people would
 61 not consider him "sick."

60 Moderate symptoms or generally functioning with some difficulty (e.g., few
    friends and flat affect, depressed mood and pathological self-doubt, euphoric
 51 mood and pressure of speech, moderately severe antisocial behavior).

50 Any serious symptomatology or impairment in functioning that most clinicians
    would think obviously requires treatment of attention (e.g., suicidal preoccupation

---

* This scale was developed by R. L. Spitzer, M. Gibbon, and J. Endicott.

or gesture, severe obsessional rituals, frequent anxiety attacks, serious antisocial be-
41 havior, compulsive drinking).

40 Major impairment in several areas, such as work, family relations, judgment,
thinking, or mood (e.g., depressed woman avoids friends, neglects family, unable
to do housework), or some impairment in reality testing or communication (e.g.,
31 speech is at times obscure, illogical, or irrelevant), or single serious suicide attempt.

30 Unable to function in almost all areas (e.g., stays in bed all day) or behavior is considerably influenced by either delusions or hallucinations or serious impairment in
communication (e.g., sometimes incoherent or unresponsive) or judgment (e.g.,
21 acts grossly inappropriately).

20 Needs some supervision to prevent hurting self or others to maintain minimal personal hygiene (e.g., repeated suicide attempts, frequently violent, manic excitement, smears faces) or gross impairment in communication (e.g., largely incoher-
11 ent or mute).

10 Needs constant supervision for several days to prevent hurting self or others, or
01 makes no attempt to maintain minimal personal hygiene.

Appendix D

Physician Questionnaire

Patient: .... Date: .... Patient code:.........

Symptom	Not present	Very mild	Mild	Moderate	Moderately severe	Severe	Extremely severe
1. Anxiety (apprehensive, tense, worried, frightened, anxious, nervous)	1	2	3	4	5	6	7
2. Depressive Mood (feelings of depression, unhappiness, sorrow, pessimism, sadness; hopelessness, tearfulness)	1	2	3	4	5	6	7
3. Irritability (easily annoyed or irritated)	1	2	3	4	5	6	7
4. Hostility (anger, animosity, contempt, belligerence, disdain for other people)	1	2	3	4	5	6	7
5. Phobia (unrealistic fears)	1	2	3	4	5	6	7
6. Obsession-compulsion (repetitive unwanted thoughts or actions)	1	2	3	4	5	6	7
7. Hypochondriasis (preoccupation with physical health)	1	2	3	4	5	6	7
8. Somatization-musculoskeletal (e.g., backache, muscle ache, heaviness of limbs)	1	2	3	4	5	6	7
9. Somatization-autonomic (e.g., GI, respiratory, sweating, trembling, heart palpitations)	1	2	3	4	5	6	7
10. Insomnia	1	2	3	4	5	6	7
11. Appetite disturbance	1	2	3	4	5	6	7
12. Headaches (frequency and intensity)	1	2	3	4	5	6	7

Table 1. Hostility scores for patients and hostility scores in reference to the patient's hostility by the psychotherapist during first psychotherapy session plus symptomatic changes in patients after 1 month of psychotherapy

Patient no.	Patient				Therapist				GAS		GAS change	PQ		PQ change			PQT
	HFP	HDP	HAP	HTP	HFT	HDT	HAT	HTT	t1	t2		t1	t2	Δcp	Δcs	Δri	
01	1.38	0.24	0.24	1.38	0.24	0.55	0.24	0.55	74	74	0	28	31	-2	-2	-1	-3
02	1.08	1.08	1.14	1.87	0.43	0.43	0.43	0.43	55	53	-2	47	52	-3	-1	-1	-5
03	2.42	1.05	1.05	2.81	1.05	0.29	0.29	1.05	70	68	-2	35	38	-1	-1	-1	-3
04	1.52	1.90	0.80	2.53	0.30	1.39	0.30	1.39	60	60	0	50	46	5	-1	0	4
05	1.78	1.64	1.41	2.76	0.91	0.90	1.41	1.64	68	75	7	48	37	3	8	0	11
06	2.19	0.99	1.53	2.82	0.27	0.27	0.27	0.27	55	68	13	46	35	7	3	1	11
07	1.63	1.11	1.11	1.16	0.32	0.18	0.18	0.32	53	56	3	50	45	4	0	1	5
08	1.79	2.16	1.16	3.02	0.19	0.19	0.63	0.63	62	64	2	46	39	4	3	0	7
09	1.24	0.84	1.71	2.21	0.37	1.24	1.87	2.21	70	73	3	24	19	1	3	1	5
10	3.40	0.38	1.38	3.65	1.01	0.38	0.38	1.01	55	70	5	35	24	6	4	1	11
11	1.18	1.13	1.03	1.90	0.62	0.92	2.10	2.35	51	60	9	58	48	1	9	0	10
12	1.59	0.86	0.92	2.00	0.80	0.59	0.59	1.11	65	67	2	22	23	-1	0	0	-1
13	0.25	1.82	1.19	1.64	0.25	0.25	0.25	0.25	50	41	-9	43	44	0	-1	0	-1
14	1.03	1.21	0.31	1.56	0.31	0.31	0.31	0.31	70	75	5	27	19	2	6	0	8
15	0.63	1.14	1.32	1.82	0.23	0.63	0.53	0.79	75	71	-4	29	30	0	-1	0	-1
16	1.92	1.11	0.34	2.22	0.20	0.20	0.28	0.28	70	70	0	25	27	-2	0	0	-2

Code of Variables

HFP, patient's hostility-outward scores; HDP, patient's hostility-inward scores; HAP, patient's ambivalent-hostility scores; HTP, patient's total hostility scores; HFT, therapist's hostility-outward scores; HDT, therapist's hostility-inward scores; HAT, therapist's ambivalent-hostility scores; HTT, therapist's total hostility scores; GAS, t1 and t2, GAS scores in time 1 (initial) and 2 (after 1 month); PQ, t1 and t2, PQ scores at time 1 (initial) and 2 (after 1 month); Δcp, Δcs, Δri, symptom variance of psychological, somatic, and interpersonal relationship clusters

20 A Preliminary Report on Antidepressant Therapy and Its Effects on Hope and Immunity[*]

Donna Lou Udelman and Harold D. Udelman

20.1 Introduction

For years, literary authors and scientific researchers have described the association between illness and losses through death, separation, divorce, or other termination of relationships. "Anniversary reactions" to dates of such events have often yielded pathophysiological responses. The field of psychoimmunology has attempted to identify the process and anatomical routes through which such events are mediated. Apparently such emotional stresses involve hypothalamic pathways leading to the complexities of the immune system. Key elements of this system include T- and B-lymphocytes, natural killer cells, macrophages, complement, and polymorphonuclear leukocytes. Current studies include all of the above components.

20.2 Current Studies

Gottschalk [1] studied a group of seven depressed patients, measuring the chemiluminescent activity of polymorphonuclear leukocytes. He found decreased chemiluminescence of leukocytes associated with greater degree of depression. Dorian [2] found significant reduction in lymphocyte response to mitogenic stimulation by phytohemagglutin and pokeweed mitogen in psychiatric residents undergoing oral examinations. Elevation of response occurred after the exams. Locke [3] found significant correlation in college students between high stress combined with poor coping and a decline in natural killer cells.

Palmblad [4] studied sleep deprivation and its effects on immune competence, hormonal concentrations, and reported feelings in healthy volunteers. Among his findings were decreased phagocytosis by neutrophils, but increased interferon production by lymphocytes. A further study indicated decrease in both lymphocyte and granulocyte function. Several days after sleep deprivation has been terminated, cellular function seems to be restored or even enhanced.

Kimzey [5] studied immune mechanisms in astronauts during the first 3 days after

[*] Reprinted from *Social Science and Medicine* (20: 1069–1072, 1985) with permission of the authors and publisher.

return to earth. He found depressed T-lymphocyte function, but unchanged serum concentrations of immunoglobulins and C3 component factor.

Stein [6] referred to immunosuppression in bereaved spouses. He found a decrease in function of both B and T cells following the death of spouses. The suppression lasted for 6 months, but normal levels of function were not obtained until 1 year post-bereavement.

20.3 Medication and the Immune System

The aforementioned studies tie together stress, psychological states, and the immune system. Depression and bereavement have clearly defined effects on lymphocytes and phagocytes. If pharmacotherapy can alter psychological states, it may well affect immune responsiveness.

Imipramine, a tricyclic antidepressant drug [7], has been shown to interact with polymorphonuclear leukocytes to enhance their chemiluminescence. This has been "attributed to the electronic excitation of the imipramine molecule resulting from a reaction of the drug with reactive oxygen species."

Lithium [8] may exert a role as a "regulator of lymphocyte responsiveness by acting on specific lymphocyte subpopulations." Although direct proof is as yet unclear, Gelfand et al. [8] performed studies, which indicated the validity of using lithium for assessing the role of the lymphocyte adenylate cyclase cyclic AMP system in the generation and expression of regulatory signals leading to modulation of the immune system.

Rheumatoid factors – an unusual group of antibodies to gamma globulin – are found in rheumatoid arthritis. Rosenblatt [9] found that "the incidence of rheumatoid factor in rheumatoid arthritis is of the same order of magnitude as in a depressed group: approximately seventy-five percent. The titers were considerably higher, though, in rheumatoid arthritis." Haydu et al. [10] noted the parallel effects of imipramine in reducing rheumatoid factor titers in depressed psychotic patients and rheumatoid patients. They questioned whether rheumatoid factor titers and energy dynamics of depression were related.

Medications that generally increase gamma globulins include: (a) anticonvulsants, (b) hydralazine, (c) oral contraceptives, and (d) phenylbutazone. Those that decrease gamma globulins include the tuberculosis vaccine (BCG) and methotrexate, an immunosuppressive drug.

20.4 Immunity and Psychological States

Various psychological states are experientially intense. Hope represents a significant emotion in human experience. Various studies have suggested that hopeful states may contribute to the maintenance of healthy physiological states under the stress of significant loss. Udelman and Udelman [11] found that hope scores on their Rheumatology

Reaction Pattern Survey predicted emotional responses and coping patterns of patients over a 2-year period. Adverse scores were more common in younger patients, raising the question of whether chronic illness affected younger people more severely.

Little has been written of the correlation between attitudes, such as hope and the incidence of illness. Less has been said of the immunological impact of hope or hopelessness. Engel's [12] early studies described anecdotally the association between these affects and illness. Although current studies are beginning to focus on immunological components and their response to psychiatric treatments, no study has as yet attempted to correlate these variables.

Several avenues of exploration regarding psychological states and immunity can be suggested. If adequate hope levels were found to correlate with greater T cell count changes over a defined period, would greater hope be a significant, measureably effective factor in prophylaxis against disease? If antidepressant therapy enhanced hope and correlated with favorable alterations in T and B cells, could such pharmacotherapy aid in disease prevention for "at risk" populations? Finally, could psychological measurements assist in predicting physiological response?

We designed a study to measure psychological states and immune responsivity in two groups of psychiatric outpatients: (1) a group administered a psychoactive drug and (2) a group not receiving any psychoactive medication. The former group would be diagnostically the same as the latter. Both groups of patients would receive psychotherapy by the same therapists. The first group would receive antidepressant therapy in addition to psychotherapy. The second group of patients would be age- and sex-matched, as well as diagnostically matched, but would receive no medication unless clinical conditions warranted it. With psychotherapy as constant as could be arranged, antidepressant therapy was expected to heighten hope, and concurrently, enhance immune responsivity in subjects. Controls were also expected to show some favorable changes in both areas, but to lesser degrees.

20.5 Antidepressant Therapy and Immunity

20.5.1 Method

The study included ten psychiatric outpatients administered Ludiomil and ten psychiatric outpatients given no medication. These patients included ten men and ten women, ranging in age from 25 to 57. The two groups of patients were age- and sex-matched. All patients were diagnosed as having dysthymic disorder (depressive neurosis) according to DSM-III. Dysthymic disorder (depressive neurosis) was chosen as the affective disorder for treatment on an outpatient basis to minimize the potential for hospitalization, polypharmacy, and potential complications in immune reactions.

Comparisons were made between predrug tests and postdrug tests in both patient groups. An effort was made to ascertain whether there was significant correlations between psychological and biochemical measurements within testing periods. The duration of the study was 3 months, with pretreatment testing and repeat posttreatment testing at 3 months.

All patients were given the following tests at the onset of the study and 3 months later:

1. *Beck Depression Inventory*
2. *Gottschalk Hope Scales,* derived from the content analysis of 5-min speech samples [13].
3. *T- and B-Lymphocyte Counts*

    Null cell counts: null cells are lymphocytes which lack readily detectable B cell or T cell membrane markers. Some investigators feel that null cells are pre-T cells. Because these cells participate in antibody-dependent cellular cytotoxic reactions, it has been suggested that they play a prominent role in the natural killer cell phenomenon. Natural killer cells carry tumor-specific receptors on their cell surface.

4. *Mitogenic Stimulation*

    Mitogens such as phytohemagglutinin (PHA) and concanavalin A (Con A) are nonspecific T cell mitogens which are used to measure the ability of cells to undergo a blastogenic response. Pokeweed mitogen (PWM) stimulates B cells. Mitogen-induced lymphocyte proliferation assay is useful in assessing cellular function.

The subjects were started on Ludiomil 50–75 mg/day following the first testing. The dosage of Ludiomil was increased over a 2- to 3-week period, as required by the clinical picture of depression, i.e., continued vegetative signs, withdrawal fatigue, and general lack of interest. The average dosage was 125 mg/day with the range varying between 100 and 150 mg. The controls were given no medication. Because this was a pilot study designed to detect immunological changes that might occur with antidepressant therapy, it was decided that placebos would not be used. Psychotherapy was a constant treatment in both groups with hourly sessions held weekly on the average. Although formal testing was done only twice, mental status assessments were monitored and crosschecked by the investigators.

Sideeffects of Ludiomil were noted in all subjects. The universal sideeffect was dryness of the mouth. Initial blurred vision was reported by two subjects, while drowsiness occurred briefly (5–10 days) in four patients. Patient compliance was felt to be excellent.

20.5.2 Results

All physiological and psychological measures were examined before and after treatment. Table 1 compares pretreatment to posttreatment test variables for patients treated with antidepressant medication (experimental group) and for patients not receiving medication (control group). Beck depression scores declined in both groups, but only Beck depression scores from the unmedicated patients decreased significantly ($P < 0.02$). No significant changes occurred in hope scores nor number of words in the 5-min verbal samples. The unmedicated group of patients had significantly higher hope scores ($P < 0.05$) than the medicated group before drug treatment was initiated. Percent T cells in medicated patients decreased significantly ($P = 0.002$), and percent null cells increased significantly ($P < 0.03$) from predrug to postdrug test. Mitogenic stimulation was significantly lower in both groups of patients from predrug to postdrug test ($P < 0.05$ to < 0.001).

Table 1. Predrug to postdrug variable comparisons for groups

Variable	Group	Predrug mean	Postdrug mean	T value	Probability
Beck					
	Control	9.2	6.3	2.89	0.02[a]
	Experimental	15.1	10.4	1.71	0.12
Number of words in a 5-min sample					
	Control	738.3	775.2	− 0.75	0.48
	Experimental	673.4	720.9	− 1.80	0.11
Hope scores					
	Control	1.04	0.74	0.33	0.75
	Experimental	− 0.33	0.17	− 0.52	0.62
Percent T					
	Control	62.2	62.2	0.30	0.77
	Experimental	63.5	51.6	4.26	0.002[b]
Percent B					
	Control	26.1	27.2	− 0.52	0.62
	Experimental	27.6	31.4	− 1.15	0.28
Percent Null					
	Control	10.7	10.6	0.03	0.98
	Experimental	9.1	17.0	− 2.56	0.03[a]
PHA					
	Control	65 234.0	27 277.6	2.97	0.02[a]
	Experimental	52 047.1	28 073.4	3.42	0.008[b]
PWM					
	Control	66 278.9	30 854.4	4.65	0.001[c]
	Experimental	68 007.4	38 003.3	5.79	0.0001[c]
Con A					
	Control	97 189.7	43 808.1	4.70	0.001[c]
	Experimental	96 849.4	47 114.1	4.61	0.001[c]

[a] $P < 0.05$;   [b] $P < 0.01$;   [c] $P < 0.001$

Table 2 shows correlations for both groups on predrug variables and predrug hope scores. Percent B cells correlated negatively with predrug hope scores ($r = − 0.51$; $P < 0.05$). PWM scores correlated positively with hope ($r = 0.25$; $P < 0.05$), and Con A scores also correlated positively with hope scores ($r = 0.32$; $P < 0.05$).

Table 3 demonstrates correlations between postdrug variables and postdrug hope scores as well as with predrug hope scores. Again, percent B cells correlated negatively with postdrug hope scores ($r = − 0.24$). Postdrug Con A scores correlated with predrug hope scores ($r = 0.28$) and with postdrug hope scores ($r = 0.31$). Finally, predrug hope scores correlated positively with postdrug percent B cells ($r = 0.38$).

The scores on the Beck Depression Inventory and on the Hope Scales became more strongly associated between predrug testing and postdrug testing. Correlations increased from $r = − 0.18$ to $r = − 0.38$. Predrug testing hope and postdrug testing hope correlated at $r = 0.35$.

Table 2. Correlations for all depressed patients ($n = 20$) between predrug hope scores and various immune response indices

Predrug immune response indices	Predrug hope scores
% T	0.10
% B	− 0.51
% null	− 0.05
PHA	− 0.17
PWM	0.25[a]
Con A	0.32[a]

[a] $P < 0.05$

Table 3. Correlations between predrug and postdrug hope scores and various immune response indices

Postdrug immune response indices	Predrug hope scores	Postdrug hope scores
% T	0.01	0.16
% B	0.38★	− 0.24★
% null	0.05	0.12
PHA	0.01	0.12
PWM	0.07	0.07
Con A	0.28★	0.31★

★ $P < 0.05$

20.6 Discussion

Several hypotheses were considered prior to beginning this preliminary study:
1. If mental depression can lead to an immunosuppressive state, can treatment of depression enhance immune competence?
2. If enhanced immunocompetence occurs with antidepressant therapy, what immune components would be affected?
3. Would a depressed group of patients fare as well in immune function with psychotherapy alone as with psychotherapy and pharmacotherapy?
4. Can psychological measurements of hope, and depression show parallel changes with physiological immune system measurements?

The hypotheses examined were not supported by this study. The capacity for mitogenic stimulation decreased significantly in both patient groups with treatment. No evidence of enhanced immune competence including T, B, and null cells occurred in either group with treatment. On the other hand, significant positive correlations between predrug hope scores and mitogenic stimulation with PWM and Con A as well as a significant positive correlation between predrug hope scores and B cell percent suggest some predictive value for hope scores with respect to immune competence.

The complexities of the immune system grow geometrically as new studies seek new answers, but often provide only new questions. The field of psychoimmunology is subject to the constant critique of observers and awareness by researchers of the need to ask the "right questions". Immune responsivity includes not only T- and B-lymphocytes, but also macrophages, natural killer cells, polymorphonuclear leukocytes, complement, and possibly even red blood cells [14]. Interactions between exogenous chemicals, such as medication, and endogeneous substances, such as catecholamines, endorphins, and encephalins, challenge researchers further.

This study was designed as a pilot program to determine potential associations between antidepressant therapy and the immune system. The authors plan to expand the scope and numbers of patients of this preliminary study.

20.7 Summary

The findings obtained in this study arouse interest in that significant changes were noted between a psychotherapy only and a pharmacotherapy plus psychotherapy group. The decrease in percent T cells along with the increase in null cells (see Table 1) suggests a possible specific action by Ludiomil on natural killer cells and suppressor cells. A change in the suppressor: helper T cell ratio could explain the significant decrease in PWM, PHA, and Con A stimulation on postdrug test assessment.

The significant correlation between hope scores and Con A mitogenic stimulation suggests a link between predrug hope scores and cellular blastogenic potential. Finally, the positive correlation between predrug hope scores and postdrug B cell percent suggest some predictive value for hope scores relative to immunoglobulin and antibody status. The declining negative correlations between predrug and postdrug test hope scores and percent B cells have yet to be explained.

References

1. Gottschalk LA, Welch WD, Weiss J (1983) Vulnerability and immune response and overview. Psychother Psychosom 39: 23–35
2. Dorian BJ, Keystone E, Garfinkel PE, Brown GM (1981) Suppression of immunity by stress: effect of a graded series of stressors on lymphocyte stimulation in the rat. Science 213: 1397–1400
3. Locke SE (1982) Stress adaptation and immunity: Studies in humans. Gen Hosp Psychiatry 4: 49–58
4. Palmblad J (1976) Fasting in man: effect on PMN granulocyte function, plasma iron and serum transferrin. Scand J Haematol 17: 217–226
5. Kimzey SL, Johnson PC, Ritzman SE, Mengel CE (1976) Hematology and immunology studies: the second manned sky lab mission. Aviat Space Environ Med 47: 383–390
6. Stein M (1982) Stress brain and immune function. Symposium American psychiatric association annual meeting, May 1982, Toronto
7. Trush MA, Reason MJ, Wilson ME, Van Dyke K (1979) Comparison of the interaction of tricyclic antidepressants with human polymorphonuclear leukocytes as monitored by the generation of chemiluminescence. Chem Biol Interact 28: 71–81
8. Gelfand EW, Cheung R, Hastings D, Dosch HM (1980) Characterization of lithium effects on two aspects of T cell function. Adv Exp Med Biol 127: 429–446
9. Rosenblatt S, et al. (1968) The relationship between antigammaglobulins activity and depression. Am J Psychiatry 124: 12
10. Haydu GG, Goldschmidt L, Drymiotis AD (1974) Effect of imipramine on the rheumatoid factor titre of psychotic patients with depressive symptomatology. Ann Rheum Dis 33: 273
11. Udelman HD, Udelman DL (1978) Rheumatology reaction pattern survey. Psychosomatics 19: 776–780
12. Engel GL (1954) Selection of clinical material in psychosomatic medicine: the need for a new physiology (special article) Psychosomatics 16: 368–373
13. Gottschalk LA (1974) A hope scale applicable to verbal samples. Arch Gen Psychiatry 30: 779–785
14. Seigel I, Gleicher N (1983) The red army. The Sciences 23: 30–34

21 The Pharmacokinetics of Some Psychoactive Drugs and Relationships to Clinical Response*

Louis A. Gottschalk

21.1 Pharmacokinetics of Single Doses of Psychoactive Drugs

Pharmacokinetic studies of single, standardized, oral, or intramuscular doses (25 mg) of chlordiazepoxide [15, 20, 22], meperidine (100 mg) [11], oral thioridazine (4 mg/kg) [14], and intramuscular mesoridazine (2 mg/kg) [18] have revealed wide individual differences in blood plasma concentrations, peak plasma levels, half-lives, and area-under-the-curve plotting blood concentration against time [4, 13].

21.2 Relationship of Pharmacokinetics of Single Doses of Psychoactive Drugs to Clinical Responses

These studies have indicated that the clinical responses to these drugs are significantly related to the magnitude of some of these pharmacokinetic indices.

For example, in *chlordiazepoxide studies,* anxiety, outward-hostility, and ambivalent-hostility scores, as measured by the method of content analysis of verbal samples, decreased over a 50 min observation period when subjects were given 25 mg oral chlordiazepoxide compared with a placebo. A statistically significant decrease in anxiety scores ($P < 0.25$) during this time period, however, occurred only in 11 subjects whose chlordiazepoxide blood levels exceeded 0.70 µg/ml. No significant decreases occurred in anxiety scores of the subjects whose blood chlordiazepoxide blood levels were less than 0.70 µg/ml.

In a *meperidine study,* there were significant correlations between meperidine plasma levels, after either oral or intramuscular administration of 100 mg, and decreases in anxiety scores.

In a single-dose (4 mg kg) oral *thioridazine study,* involving the administration of this major tranquilizer to 25 acute schizophrenic patients, significant decreases occurred in measures of the schizophrenic syndrome 24–48 h postdrug among the schizophrenic patients, as assessed by the following: Overall Gorham Brief Psychiatric Rating Scale (BPRS) [28]; Hamilton Depression Rating Scale [25], and Wittenborn Rating Scale [24]

* Reprinted from *Methods and Findings in Experimental and Clinical Pharmacology* (1985) 7: 275–282 with permission of the author and publisher.

Table 1. Relationships of plasma pharmacokinetic indices after single doses of psychoactive drugs to clinical responses

Drug	Dose	Clinical responses
Chlordiaze-poxide	25 mg oral	Significant decreases in anxiety scores ($t=2.25$, $P<0.025$) only in those 11 subjects (of 18) whose chlordiazepoxide blood levels exceeded 0.70 µg/ml
Meperidine	100 mg oral	Significant correlations between meperidine plasma levels and decreases in anxiety scores ($n=6$; $r=0.72$; $P<0.05$) after a 100 mg oral dose, decreases in hostility-inward scores ($n=12$; $r=0.57$; $P<0.05$) after 100 mg oral or i.m. doses, and significant negative correlations between meperidine plasma levels and hostility-out (overt) scores ($n=6$; $r=0.74$; $P<0.05$) and hostility-in scores ($n=6$; $r=0.67$; $P<0.05$) after a 100 mg oral dose
Thioridazine	4 mg/kg oral	Significant correlations 48 h after administration between plasma pharmacokinetic thioridazine indices (plasma level, half-life, area-under-the-curve) (by fluorometric and gas chromatographic methods) and decreases in scores on: *brief psychiatric rating scale (BPRS)* Depression factor ($r=0.42$–0.46; $P<0.05$; $n=25$) Thinking disorder factor ($r=0.41$; $P<0.05$; $n=25$) Excitement-disorientation factor ($r=0.42$; $P<0.05$; $n=25$) *Hamilton Rating Scale* Sleep disturbance factor ($r=0.46$–0.50; $P<0.05$; $n=25$) Anxiety/depression factor ($r=0.44$–0.45; $P<0.05$; $n=25$) *Wittenborn Rating Scale* Excitement factor ($r=0.41$; $P<0.05$; $n=25$) Paranoia factor ($r=0.47$; $P<0.05$; $n=25$) *Gottschalk-Gleser Social Alienation-Personal Disorganization Scale* (16 of 19) negative individual correlations between plasma thioridazine level and "schizophrenic" scores over four occasions during 24 h after drug ingestion; $P<0.03$)
Mesoridazine and sulfo-ridazine	Single dose of 2 mg/kg i.m.	Significant correlations between plasma pharmacokinetic indices (by fluorometric and gas chromatographic methods) and decreases in scores on: *BPRS* (48 h postdrug) Anergic factor ($r=0.68$; $P<0.05$; $n=9$, plasma mesoridazine conc. by UV), ($r=0.57$; $P<0.10$; $n=9$, plasma mesoridazine area-under-curve by UV), ($r=0.67$; $P<0.05$; $n=9$, plasma mesoridazine conc. by GC), ($r=0.76$; $P<0.05$; $n=9$, plasma sulforidazine by GC), ($r=0.75$; $P<0.05$; $n=9$, plasma mesoridazine area-under-curve by GC), ($r=0.68$; $P<0.05$; $n=9$, plasma sulforidazine area-under-curve by GC) *Wittenborn Scale* Somatic-hysterical factor (48 h postdrug) ($r=0.66$; $P<0.05$; $n=9$, plasma mesoridazine area-under-curve by UV) ($r=0.76$; $P<0.05$; $n=9$, plasma mesoridazine area-under-curve by GC), ($r=0.68$; $P<0.05$; $n=0$, plasma sulforidazine area under curve by GC)

UV, spectrophotofluorometer; GC, gas chromatograph

and in Gottschalk-Gleser [19] Content Analysis Scale scores measuring the severity of the schizophrenic syndrome in terms of social alienation-personal disorganization. Also, thioridazine plasma pharmacokinetic indices (plasma level, plasma half-life, area-under-the-curve) correlated significantly with improvement in the depression, thinking disorder, and excitement-disorientation factors of the BPRS; with sleep disturbance and anxiety/depression factors of the Hamilton Depression Scale; and with the excitement factors of the Wittenborn Scale. Also, the higher the thioridazine plasma levels the lower the social alienation-personal disorganization scores derived from speech samples at regular intervals (1–24 h later) in 80% of the patients .

In a single-dose *mesoridazine study,* in which the drug was administered intramuscularly (2 mg/kg) to ten acute schizophrenic patients, again there was a significant improvement in the rating scale and content analysis scale indices of the schizophrenic syndrome. Moreover, significant correlations of the same drug concentration indices occurred with improvement in anergia factor scores derived from the Brief Psychiatric Rating Scale (BPRS) and the somatic-hysterical factor scores of the Wittenborn-Scale. These differences in correlations between pharmacokinetic indices and clinical response in the thioridazine and mesoridazine studies strongly suggested that the parent drug, thioridazine, has somewhat different pharmacological effects, either quantitatively or qualitatively, than its metabolites mesoridazine and sulforidazine, the latter being another metabolite of thioridazine and mesoridazine detectable after a single dose of these drugs [9, 23] (Table 1).

21.3 Neuropsychological Questions Unanswered by Single-Dose Psychoactive Drug Studies

Although these single-dose psychoactive drug studies were very useful in that they demonstrated conclusively the wide individual variations in the pharmacokinetics of psychoactive drugs, as well as the relationships of various pharmacokinetic indices to antianxiety and antischizophrenic manifestations, there were certain important questions they could not answer. They did not provide information on what the drug concentrations in the blood were likely to be during continuous dose drug administration, and they did not indicate to what extent a favorable response to a single dose of a phenothiazine is predictive of the kind and degree of clinical response with continuous drug dosage.

With respect to the latter issue, psychoactive drug treatment of acute schizophrenia has been considered by some investigators to require weeks to be able to make its effect manifest in the schizophrenic syndrome. Many of our acute schizophrenic patients in the single-dose thioridazine and mesoridazine studies had, however, marked beneficial responses within 24 h with a single dose of these phenothiazines, although some patients had little or no favorable clinical response.

Combining single-dose and multiple-dose phenothiazine studies in the same schizophrenic patients would permit determining whether examining the single-dose pharmacokinetic and clinical response in each patient might be of practical significance in providing an approximation of optimal drug dose and probable clinical response in long-term pharmacotherapy of the schizophrenic syndrome.

21.4 Research Relating The Relevance of a Single-Dose Major Tranquilizer to Continuous Dose Psychoactive Drug Administration

21.4.1 Single Intramuscular Dose, Mesoridazine Followed by Continuous Oral Thioridazine

In this study, ten acute schizophrenic patients initially received a single dose of intramuscular mesoridazine (2 mg/kg) and 4 days later a daily dose of oral thioridazine (4 mg/kg) over a 3- to 8-week period. The levels of thioridazine and its metabolites were measured by the spectrofluorometric method of Pacha [29] and the gas chromatographic (GC) method of Dinovo et al. [8].

The aims of this combined single dose followed by continuous dose drug study were as follows:

1. To determine whether those who responded to a single dose of mesoridazine were more likely to respond favorably during continuous dosage with thioridazine.
2. To determine whether any pharmacokinetic indices observed during the single dose study were predictors of the average blood levels during continuing daily doses of thioridazine.
3. To look for any relationship between the plasma level of the parent drug or its metabolites and the development of any adverse side-effects associated with administration of thioridazine.
4. To examine the equilibrium established between blood and spinal fluid concentration of thioridazine and its metabolites in patients receiving continuous daily administration of this drug.

Previous studies with single dose oral thioridazine [14] and intramuscular mesoridazine [18] had demonstrated that thioridazine is first metabolized to the pharmacologically active mesoridazine (thioridazine-S-sulfoxide), which is in turn metabolized to the pharmacologically active sulforidazine (thioridazine-S-sulfone) [9, 23]. No other metabolites had been positively identified after a single dose by gas chromatography. After continuous daily dosage with thioridazine (4 mg/kg), however, another metabolite was detected. It has been identified as thioridazine-R-sulfoxide [23]. It was of interest whether these very similar phenothiazines, thioridazine and mesoridazine or their metabolites, might have some similarities after a single dose in certain aspects of their pharmacokinetics (peak concentration, peak hours, half-life, area-under-the-time-concentration-curve, absorption constant, elimination constant) within each individual. Also of interest was whether one or more of these indices might serve as a predictor of the steady-state drug concentration with daily continuous dose treatment with thioridazine. What answers were obtained to these questions?

Do acute schizophrenic patients who respond favorably to a single dose of intramuscular mesoridazine respond more favorably to continuous oral thioridazine?

In the group of ten acute schizophrenic patients, seven patients were responders and three were nonresponders to both mesoridazine and thioridazine. All three patients who were nonresponders had marked disturbances in thought disorder, were apathetic or anergic, and had hallucinatory or delusional manifestations typical of acute schizophrenia. They appeared to be symptomatically indistinguishable from the seven patients who were quite responsive to phenothiazine therapy.

Analysis of the data with all ten patients in this study indicated that the kind and degree of psychological response to a single-dose of intramuscular mesoridazine could predict the likelihood of a favorable psychological response with continuous daily treatment of oral thioridazine. Specifically, a patient's clinical status 24 h after a single drug dose was used to predict his clinical status during the continuous dose phase, over and above what his predrug clinical status would predict. Toward this end, partial correlations were calculated between clinical rating scale scores 24 h after a single dose of mesoridazine with rating scale scores obtained after 3 weeks of continuous daily doses with thioridazine, while partialling out or eliminating the effect of initial clinical status as measured just before the administration of the single dose of mesoridazine. The results of these statistical evaluations were as follows:

1. Social alienation-personal disorganization scores 24 h after the single mesoridazine dose correlated 0.77 ($n = 10$; $P < 0.05$) with the average social alienation-personal disorganization score during the 3 weeks of daily thioridazine administration.
2. The BPRS thinking disorder factor score 24 h after the single drug dose correlated 0.76 ($n = 10$; $P < 0.05$) with the average BPRS thinking disorder factor score during the 3 weeks of daily drug dose.
3. The Wittenborn somatic-hysterical factor score 24 h after the single drug dose correlated 0.80 ($n = 10$; $P < 0.009$) with the average Wittenborn somatic-hysterical factor score during the 3 weeks of daily thioridazine administration.
4. The Wittenborn obsessive-compulsive-phobic factor score 24 h after the single drug dose correlated 0.92 ($n = 10$; $P < 0.001$) with the Wittenborn factor score during the 3 weeks of daily thioridazine administration.

Were there any pharmacokinetic indices during the single intramuscular dose study which might predict average blood levels during continuous daily doses of thioridazine?

The answer was yes. Following a single dose of intramuscular mesoridazine, mesoridazine half-life (by GC) correlated 0.86 ($n = 10$; $P < 0.01$) and mesoridazine area-under-the-curve correlated 0.86 ($P < 0.01$) with the average mesoridazine blood concentration over the first 3 weeks of daily oral thioridazine administration.

Following a single dose of intramuscular mesoridazine, sulforidazine area-under-the-curve (by GC) correlated significantly positively ($r = 0.88$; $n = 10$; $P < 0.01$) with the average sulforidazine blood concentration over the first 3 weeks of daily oral thioridazine administration.

Were there any pharmacokinetic indices occurring with the single dose of mesoridazine that predicted the behavioral response after continuous daily doses of thioridazine?

Yes. The mesoridazine area-under-the-curve (for the first 24 h postdrug measured by the fluorometric method) correlated significantly ($n = 10$) with improvement in many different average psychiatric measures over 3 weeks following daily administration of oral thioridazine:

Gottschalk social alienation-personal disorganization score ($r = 0.75$; $P < 0.01$)
BPRS depression factor score ($r = 0.67$; $P < 0.04$)
BPRS thinking disorder factor score ($r = 0.78$; $P < 0.007$)
BPRS anxiety-depression factor score ($r = 0.94$; $P < 0.001$)

Hamilton anxiety-depression score ($r = 0.65$; $P < 0.05$)
Hamilton apathy factor score ($r = 0.84$; $P < 0.003$)
Wittenborn anxiety factor score ($r = 0.84$; $P < 0.05$)
Wittenborn depression-retardation factor score ($r = 0.65$; $P < 0.05$)

Sulforidazine half-life (by GC), following a single dose of intramuscular mesoridazine, correlated significantly negatively ($r = 0.65$; $n = 10$; $P < 0.04$) with the average BPRS excitement-disorientation factor score during the first 3 weeks after daily continuous oral thioridazine, that is, the longer the sulforidazine half-life after a single dose of mesoridazine, the lower the BPRS excitement-disorientation factor score with daily continuous oral thioridazine.

Table 2. Relationships of plasma pharmacokinetic indices after a single drug dose to clinical responses over a period 3–8 weeks later during a continuous daily dose of a psychoactive drug

Drug	Dose	Clinical responses
Mesoridazine	2 mg/kg i.m. dose over 24 h	Significant correlations 24 h after drug administration between plasma pharmacokinetic indices and behavioral responses ($n = 10$)
Thioridazine	4 mg/kg daily oral dose for 3–8 weeks	Mesoridazine area-under-the-curve (measured by the fluorometric method for first 24 h postdrug) correlated significantly ($n = 10$) with improvement in average behavioral measures over 3–8 weeks during daily administration of oral thioridazine with:
		Gottschalk-Gleser Social Alienation-Personal Disorganization Scale ($r = 0.75$; $P < 0.05$)
		Anxiety depression factor score ($r = 0.95$; $P < 0.001$)
		Depression factor score ($r = 0.67$; $P < 0.04$)
		Thinking disorder factor score ($r = 0.78$; $P < 0.007$)
		Hamilton Rating Scale
		Anxiety depression factor score ($r = 0.65$; $P < 0.05$)
		Apathy factor score ($r = 0.84$; $P < 0.003$)
		Wittenborn Scale
		Anxiety factor score ($r = 0.84$; $P < 0.05$)
		Depression-retardation factor score ($r = 0.65$; $P < 0.05$)
		Sulforidazine half-life (by gas chromatography) following a single i.m. dose of mesoridazine (2 mg/kg) significantly correlated with the average behavioral measures over 3–8 weeks during daily oral administration of thioridazine (4 mg/kg) with:
		Gottschalk-Gleser Social Alienation-Personal Disorganization Scale scores ($r = 0.72$; $P < 0.02$)
		Excitement-disorientation ($r = 0.65$; $P < 0.04$)
		On four patients within-patient correlations of plasma thioridazine levels on 16–43 occasions (by UV assay) and social alienation-personal disorganization scores over 3–8 weeks was 0.34–0.75; $P < 0.025$–0.005. Using a GC assay, these within-patient correlations were 0.38–0.52; $P < 0.05$–0.005 between mesoridazine plasma levels and social alienation-personal disorganization scores.

Sulforidazine half-life, after a single dose of intramuscular mesoridazine, did correlate significantly negatively with the average social alienation-personal disorganization scores derived from 5-min speech samples ($r = 0.72$; $n = 10$; $P < 0.02$) during daily continuous oral thioridazine treatment.

Mesoridazine peak (by GC) following a single intramuscular dose of mesoridazine, correlated negatively with the average BPRS thought disorder factor score ($r = 0.64$, $n = 10$; $P < 0.05$) during daily continuous oral thioridazine administration.

These findings correspond to those of May et al. [27] who reported that plasma thioridazine levels in 23 male schizophrenic patients at 3 and 6 h after an initial dose of 50 mg of thioridazine were predictive of subsequent clinical outcome (Table 2).

Were there any adverse side effects observed and were these noted to be associated with any pharmacodynamic variables?

One patient developed abnormal EKG changes, and this patient had unusually high thioridazine-R-sulfoxide plasma levels about 1 week before these EKG changes appeared. On the basis of this preliminary finding, a more thorough study following five acute schizophrenic patients receiving daily treatment with thioridazine showed that high plasma levels of thioridazine-R-sulfoxide were associated with EKG abnormalities, specifically, malformation of the T-wave or lengthening of the repolarization time [16]. Although thioridazine-R-sulfoxide is not considered to be psychoactive, this investigation revealed that it was cardioactive.

What were the relationships between blood and spinal fluid concentrations of thioridazine and its metabolites?

On three of our acute schizophrenic patients whose social alienation-personal disorganization scores and other measures of schizophrenia improved significantly after thioridazine administration, lumbar punctures were done to obtain cerebrospinal fluid (CSF) samples for assay of the concentration of thioridazine and its metabolites, specifically, 3 and 5 weeks after daily administration of oral (4 mg/kg) thioridazine [17]. The purpose of this was to determine whether there were fixed individual or group ratios between plasma concentrations and spinal fluid concentrations of these pharmacological substances. No traces of these chemical substances could be detected in the spinal fluid using the GC method of Dinovo et al. [8], which is sensitive to 0.05 µg/ml. By the spectrofluorometric method [29], however, thioridazine and its metabolites were detected at just below the level of sensitivity of the method, that is, 0,05 µg/ml. Since the fluorometric method is nonspecific and assays thioridazine plus its metabolites, whereas the GC method assays thioridazine and its metabolites separately, the fluorometric method can more easily detect these pharmacological agents.

The ratio of drug concentrations in CSF and plasma, for thioridazine and metabolites, ranged from 1.3% to 3.4% by spectrofluorometric assay. This is certainly less than the CSF/plasma ratio for nortriptyline (range 4% to 10%) reported by Kragh-Sorensen [26].

Why were the levels of thioridazine and its metabolites so low in CSF? Certain substances are slow penetrators of CSF by comparison, for example, with ethyl alcohol, and they do not complete the process of penetration. There is an inverse relationship between the lipid solubility of a drug and its penetration into the CSF [7]. Thioridazine is more lipid soluble than other psychoactive drugs, and therefore it enters the CSF very slowly if at all. Moreover, thioridazine occurs in biological fluids primarily in protein-bound form. Only in the free forms does it cross the blood-brain barrier, and this perhaps applies to its passage through the brain-CSF barrier. Also, thioridazine is very hydrophobic and, thus, becomes tightly bound to brain tissue and its receptors. Since there is relatively little protein in CSF, thioridazine does not readily enter the CSF, which is an essentially aqueous medium. More information is needed to ascertain the precise significance of these preliminary findings.

21.4.2 Administration of Daily Oral Thioridazine (4 mg/kg) and Correlations Between Thioridazine Plasma Levels and Clinical Response with Schizophrenic Patients

Significant correlations, within patients, were found in four of five schizophrenic patients between plasma thioridazine (and/or metabolite) levels as measured by both a fluorometric and gas chromatographic assay, in the relative severity of the schizophrenic syndrome [21] as measured by the Gottschalk-Gleser Social Alienation-Personal Disorganization Scale. This significant within-subject correlation occurred even in the one schizophrenic patient who could not be considered a drug responder, for his manifestations of the schizophrenic syndrome fluctuated around a grossly psychotic mean as adjudged from BPRS ratings as well as from social alienation-personal disorganization scores. With this nonresponder, there was no improvement in thought disorder and interpersonal reference subscores of the Social Alienation-Personal-Disorganization Scale with plasma thioridazine levels, but improvement did occur in the subscores dealing with personal complaints.

21.5 Discussion

A major issue in single-dose psychoactive drug studies of pharmacokinetics is the extent to which such research gives information on what the pharmacokinetics and the clinical response are likely to be during continuous and multiple-dose drug administration. Other investigators have reported promising evidence that the immediate pharmacokinetic response to a single drug dose (e.g., peak level, half-life, area-under-the-curve) can predict steady-state blood levels [1, 3, 4, 6, 13, 14, 30, 33]. This study corroborates these findings and extends the applications of single-dose psychoactive drug administration.

The relationship between pharmacokinetic variables and therapeutic efficacy in the pharmacotherapy of psychiatric disorders has remained problematic, however, because of a number of methodological difficulties. Among these are (a) the failure in many studies to differentiate between placebo responders, placebo nonresponders, drug responders, and drug nonresponders [18, 21], (b) the confounding of plasma drug levels by the adjustment of doses to clinical response instead of the administration of a constant dose and (c) measurement deficiencies involving both drug assays and psychological and behavioral variables. Our studies aimed to deal with these problems.

Another problem in this research area is where to measure the drug among the various blood fractions? Some investigators have criticized using plasma levels of psychoactive drugs to assess central nervous system effects [2, 5, 12, 31, 32]. The use of phenothiazine red cell levels instead of plasma levels in such research has been said to hold some promise [12].

In a recent in vivo study [10], greater than 99% of tritiated labeled thioridazine and mesoridazine was bound to red blood cells and plasma proteins. For thioridazine, 59% was bound to red blood cells, 41% was bound to plasma protein, and 0,7% was free; for mesoridazine, 63% was bound to red blood cells, 37% was bound to plasma protein, and 0.9% was free. There was no statistically significant relationship between the amount of drug bound to the red blood cell, plasma protein, and the percent of free drug. The free drug is the pharmacologically active portion and, presumably, is in equilibrium with the drug in the bound state. At this point it is not clear what these findings mean concerning the preferential use of serum, plasma, or red cell levels in the prediction of clinical response.

Our studies clearly demonstrate that psychoactive drug levels, under appropriate circumstances, including the constant clinical reminder that there are many different kinds of schizophrenia and depression, provide definitely useful guidelines for successful pharmacotherapy.

References

1. Alexanderson B (1972) Pharmacokinetics of nortriptyline in man after single and multiple oral doses: the predictability of steady-state plasma concentrations from single-dose plasma level data. Eur J Clin Pharmacol 4: 82–91
2. Bergling R, Mjorndal T, Oreland L, Rapp W, Wold S (1975) Plasma levels and clinical effects of thioridazine and thiothixine. J Clin Pharmacol 15: 178–186
3. Cooper TB, Simpson GM (1976) Plasma techniques in psychiatric blood level monitoring. In: Gottschalk, Merlis S (eds) Pharmacokinetics of psychoactive drugs: blood levels and clinical response. Spectrum, New York, 23–31
4. Curry SH, Davis JM, Janowsky DS, Marshall JHL (1970) Factors affecting chlorpromazine plasma levels in psychiatric patients. Arch Gen Psychiatry 22: 209–215
5. Curry SH, Mould GD (1969) Gas chromatographic identification of thioridazine in plasma and method for routine essay of the drug. J Pharm Pharmacol 21: 674–677
6. Davis JM, Janowsky DS, Sekerke I, Manier H, El-Yousef MK (1974) The pharmacokinetics of butaperazine in plasma. In: Forrest IS, Usdin E (eds) The phenothiazines and structurally related drugs. Raven, New York
7. Davson H (1967) Physiology of the cerebrospinal fluid. Little Brown, Boston, pp 67–68
8. Dinovo EC, Gottschalk LA, Nandi BR, Geddes PG (1976) GLC analysis of thioridazine mesoridazine, and their metabolites. J Pharm Sci 65: 667–669
9. Dinovo EC, Gottschalk LA, Noble EP, Biener R (1974) Isolation of a possible new metabolite of thioridazine and mesoridazine from human plasma. Res Comm Chem Pathol Pharmacol 7: 489–496
10. Dinovo EC, Pollak H, Gottschalk LA (1984) Partitioning of thioridazine and mesoridazine in human blood fractions. Methods Find Exp Clin Pharmacol 6 (3): 143–146
11. Elliott H, Gottschalk LA, Uliana RL (1974) Relationships of plasma meperidine levels to changes in anxiety and hostiliy. Compr Psychiatry 15: 57–61

12. Garver DL, Dekirmenjian H, Davis JM (1979) Phenothiazine red cell levels and clinical response. In: Gottschalk LA (ed) Pharmacokinetics of psychoactive drugs: further studies, chapter 1. New York, pp 3–21

13. Goldstein A, Aronow L, Kalman SM (1974) Principles of drug action: the basis of pharmacology, 2nd edn. Wiley, New York

14. Gottschalk LA, Biener R, Noble EP, Birch H, Wilbert DE, Heiser JF (1975) Thioridazine plasma levels and clinical response. Compr Psychiatr 16: 323–337

15. Gottschalk LA, Dinovo EC, Biener R (1974) Effect of oral and intramuscular routes of administration on serum chlordiazepoxide levels and the prediction of these levels from predrug fasting serum glucose concentrations. Res Comm Chem Pathol Pharmacol 8: 697–702

16. Gottschalk LA, Dinovo E, Biener R, Nandi BR (1978) Plasma concentrations of thioridazine metabolites and ECG abnormalities. J Pharm Sci 67: 155–157

17. Gottschalk LA, Dinovo EC, Nandi BR (1978) Cerebrospinal fluids concentration of thioridazine and its metabolites in schizophrenic patients. Res Comm Psychol Psychiatry Behav 3: 83–87

18. Gottschalk LA, Dinovo E, Biener R, Birch H, Syben M, Noble EP (1975) Plasma levels of mesoridazine and its metabolites and clinical response in acute schizophrenia after a single intramuscular dose. In: Gottschalk LA, Merlis S (eds) Pharmacokinetics, psychoactive drug levels, and clinical response. Spectrum, New York.

19. Gottschalk LA, Gleser GC (1969) The measurement of psychological states through the content of verbal behavior. University of California Press, Los Angeles

20. Gottschalk LA, Kaplan SA (1972) Chlordiazepoxide plasma levels and clinical response. Compr Psychiatry 13: 519–528

21. Gottschalk LA, Mennuti SA, Cohn JB (1979) Thioridazine plasma levels and clinical response in five schizophrenic patients receiving daily oral medication: correlations and the prediction of clinical response. In: Gottschalk LA (ed) Pharmacokinetics of psychoactive drugs: further studies. Spectrum, New York, pp 83–96

22. Gottschalk LA, Noble EP, Stolzoff GE, Bates DE, Cable CG, Uliana RL, Birch H, Fleming EW (1973) Relationships of chlordiazepoxide blood level to psychological and biochemical responses. In: Garattini S, Mussini E, Randall L (eds) The Benzodiazepines. New York

23. Gruenke LD, Craig JC, Dinovo EC, Gottschalk LA, Noble EP, Biener R (1975) Identification of a metabolite of thioridazine and mesoridazine from human plasma. Res Comm Chem Pathol Pharmacol 10: 221–225

24. Guy W, Bonato RR (1970) Manual for the ECDEU assessment battery, 2nd revision, chevy chase. In: National Institute of Mental Health (ed) Education and welfare, US Department of Health, Maryland

25. Hamilton M (1967) Development of a rating scale for primary depressive illness. Brit J Soc Clin Psychol 6: 278–296

26. Kragh-Sorensen P, Hansen E, Baastrup PC, Hvidberg EG (1976) Self-inhibiting action of nortriptyline's antidepressive effect at high plasma levels. Psychopharmacologia 45: 305–312

27. May PRA, Tokar JT, Davis JM, Yale C, Dekirmenjian H (1979) Plasma thioridazine and therapeutic response in schizophrenia. In: Gottschalk LA (ed) Pharmacokinetics of psychoactive drugs: further studies. Spectrum, New York, pp 97–114

28. Overall JE, Gorham DP (1972) The brief psychiatric rating scale (BPRS) Psychol Rep 10: 799–812

29. Pacha WLA (1969) A method for the fluorometric determination of thioridazine or mesoridazine in plasma. Experientia 103–104

30. Potter WZ, Zavadil AP, Goodwin FK (1979) Prediction of steady-state plasma concentrations of imipramine. In: Gottschalk LA (ed) Pharmacokinetics of psychoactive drugs: further studies. Spectrum, New York, pp 37–48

31. Sakalis G, Curry SH, Mould GP, Lader MH (1972) Physiologic and clinical effects of chlor-promazine and their relationship to plasma level. Clin Pharmacol Ther 13: 931–946
32. Rivera-Calimlim L, Nasrallah H, Strauss J, Lasagna L (1976) Clinical response and plasma levels: effect of dose, dosage schedules and drug interaction on plasma chlorpromazine levels. Am J Psychiatry 133: 646–652
33. Van Putten T, May PRA (1978) Subjective response as a predictor of outcome in pharmaco-therapy. Arch Gen Psychiatry 35: 477–480

Author Index

Subject Index